Health & Medical Year Book

1992

P. F. COLLIER, INC.

NEW YORK   TORONTO   SYDNEY

Lauren S. Bahr, *Editorial Director*
Robert Famighetti, *Editor in Chief*
Christine Martin Grove, *Senior Editor*
Mary Ann Albanese, *Design Director*

EDITORIAL STAFF

Joseph Gustaitis, *Senior Editor*
Richard Hantula, *Senior Editor*
William A. McGeveran, Jr., *Senior Editor*
Louise A. Bloomfield, *Editor*
Ingrid J. Strauch, *Editor*
Carol R. Nelson, *Editorial Technology Specialist*
Andrew N. Lee, *Editorial Assistant*
Jordan Erdos, *Administrative Assistant*

AEIOU Inc., *Indexing*

ART/PRODUCTION STAFF

Jill Hoffman, *Design Supervisor*
Gerald Vogt, *Production Supervisor*
Marvin Friedman, *Senior Designer*
Emil Chendea, *Designer*
Brian Boerner, *Color Coordinator*
Elnora Bode, *Photo Editor*
Joyce Deyo, *Photo Editor*
Jerry Miller, *Photo Editor*
Michele Carney, *Senior Production Assistant*
Virginia Malagon, *Production Assistant*

The 1992 Health & Medical Year Book is not intended as a substitute for the medical advice of physicians. Readers should regularly consult a physician in matters relating to their health and particularly regarding symptoms that may require diagnosis or medical attention.

COPYRIGHT © 1992 BY P. F. COLLIER, INC.

All rights reserved. No part of this book may be reproduced or transmitted in any form or by any means, electronic or mechanical, including photocopying, recording, or by any information storage and retrieval system, without permission in writing from the publisher.

P. F. Collier, Inc.
866 Third Avenue
New York, N.Y. 10022

P. F. Collier & Son Ltd.
7 Taymall Avenue
Etobicoke, Ontario
Canada M8Z 6A5

ISBN 0-02-944092-0

Library of Congress Catalog Card Number 82-645223

Manufactured in the United States of America

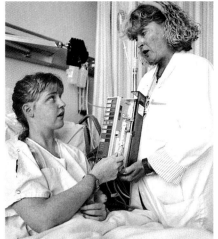

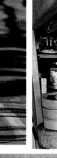

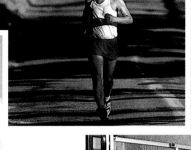

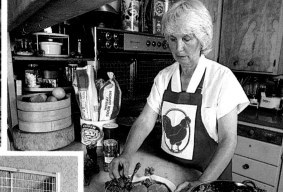

FEATURE ARTICLES

(Contents Continues)

SPOTLIGHT ON HEALTH

A series of concise reports on practical health topics.

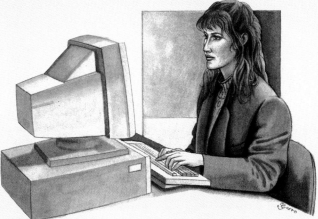

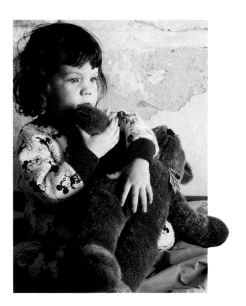

Health & Medical News

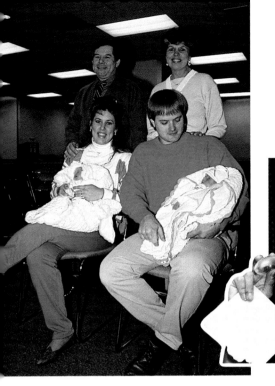

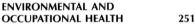

ACKNOWLEDGMENTS

Page 6: Reprinted from *Mayo Clinic Health Letter* with permission of Mayo Foundation for Medical Education and Research, Rochester, Minnesota 55905.

Page 54: Reprinted from *FDA Consumer.*

Page 63: Reprinted with permission of the author; article originally appeared in the Summer 1991 issue of *Columbia.*

Page 72: Reprinted from *FDA Consumer.*

Page 80: Copyright © 1991 by The New York Times Company. Reprinted by permission.

Page 88: Reprinted with permission. Copyright © June 1991 by Scientific American, Inc. All rights reserved.

Page 98: Reprinted with permission of *Tufts University Diet & Nutrition Letter;* article originally appeared in the February 1991 issue.

Page 107: Excerpted from the July and August 1991 issues of the *HARVARD HEALTH LETTER,* © 1991, President and Fellows of Harvard College.

Page 126: Reprinted with permission of the Health Policy Advisory Center.

Page 134: Reprinted permission of: *Johns Hopkins Medical Letter Health After 50* © Medletter Associates, 1992.

Page 138: Reprinted with permission from *The University of Texas Lifetime Health Letter,* Houston.

Page 142: Reprinted from *FDA Consumer.*

Page 150: Reprinted by permission of Karen Levine. Copyright © 1991 by Karen Levine.

Page 158: Reprinted from *Mayo Clinic Health Letter* with permission of Mayo Foundation for Medical Education and Research, Rochester, Minnesota 55905.

Page 170: Reprinted from *FDA Consumer.*

Page 180: Reprinted from *FDA Consumer.*

Page 184: Copyright © 1991 by Felicia E. Halpert. Reprinted by permission of McIntosh and Otis, Inc.

Page 187: Bruce Dobkin/© 1991 Discover Publications.

Page 190: Copyright 1991 by Consumers Union of United States, Inc., Yonkers, NY 10703. Reprinted by permission from *CONSUMER REPORTS HEALTH LETTER/CONSUMER REPORTS ON HEALTH,* June 1991.

Page 192: Excerpted from the February, March, and June 1991 issues of the *HARVARD HEALTH LETTER,* © 1991, President and Fellows of Harvard College.

Page 197: By Laura Fraser. Reprinted from *IN HEALTH.* (Sept./Oct. 1991). Copyright © 1991.

Page 199: By Linda Heller. Reprinted from *IN HEALTH.* (July/Aug. 1991). Copyright © 1991.

Page 202: Copyright © 1991 by The New York Times Company. Reprinted by permission.

Page 204: Reprinted with permission from *The University of Texas Lifetime Health Letter,* Houston.

Page 207: Reprinted from *Mayo Clinic Health Letter* with permission of Mayo Foundation for Medical Education and Research, Rochester, Minnesota 55905.

Page 209: Reprinted from *The Journal of the American Medical Association,* September 11, Volume 266, pp. 1322-1324 and 1329. Copyright 1991, American Medical Association.

Page 212: Excerpted from the April 1991 issue of the *HARVARD HEALTH LETTER,* © 1991, President and Fellows of Harvard College.

Page 215: Reprinted permission of: *University of California, Berkeley Wellness Letter,* © Health Letter Associates, 1992.

Page 219: Reprinted by permission of *PREVENTION.* Copyright 1991 Rodale Press, Inc. All rights reserved.

Page 223: Copyright © 1991 by The New York Times Company. Reprinted by permission.

Page 225: By Jamie Tallan © 1991 Newsday, Inc.

Page 232: Reprinted permission of: *Johns Hopkins Medical Letter Health After 50* © Medletter Associates, 1992.

Page 234: Reprinted with permission from *The University of Texas Lifetime Health Letter,* Houston.

Page 236: Copyright © 1991 by The New York Times Company. Reprinted by permission.

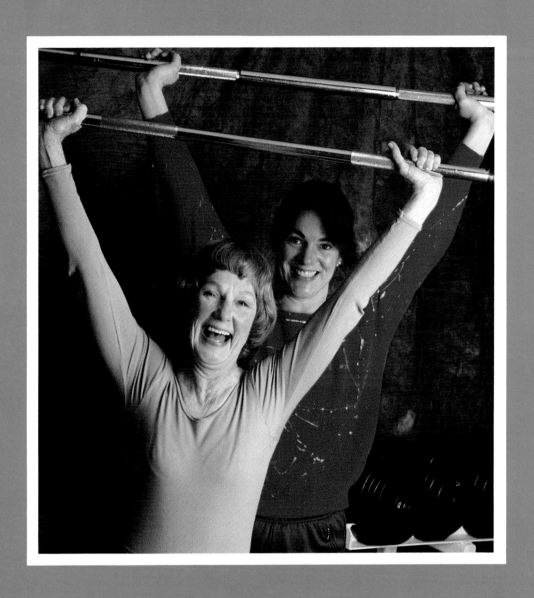

FEATURE
ARTICLES

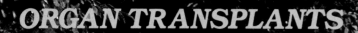

The Gift of New Life

Transplantation—"healthy organs for damaged ones"— is fostering a revolution not only in the technology of medicine, but in the basic philosophy of healthcare.

From earliest times, medicine has sought to treat

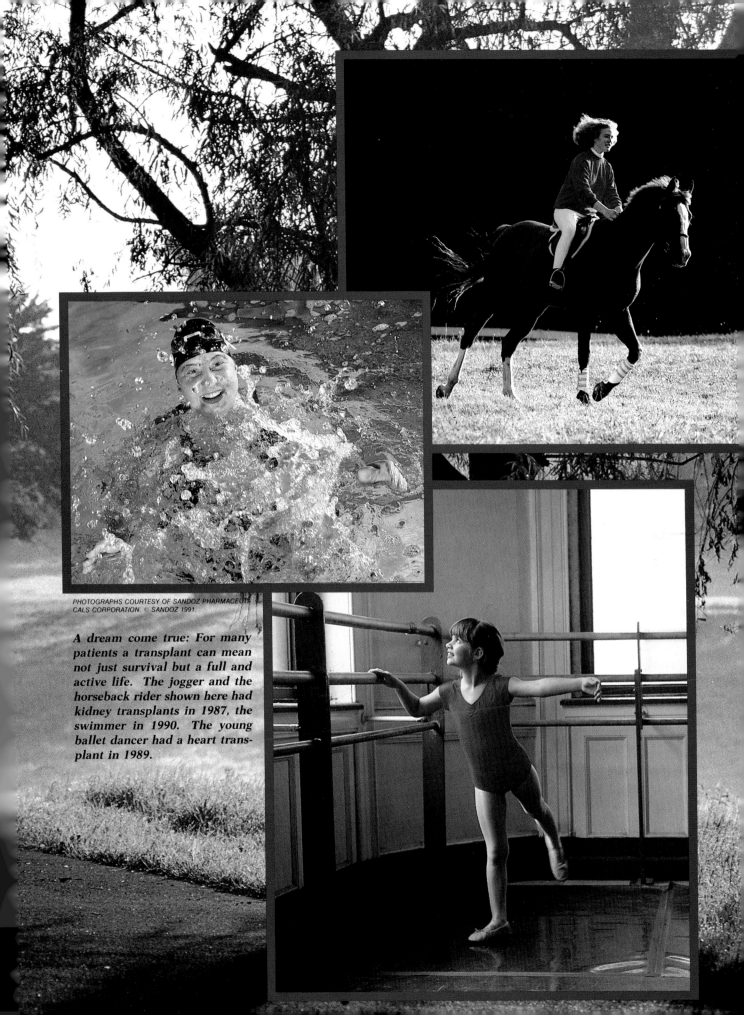

PHOTOGRAPHS COURTESY OF SANDOZ PHARMACEUTI
CALS CORPORATION. © SANDOZ 1991.

A dream come true: For many patients a transplant can mean not just survival but a full and active life. The jogger and the horseback rider shown here had kidney transplants in 1987, the swimmer in 1990. The young ballet dancer had a heart transplant in 1989.

malfunctioning parts of the body or remove those that no longer work properly. When these approaches failed, death often was swift and sure.

To a large extent, that scenario remains true. But a new approach now offers an increasingly successful alternative. Today, an expanding number of diseased organs and body tissues can be replaced with healthy equivalents.

When an organ is removed from one person and put into another, the procedure is called an allogenic transplantation. It is by far the most common form of transplantation.

In a newer procedure that shows promise, doctors reposition tissue within an individual's own body. This form of transplantation is known as an autologous transplant.

Transplant surgery can restore the body to near-normal. It can postpone death and vastly improve the quality of life.

Yet with new hope comes a series of difficult questions. The formidable expense and scarcity of organs make transplantation both an ethical and scientific challenge.

If you are in good health, the topic for this article might seem esoteric. But a change in health, from illness or an accident, can transform the subject into one of sudden and vital importance to you or to someone you care about.

Even if you never personally require a transplant, there's a simple but important way you can help others. You can become an organ donor.

An ancient idea, organ transplantation has been a reality for only about three decades. Today, we're standing on the threshold of the greatest advances yet in this field.

The Team Approach

Depending upon the organ involved, procedures for transplantation vary; but the overall approach does not. This clearly requires a team effort. And the patient is a member of the team, which includes an array of surgeons, physicians, nurses, and other allied health professionals. In fact the patient, in some ways, is the key member.

The need for transplantation rarely comes without warning. Typically, a recipient experiences a

The text of this article originally appeared in the Mayo Clinic Health Letter.

period of declining health, sometimes lasting for years, until the cumulative effects of disease, or a health crisis, rule out other forms of treatment.

Medical Assessment. The first step to becoming a candidate for transplantation, the initial evaluation, is fairly routine. In fact, conventional treatment will continue because transplantation is by no means assured—soon or ever. Next comes a thorough workup to be sure you have a good chance of benefiting from transplantation.

If you are accepted as a transplant candidate, you will undergo additional testing. Information about your blood and body tissue will be entered into a national registry. This information is of vital importance because it enhances your chance of securing the best possible organ match.

Before surgery, you and your family or friends may get a complete tour of the medical center's facilities. This knowledge can help to offset anxiety.

Personal Factors. The "human factor" also is vital. Your attitude and willingness to follow directions—including taking powerful antirejection drugs for life—help determine whether you will become a transplant candidate. Also, the emotional support you receive from loved ones plays an important role. Most medical centers include support groups of other patients as well as clergy and social workers to help you through the transplant process.

Organ Availability. In the United States statistics on every potential organ recipient are entered into the United Network for Organ Sharing (UNOS). This national network of data was created out of the 1984 National Organ Transplantation Act to assure equitable distribution of available organs throughout the country. To be eligible for federal funding, all transplant centers must belong to and abide by the rules of UNOS.

Organs are distributed on a priority basis. Every day, UNOS updates the number of people waiting for each type of organ. The numbers vary widely among different organ systems. When an organ becomes available, time is of critical importance. A pancreas, for example, must be transplanted within 24 hours of its removal from a donor if it is to function successfully in the recipient's body.

Transplants and the Immune System

The major challenge to organ transplantation is rejection by the body's immune system. Programmed to defend your body against disease-causing bacte-

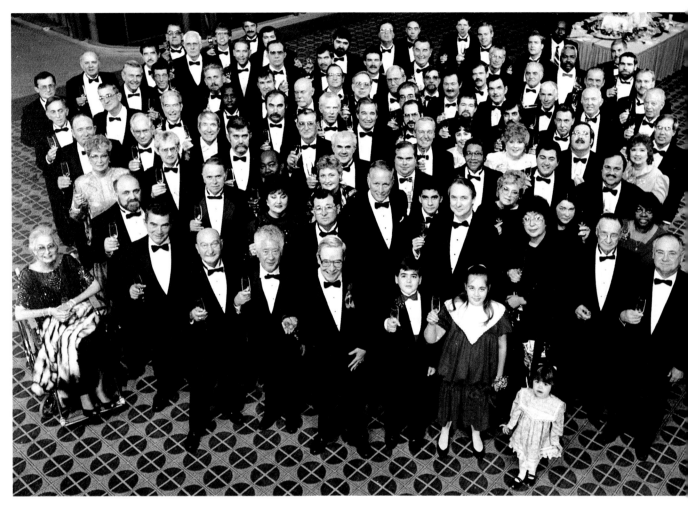

In a rare assembly, 103 recipients of heart transplants gathered at the Texas Heart Institute in Houston to celebrate their success. In the center of the second row is the institute's renowned transplant pioneer, Dr. Denton Cooley.

ria, viruses, and fungi, your immune system also regards the cells of transplanted tissue as foreign.

If you were to have a transplant and preventive steps were not taken, your immune system immediately would set out to destroy the new tissue by activating release of white blood cells called T lymphocytes. If unchecked, T cells would attack and eventually destroy the transplanted organ.

Kidney, heart, lung, liver, pancreas, and allogenic skin transplants are particularly vulnerable to rejection. The cornea and bone usually are less susceptible to rejection. Because bone marrow contains its own T cells, it is unique in its ability to identify the recipient's tissues as "foreign," leading to what specialists in blood disorders call a graft vs. host disease (GVHD).

To minimize rejection and the eventual destruction of transplanted tissue, doctors use a number of techniques.

Cross-matching Blood. Your immune system regards proteins in your blood as foreign only if they differ from your own proteins. By matching the recipient's and donor's ABO blood types, doctors greatly increase chances for acceptance of the organ.

Tissue Typing. If you need an organ transplant, the ideal donor is your identical twin. That's because identical twins have identical blood proteins. To further enhance compatibility, doctors match another protein in the blood. This protein is called the human leukocyte antigen (HLA) system.

Because most transplant candidates don't have an

identical twin, doctors use the HLA system to judge whether there's a good match between donor and recipient. The more compatible the HLA antigens between donor and recipient, the less chance of rejection. Among brothers and sisters, about one in four inherit identical HLA proteins, making a brother or sister the next best match when there's no identical twin. Two out of four brothers and sisters share half their HLA antigens; one in four are completely mismatched.

Immune-suppressing Therapy. Before operating, physicians use a variety of drugs and techniques to suppress the immune response and thus prepare the individual for surgery. Because every approach weakens the body's normal defense against illness, doctors must strike a delicate balance between preventing rejections and allowing a fatal infection.

During the past decade, an antirejection drug called cyclosporine (brand name, Sandimmune) has gained wide acceptance. Unlike other drugs, it has a more focused impact on the immune system. Another family of drugs, called corticosteroids, also helps prevent rejection. Prednisone, for example, is widely prescribed for this purpose.

Transplantable Organs and Tissues

The field of transplantation has expanded to include a variety of organs and tissues. Some, including the heart, lung, liver, pancreas, and kidney, are

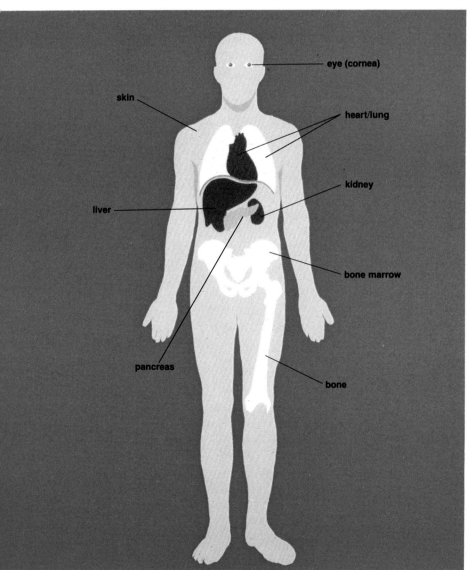

Shown here are the organs and tissues most commonly transplanted in the United States today.

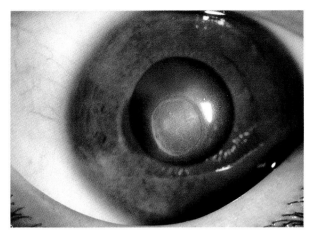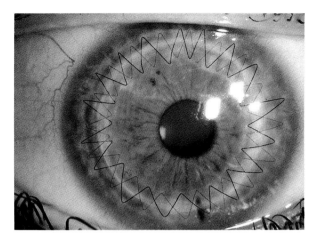

When the cornea—the eye's normally clear "front window"—is clouded (left), normal vision is impossible. A cornea transplant restores clarity (right). (The stitches from the surgery can still be seen.)

homovital transplants—expected to function permanently in the recipient's body.

Others are homostatic. They serve as a type of "scaffolding" for growth and repair by the recipient's cells. Examples include the cornea, as well as the large blood vessels, tendons, bones, and cartilage. Homostatic transplants provoke minimal or no response from the immune system.

The organs and tissues most commonly transplanted today are the cornea, liver, kidney, pancreas, heart and lung, bone marrow, skin, and bone.

Cornea

The Organ. The cornea is more than the clear "front window" of the eye. It also plays an important role in focusing images on your retina and allows you to see clearly.

Injury and Disease. Injury to the cornea can cause severe pain. Protection of the cornea is the main reason it's essential to wash your eyes promptly if you're accidentally exposed to toxic chemicals, especially alkalis. You can prevent most injuries by wearing protective glasses and by following safety instructions.

Many conditions can cause swelling or scarring of the cornea. Bacterial, viral, and fungal infections can lead to ulcers on the cornea. Infections also can cloud your cornea, diminishing your sight to the point of blindness. A small percentage of people who undergo cataract removal may develop clouding and swelling of the cornea.

The Procedure. Corneal transplantation can be either an inpatient or outpatient procedure, requiring only local anesthetic. The operation usually takes less than two hours.

Unlike with many forms of organ transplantation, the body endures minimal stress, there is no blood loss, and it's not necessary to obtain a match between donor and recipient.

First, the surgeon uses a circular cutting instrument to remove the center of the recipient's cornea, which is about the size of a pencil eraser. Then the surgeon stitches a donor cornea, sometimes called a "button," into place.

Frequency. Corneal replacement is one of the oldest forms of transplant surgery. Today, it's the most common form of transplant; in the United States, about 30,000 were done in 1989.

Donor. Most donors are age 70 or younger at the time of death. Donors must not have had a history of systemic (generalized) infections or neurologic conditions such as Alzheimer's disease.

Recipient. If the cornea becomes cloudy, transplantation is the only way to restore sight.

Although other types of transplant surgery have requirements relating to age, health, and tissue compatibility, this is not so for a corneal replacement. The procedure is available to people from childhood to age 80 and beyond.

Outcome. Corneal transplantation does not guarantee 20-20 vision. But in up to 95 percent of cases, it can improve sight, although you may need to wear glasses or contact lenses. After the surgery, it can take three months to a year to achieve optimal vision. Occasionally, following surgery, astigmatism can occur.

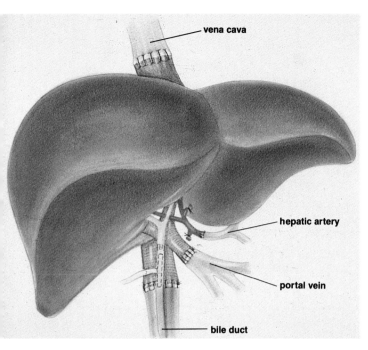

The transplanted human liver is attached to the recipient's vena cava (the main vein returning blood to the heart), portal vein (the vessel that brings blood containing absorbed nutrients to the liver), the hepatic (liver) artery, and the bile ducts.

As with any kind of organ transplant, rejection of the new tissue may take place. The leading signs of rejection are redness of the eye, a worsening of vision, and an increase in light sensitivity. If these problems occur—even years after the transplant— consult an ophthalmologist promptly.

Treatment of graft rejection within 48 hours usually serves to reverse the process and maintain a clear cornea.

Success of the transplant often hinges on why the cornea grew cloudy in the first place. For example, transplants for chemical burns have a low success rate while replacement following cataract surgery or distortion of the cornea have the best outcomes.

Future. Researchers are combating the development of posttransplant astigmatism, a vision ailment that sometimes occurs following cornea transplant surgery. Also, new techniques are extending the preservation and storage time for donated corneas. In the mid-1980s, it was possible to keep the organs for only two or three days. Current methods allow preservation for up to a week, and researchers hope to extend this time frame.

Studies also are under way to find ways to in-

crease the likelihood of graft survival in people at high risk of graft rejection.

Liver

The Organ. Life is not possible without the liver, one of your body's largest organs. Located in the upper right side of your abdomen, beneath your ribs, your liver weighs about three pounds.

Your liver converts food to energy. It also manufactures blood clotting factors, processes medications, produces bile that breaks down fatty foods, and helps excrete toxins removed from your bloodstream.

Disease. Liver disease is the fourth-leading cause of death among Americans age 65 and younger, resulting in about 50,000 deaths annually. Researchers suggest that chemicals, environmental pollutants, and increased use of drugs, including alcohol, may account for rising rates of liver disease.

Transplantation in adults has been particularly effective for three forms of chronic liver disease: chronic active hepatitis, which is a long-term inflammation of the liver; primary biliary cirrhosis, a usually progressive liver disease that mainly affects women; and primary sclerosing cholangitis, a disease affecting bile ducts within the liver and those connecting the liver to the intestine.

Most people who develop cirrhosis of the liver from abusing alcohol are not candidates for liver transplantation. Instead, physicians recommend treatment for alcoholism, including total lifelong abstinence. This single step can markedly improve the condition of the liver.

The Procedure. It takes three to four hours for a transplant team to remove a donor liver. With modern preservation techniques, the donor organ remains undamaged for up to 18 hours after "harvesting."

Transplantation takes about seven hours. Surgeons remove the diseased liver and gallbladder and place the donated organ in its position.

Frequency and Cost. The first liver transplant took place in 1963 at the University of Colorado. By early 1991, about 75 medical centers were performing liver transplants. In 1989, approximately 2,100 procedures were done in the United States.

The cost ranges from $120,000 to $250,000. Medicare does not yet cover the operation. State funding through Medicaid varies around the country, but usually covers only a portion of the cost. Private insurance programs cover most costs for about 80 percent of liver transplant patients.

Donor. Donors can be up to 60 years of age. They cannot have liver disease or a bacterial or viral infection, including the human immunodeficiency virus (HIV), or cancer. Other illnesses may be acceptable if liver function is normal.

Donor livers are obtained primarily from individuals who died from brain damage. Almost all liver donors are considered for multiple organ donation, including the heart, pancreas, lungs, and kidneys.

Recipient. Candidates for liver transplantation have chronic, progressive liver disease for which no other medical or surgical treatment exists. Conditions that preclude liver transplantation include active infection, severe heart or lung disease, and the presence of cancer elsewhere in the body.

Outcome. About 85 percent of liver transplant recipients are alive one year after the operation. Half of all patients have no physical problems. Most recipients enjoy an excellent quality of life and return to normal activities within a year.

Future. Mayo Clinic researchers are involved with several projects that may advance the success of liver transplants. Two examples of research now under way are:

• Drug evaluation—FK 506 is a new antirejection drug. Under a grant from the National Institutes of Health (NIH), Mayo and several other centers are evaluating FK 506 in liver transplant patients. Eventually, the drug may be recommended as a treatment for liver disease in certain people who have not had a transplant.

• Computer model—This computer program helps determine probable survival for people with chronic liver disease. The model analyzes a person's age, degree of jaundice, amount of the bodybuilding protein, albumin, blood-clotting ability, and extent of edema (fluid retention).

The tests that provide this information are inexpensive, available in most hospital laboratories, and do not require a liver biopsy. Mayo is making the program available to liver transplant centers worldwide. It is designed to help doctors make better decisions about the selection and timing of a liver transplant.

Kidney

The Organ. Your kidneys are located at the back of your abdominal cavity, just above your waist, on either side of your spine. Each kidney is about five

Help Save a Life: Be a Donor

Every 30 seconds, another person needs an organ transplant; 18,000 people are on waiting lists for transplants. Thousands die waiting.

Improvements in drugs and techniques have transformed organ transplantation from experimental to conventional treatment. Still, transplantation has yet to overcome its major hurdle—lack of donors.

Because of the critical shortage of organ donors, only 4 of 10 Americans who need a transplant receive one. Reasons people give for not donating organs range from fear that doctors will worry more about procuring their organs than saving their lives to financial concerns.

The fears are unfounded. Here are answers to common questions:

● Will becoming a donor affect my medical care?—No. Doctors do not consider organ or tissue donation until a person's condition is irreversible and death is imminent.

● Am I too old to donate?—Your age or health need not affect your decision. Donors range in age from a few months to age 65 and beyond.

● Will my family have to pay a fee?—Donor families are neither charged nor paid.

● If I sign up as a donor, can I change my mind?— Certainly. Just tell your family of your decision. Even if you carry a donor card, new laws require hospital personnel to discuss the possibility of organ or tissue donation with your next of kin.

Becoming a donor is easy. Just sign a Uniform Donor Card and carry it in your wallet. Donor cards are available by contacting the transplant program at your local hospital or medical center. Or the next time you renew your driver's license, note on the license that you desire to be a donor.

Then talk to your family and make sure they understand your commitment to donate. Organs and tissues will not be removed without the written consent of the next of kin.

UNIFORM DONOR CARD

OF _____
PRINT OR TYPE NAME OF DONOR

In the hope that I may help others, I hereby make this anatomical gift, if medically acceptable, to take effect upon my death. The words and marks below indicate my desires.

I give: (a) — any needed organs or parts

          (b) — only the following organs or parts

_____
SPECIFY THE ORGAN(S) OR PART(S)

for the purposes of transplantation, therapy, medical research or education.

          (c) — my body for anatomical study if needed

Limitations or
special wishes, if any: _____

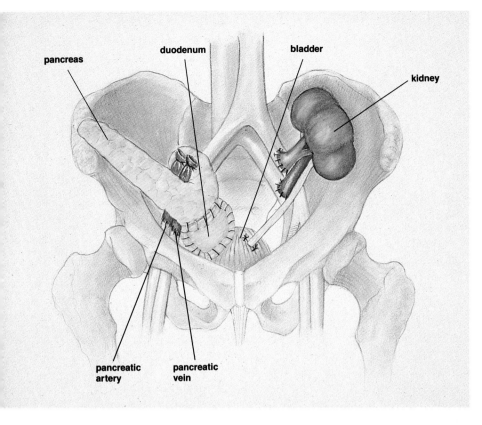

pancreas

duodenum

bladder

kidney

pancreatic artery

pancreatic vein

The transplanted human pancreas is placed within the pelvis. A portion of the donor duodenum (first part of the small intestine) is attached to the recipient's bladder to permit elimination of pancreatic digestive juices. The pancreatic artery and vein are attached to the major blood vessels that bring blood to and from the legs. This routing of blood supplies the pancreas with blood and delivers the organ's hormones to the recipient. (A transplanted kidney appears in the diagram because people who undergo a pancreas transplant also undergo a kidney transplant).

inches long and weighs roughly six ounces. These remarkable organs help to regulate blood pressure, control your body's water and salt balance, filter waste products from your blood, and excrete waste and excess water in urine.

You can live normally with just one kidney. This means that living relatives can donate a kidney in addition to organs that become available when a donor dies.

Disease. Total kidney (renal) failure once meant death. Today, patients may receive dialysis or transplantation. Both are acceptable approaches. Compared to long-term dialysis, a successful kidney transplant leads to an improved quality of life as well as greater life expectancy at less cost.

Sudden kidney failure usually responds to medical treatment. Chronic or gradual failure tends to be irreversible. Causes include chronic glomerulonephritis (glo-mer-u-lo-ne-fri′tus), polycystic kidney disease, and diabetes mellitus.

The Procedure. When a living relative donates a kidney, surgeons remove the organ via an incision under the ribs and transplant the kidney immediately. Cadaver kidneys are removed through an abdominal incision, along with other transplantable

organs. The donor organ can be preserved for up to 72 hours but is usually transplanted within 36 hours.

Transplant surgeons place the new kidney into the pelvis, connect blood vessels, and attach the donor kidney's ureter (a tube through which urine passes) to the recipient's bladder. The procedure takes about three hours.

Frequency and Cost. Since the first kidney transplant, which was performed in 1954, more than 100,000 people around the world have had the procedure. Kidney transplants and cornea transplants now are the two most common types of transplant surgery. Medicare and private insurance usually cover the $50,000 to $60,000 cost of a kidney transplant.

Donor. A living relative who makes a donation must be in excellent health. Tests must assure that the donor's remaining kidney will be able to support a full, active life without need for medication. In the United States, approximately 30 percent of kidney transplants are from related donors.

Because of the large and increasing list of patients who need kidney transplants, the current waiting time may be one to three years.

14

Almost all cadaver kidney donors are considered for multiple organ donation, including the pancreas, liver, and heart.

Recipient. Annually, about 50,000 Americans with end-stage kidney disease receive dialysis; one-fourth are candidates for kidney transplantation. Recipients range from infants to adults up to age 70. People who have cancer, active bacterial infection, severe heart disease, or HIV infection are not candidates.

Outcome. In addition to the restoration of normal kidney function, men may regain sexual potency. Women have conceived children following a kidney transplant. Restrictions on diet or activity are few.

One-year survival for recipients of a kidney from a nonliving related donor is about 85 percent. About 95 percent of people who receive a kidney from a living relative survive a year or more.

Pancreas

The Organ. Your pancreas is a slender gland between your stomach and spinal column. It secretes many hormones. For example, insulin and glucagon help control the level of sugar in your blood. Your pancreas also produce enzymes for digestion.

Disease. Transplantation of the pancreas is a treatment—not a cure—for some people with Type 1 (insulin-dependent) diabetes mellitus (previously known as juvenile diabetes). In this case, the pancreas produces little or no insulin, and the body cannot control its level of blood sugar. About 5 million Americans have diabetes; 20,000 new cases are diagnosed each year. Type 1 diabetes, affecting 25 percent of all diabetics, usually arises in childhood or young adulthood. Insulin shots are necessary to control blood sugar. Type II diabetes occurs after age 40 and usually responds to exercise, change in diet, and oral medication.

Compared to people whose pancreas works normally, those with diabetes are: 25 times more likely to become blind; 17 times more likely to develop kidney disease; 5 times more likely to experience gangrene in an extremity; and twice as likely to develop heart disease and stroke.

The Procedure. Pancreas transplantation is reserved for people with Type 1 diabetes who also undergo a kidney transplant.

Surgeons remove the donated pancreas and a connecting portion of the bowel. The donor organ is cleaned and stored in a cold preservative. Transplantation usually takes place within 18 hours. Surgeons leave the recipient's own pancreas intact. Although insulin production has failed, the organ's other functions remain.

Surgeons place the transplanted pancreas low in the abdomen. Enzymes from the new pancreas flow through the attached segment of bowel into the bladder and exit the body in urine.

The procedure takes four to six hours. Doctors test urine and blood for enzymes that show early signs of rejection; increased levels of blood sugar are a late signal.

Frequency and Cost. The first pancreas transplant took place in 1966 at the University of Minnesota. By early 1991 about 50 medical centers were performing the operation; 412 procedures were done in 1989. The cost ranges from $35,000 to $45,000. Medicare or private insurance carriers do not provide blanket coverage. An estimated 50 percent of Blue Cross/Blue Shield plans and 80 percent of other plans cover the operation. Medicare covers a kidney transplant in conjunction with transplant

James McManus, seen here greeting a well-wisher upon leaving the hospital, received a rare "domino" transplant. His donor, who was ill with fatal lung disease, received a new heart and lungs, and McManus received the donor's original, but still healthy, heart.

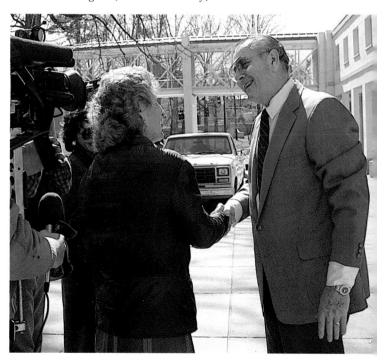

of the pancreas. Antirejection medications cost about $5,000 a year. Insurance covers much of this expense.

Donor. The standard practice is to use an entire pancreas from a cadaver donor. Cadaver donors must have had normal organ function and no evidence of infection. Partial pancreas transplants from living related donors have been performed with some success.

Recipient. People with Type I diabetes who have kidney failure are candidates for pancreas transplantation. Most are younger than 40.

Before having a pancreas transplant, some recipients have had a successful kidney transplant. Be-

cause these people already are taking powerful drugs to ward off infection, they face the least additional risk. Other recipients need a simultaneous kidney and pancreas transplant. Candidates cannot have: uncontrolled high blood pressure, heart disease or a history of heart attack, obesity, allergy to insulin, infection, recent bleeding in the retina, a history of stroke, amputation of a limb (due to circulatory disease), or HIV infection.

Outcome. About 85 percent of patients survive the first year. After a successful operation, the new pancreas goes to work immediately, allowing the recipient to enjoy a normal diet. Also, insulin injections are no longer necessary. Researchers are studying whether a pancreas transplant can prevent, stop, or reverse the complications of diabetes.

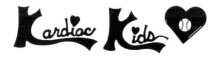

The "Kardiac Kids," a Michigan softball team composed entirely of players who have had some form of heart surgery, including transplants, prove that a new heart can indeed bring new life. Their motto: "The Beat Goes On."

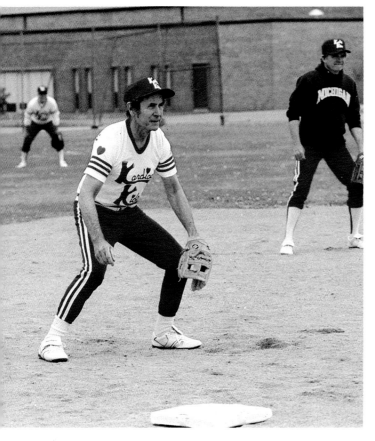

Heart/Lung

The Organs. Your heart is a muscular pump that circulates blood. Your lungs exchange the carbon dioxide produced by your body's metabolism for the oxygen necessary to sustain life.

The right side of your heart receives blood from throughout your body and sends it to your lungs to be cleared of carbon dioxide and replenished with oxygen. The left side of your heart receives the oxygenated blood and returns it to your body. During a typical lifetime, the heart beats 2.5 billion times.

Disease. Heart transplantation is necessary if the heart muscle cannot contract adequately and fails to respond to medication. The usual cause is cardiomyopathy, resulting from coronary artery disease, viral infection, or unknown factors.

Lung transplantation becomes necessary if emphysema, cystic fibrosis, or pulmonary fibrosis prevents the lungs from exchanging oxygen. Also, if pressure in the blood vessels of the lungs causes the right side of the heart to fail (this condition is called pulmonary hypertension), a transplant is necessary.

Key Concerns. Timing is critical—the right donor organ must be available at the right time. No technique can maintain the health of a person whose heart has failed. Following heart transplantation surgery, no "fallback" system exists. If the heart is rejected, the only hope for survival is another transplant. Recently, ventricular assist devices have been used to sustain dying patients until donor hearts became available. Long-term mechanical assistance or replacement of the heart is not now feasible, but several promising devices are being developed.

The Procedures. A heart transplant is no more or less difficult than other types of heart surgery. The first step is to connect the individual's major blood vessels to a heart-lung bypass machine, which pumps oxygenated blood to the body while surgeons remove the heart.

The back walls of the upper chambers (atria) remain in place to help anchor the donor organ. After it is connected to the major blood vessels, the heart is ready to pump. Surgery destroys the nerves that help control heart rate, but the heart can beat without them because heart muscle can regulate its own rhythm.

Surgeons are assessing the various uses for lung transplantation. Originally, single-lung transplants were recommended for people with pulmonary fibrosis, while double-lung and heart-lung procedures served people with emphysema and pulmonary hypertension. Recent data indicate that single-lung transplants may be effective for these latter conditions as well.

Today, donor organs are more readily available, and patients have more treatment options. The number of single-lung transplants performed is rapidly increasing.

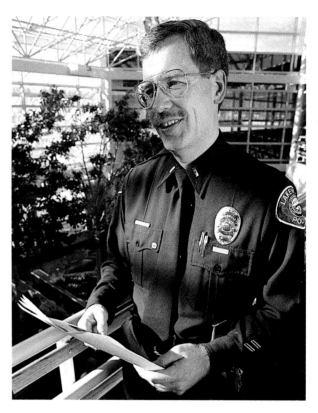

A heart transplant not only restored this policeman's health, it also enabled him to return to his job.

Notes on Cost

Transplantations are expensive. Hospitals cannot ethically pass along these costs to other patients. Thus, before performing the procedure, most medical centers require proof of ability to pay. Costs include harvesting and transplanting the organ, hospital care, extensive laboratory work, and blood products. Also, complications can occur.

The cost of transplantation varies widely. Procedures differ, as do financial provisions from government or private insurance programs.

Most medical centers have administrators, social workers, and patient representatives who can advise on available resources. Some patients also turn to grass-roots funding campaigns among hometown friends, neighbors, and townspeople.

The financial picture may improve as various forms of transplantation evolve from experimental to conventional treatments. Similarly, insurance coverage may become more readily available as transplantation emerges as a treatment of choice for more people. Even today, however, transplantation is cost-effective when compared to the expense of treating major organ failure over the course of a person's lifetime.

Frequency and Cost. The first heart transplant was performed in 1967. Since that time, about 13,000 people have received new hearts. In 1989, approximately 2,500 heart transplants were performed worldwide.

Within the United States, 148 medical centers were offering heart transplants by early 1991; 30 were performing lung transplants. The cost for a heart transplant ranges from $75,000 to $150,000, and for a lung transplant from $100,000 to $150,000.

As with other types of transplants, demand far exceeds supply. About 25 percent of patients die while waiting for a donor heart. As lung transplantation becomes increasingly common, more people also will die while waiting for this surgery.

Donor and Recipient. When heart and lung transplantations are performed, the new organs must work well immediately or the person will die. Surgical criteria, therefore, are tighter than for other transplants.

Most donors are age 50 or younger and were in good general health. Recipients may be up to age

17

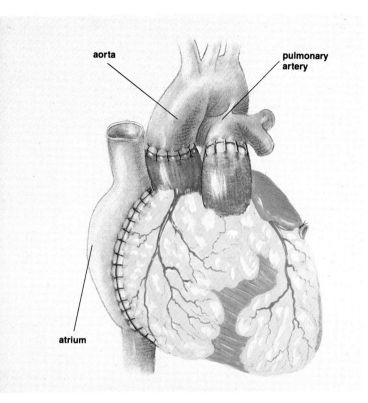

In this view, the transplanted human heart is connected to the recipient's aorta (the main artery delivering oxygenated blood to the body), the pulmonary artery (the vessel delivering blood to the lungs, where oxygen and carbon dioxide are exchanged), and a small remnant of the right atrium (the heart chamber that receives blood from the veins of the body).

65, with no other disease that would limit life expectancy. Ideally, the donor heart is retrieved while it is still beating. The heart remains viable only for four to six hours.

Outcome. Successful transplantation can lead to a near-normal quality of life. Heart transplant recipients often adjust very well. Some have even run in marathon races. The one-year survival rate is between 80 and 85 percent. Survival rates for recipients of heart-lung transplants and single-lung transplants are around 60 percent.

Bone Marrow

The Substance. This soft, spongy, semiliquid tissue produces most of your body's blood cells—red blood cells, white blood cells, and platelets—and antibodies to help fight infection. It is found in cavities of bone.

Disease. Several conditions, such as leukemia, aplastic anemia, lymphoma, multiple myeloma, and Hodgkin's disease, may destroy bone marrow.

The Procedure. To kill all diseased cells prior to transplantation, large doses of chemotherapy or radiation (sometimes both) are administered to the bone marrow of the recipient. In the process, any remaining normal cells also are destroyed.

The donor receives a general anesthetic, and doctors remove about a pint of bone marrow from bone in the person's pelvis. The recipient receives the marrow through a vein in a manner similar to a blood transfusion. The marrow cells find their way to the recipient's bone marrow. In about three weeks, they begin to grow and reproduce.

Risk. Because the blood (HLA) match is perfect, the person who receives donor marrow from an identical twin has the greatest chance for a successful transplant. The fewer antigens a donor and recipient share, the greater the risk of the life-threatening graft vs. host disease (GVHD).

Frequency and Cost. About 4,000 people in the United States receive a bone marrow transplant each year. Costs vary widely. The range is around $70,000 to $200,000.

Donor and Recipient. Usually a sibling donates the bone marrow. A parent also may be a donor. In some cancer cases the patient may donate his or her own marrow. (In these autologous transplants, marrow is removed from the patient, who is then treated with whole-body radiation or with high doses of chemotherapy to wipe out any cancer cells in the body. After the stored marrow has been examined for cancer cells and, if necessary, treated with drugs to kill them, the marrow is reinfused into the patient.)

Each year, about 3,000 persons donate bone marrow for transplantation. And that's not enough. Experts say 11,000 persons could benefit from bone marrow transplants if compatible donors were available.

Still, the number of donors and transplants is increasing, partly due to efforts of the National Bone Marrow Registry and the National Marrow Donor Program, which make the search for compatible donors more efficient.

Outcome. About 69 percent of persons with a bone marrow transplant survive the first year, and 50 percent live for at least five years. In the absence of GVHD, a person may resume a normal life-style after about three months.

Future. Throughout the United States, researchers are developing new techniques to improve the success of bone marrow transplants. Mayo doctors are studying the use of growth factors (proteins that stimulate growth and development of cells in bone marrow) to speed recovery after marrow transplantation and to help prevent rejection. They are also experimenting with a special antibody linked to a toxin that can destroy cells that accentuate GVHD.

Skin

The Organ. Skin is the largest of your body's organs. It provides your sense of touch and also serves as a barrier against the environment. Skin stops microorganisms from invading and infecting your body. It regulates temperature and fluid balance, helps make hormones, and offers protection from the sun's ultraviolet radiation.

Injury or Disease. Loss of skin following a disease, an injury, or a burn, may require a skin transplant. The new skin may come from another area of the person's own body or, in rare instances, from a cadaver donor. Transplanting skin from one person to another offers only a temporary solution. Skin from another person is even more likely than other organs to be rejected by the recipient's immune system.

Whenever possible, doctors cover the injured area with healthy skin taken from the recipient's own body (an autologous transplant).

If skin loss is extensive, or if a person needs repeated skin grafting, physicians at some medical centers can perform an autologous cultured skin transplantation. This remarkable new approach grows (cultures) a small piece of the person's own skin for transplantation. Cells from a piece of the outer layer of skin (epidermis), no larger than a postage stamp, can be grown in a laboratory. In about four weeks, the cells combine to form multiple sheets of skin capable of covering an area of the body greater than one square yard.

Mayo dermatologists developed some of the original techniques required to grow new skin in the laboratory. The work has been done within the last few years. Today, the procedure is available at fewer than 10 medical centers.

The Procedure. For most skin transplantations, a thin layer of healthy skin is removed and placed over the wound. After several weeks, the transplanted skin adheres, develops a new blood supply, and matures.

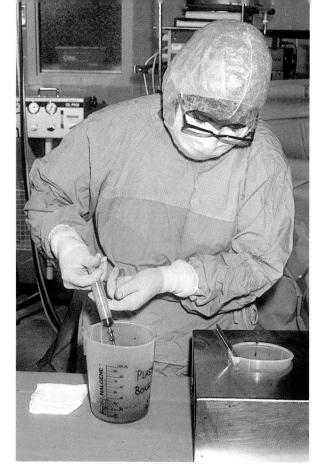

Above, a surgeon transfers bone marrow harvested from a donor into a container prior to transplantation. Below, a young bone marrow patient at the University of Minnesota Hospital. The word "Host" on her shirt indicates that she is the recipient of the transplant.

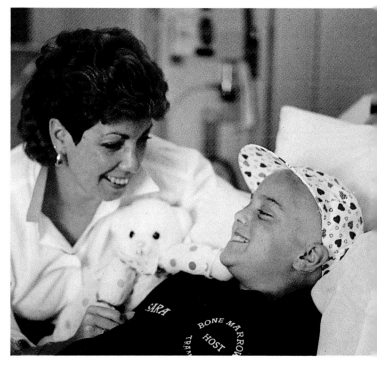

19

New Approaches to an Ancient Idea

Can animal organs be transplanted into a human being?

The concept of xenografting (ze'-no-graft-ing) holds exciting promise. Animal organs could help many people who now wait for the scarce supply of donated human organs. Presently, biological differences among species rule out the permanent use of animal tissue in humans. Researchers are looking for ways to suppress the immune system to make this form of transplantation possible. This concept also raises some questions of medical and social ethics.

The idea of organ transplantation is at least 4,000 years old. Egyptian tile makers transplanted skin grafts from one part of a patient's body to another.

In 1597 an Italian surgeon tried using the flesh of other persons to restore the appearance of patients who had lost their noses. He blamed his failure on the power of human individuality.

By highlighting the differences among individuals and species, these early efforts pioneered today's understanding of the immune system—and how it can be adjusted to permit the transplantation of different organs and tissues.

Cultured, autologous skin transplants are applied in the same manner.

Frequency and Cost. Every year, surgeons perform thousands of routine skin transplants; but autologous cultured skin transplants remain experimental. Mayo physicians performed seven of the several dozen done in the United States in 1989.

Donor and Recipient. Virtually anyone can receive a skin transplant. Age is not a limitation. Younger recipients usually fare better.

You can donate your skin just as you can any other organ. Skin donor banks, similar to blood banks, operate in several regions around the United States.

Outcome. Skin grafted from a donor typically lasts only several weeks. When a person's own skin is transplanted, growth and maturation of the new skin is excellent—autologous transplants have an average success rate of 95 percent. Autologous cultured skin is more susceptible to loss from infection and other wound factors, reducing the success rate to between 50 and 60 percent.

During the years immediately following a skin transplant, the graft continues to mature and eventually resembles normal skin. But grafted skin remains more vulnerable to injury. It sometimes heals more slowly and doesn't tan as readily.

Skin cultured in the laboratory doesn't contain hair or sweat glands. If a large surface of the body is covered with an autologous cultured graft, a person may have trouble regulating body temperature.

Future. To overcome immunological barriers to skin transplantation from unrelated donors, scientists at Mayo and other medical centers are seeking ways to selectively alter the immune system, thus creating a "tolerant immune state." Also, if skin can be grown in a laboratory and preserved, it could serve to make emergency skin transplants more feasible than they are at present.

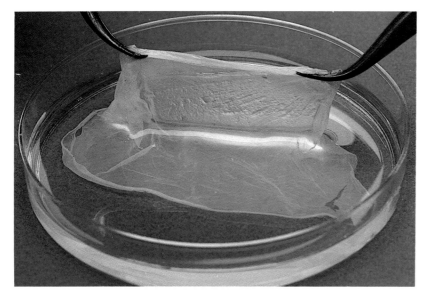

Skin can be grown in the laboratory from a small piece of a patient's own skin. Starting at postage-stamp size, several sheets can be grown and connected to cover an area greater than a square yard.

Bone

The Substance. Bone is made up of collagen, which gives it its form, and calcium phosphate, which provides strength. Like all living tissues, bone constantly breaks down and is replaced with new bone.

Injury or Disease. Bone transplantation is an established treatment for people with serious bone injuries, infections, or certain types of malignant bone tumors.

The Procedure. Surgeons replace damaged bone with bone tissue harvested from cadaver donors, or they graft bone taken from another site within the recipient's body. Bone taken from a cadaver usually is frozen prior to the transplantation surgery.

Cells and blood vessels in the recipient's bone unite with the transplanted bone to form a new column of bone. The healing process requires about 12 months, after which the recipient's original bone is firmly bonded to the transplanted bone. However, complete assimilation of the bone is uncommon. When surgeons use autologous bone for the transplantation, it may be unnecessary to reattach the blood supply of the donated bone. Whether the blood supply must be repaired depends upon the size of the bone involved and other factors. If a blood supply is necessary, microsurgery can be performed to reconnect the vessels.

Risk. Freezing donor bone reduces the chance for rejection due to an immune response. Typically, immune-suppressive medications aren't needed.

Donor and Recipient. The sex of the donor is not a factor, but age is. Donors generally must be older than age 19 to ensure that bone growth is complete. Ideally, donors should be younger than age 50. They also must be free of infection. Unsuitable donors include people with a history of hepatitis, or those who have had a malignant tumor or disorders of normal bone chemistry.

Outcome. From 70 to 90 percent of bone transplantations are successful. People who receive new bone typically can use the treated limb within 6 to 12 months. If a leg bone is involved, bearing full weight on the limb is, of course, restricted during this time.

Future. To enhance long-term results, doctors hope to refine bone storage techniques and to speed the union of new with old bone.

Wide-ranging Benefits

Research into organ transplantation is yielding benefits that someday may outweigh the obvious advantages of organ replacement itself. Transplantation offers a unique "proving ground" for research in biology, immunology, and medicine. Each year, physicians learn more about the ways organs function and about the process by which disease begins and spreads. For example, new findings suggest that the rejection response that helps to protect you from infection also may ward off cancer.

Your immune system may be linked to a sophisticated surveillance system that marks and destroys cancer cells continually produced by your body as part of its normal function. If physicians can understand more precisely why the body identifies and rejects transplanted organs, they may learn why some individuals lose this protective ability and die of various forms of cancer.

These encouraging advances in experimental medicine and biology are emerging at the same time that surgical procedures become safer and available to more people. These factors may hold the greatest promise for organ transplantation in the future. □

21

DOCTORS ON TV

Dr. Anthony Pagano, a young surgeon in Syracuse, N.Y., was performing an operation when an aneurysm in one of the patient's blood vessels suddenly burst. Instead of immediately confronting this unexpected complication, Pagano froze, and the patient nearly died.

As a result, Pagano lost his position in the hospital. He moved to San Francisco, bought a helicopter, and set up a medical rescue service, vowing never to enter an operating room again. But when his co-pilot was injured in a crash and no other surgeon was available, Pagano had to take up the scalpel. Fortunately, a senior physician was there to bolster his confidence. Pagano performed the operation and then joined the hospital staff.

If Dr. Pagano were real, his story could make a good movie. He is, of course, as the tidy symmetry of his comeback reveals, fictional. The senior physician was Trapper John, M.D., and the story was an episode on the television series of the same name.

If you think that's an unlikely tale, consider Dr. Joel Fleischman, protagonist of the CBS series *Northern Exposure*, set in an Alaskan town "somewhere between the end of the line and the middle of nowhere." This is the kind of place where a hiker gets killed by a falling satellite, an Inuit woman cures the Russian flu (after the doctor has failed) with a mixture made of moose droppings, and the same poor fellow shows up dripping blood in Dr. Fleischman's clinic virtually every day bearing a gunshot or stab wound inflicted by his wife.

Then there's nurse Jessie Brewer of the soap opera *General Hospital*. After the death on April 26, 1991, of actress Emily McLaughlin, Jessie's portrayer, *People* magazine calculated that during her 28 years on the show, nurse Brewer endured "five marriages, the loss of two infants, an 11-month pregnancy, a nervous breakdown, a hysterectomy, and potentially fatal spots on her lungs."

Welcome to the wonderful world of television medicine, where ratings outrank realism every time and audiences love it. Along with westerns, soap operas, whodunits, and sitcoms, medical television shows have become programming staples—a genre of their own. And whether we're watching another

Opposite page: A scene from M*A*S*H.

accident victim being rushed into the emergency room, another difficult old codger refuse medical advice, or another vibrant teenager confront a rare, enervating disease, we may wonder: why have audiences remained so fascinated with media medicine? How accurate is what we see? Is this the way medicine is practiced? And is this how doctors are—or how we would *like* them to be?

The Golden Age

One of the first memorable television medical shows was *Medic*, which went on the air in 1954 with Richard Boone as Dr. Konrad Styner. Drawing on case studies and unleavened by humor, the show was a serious attempt to discuss medical issues, and its realism was often uncomfortably intense. Dr. Michael Yogman, now an assistant professor of pediatrics at Harvard Medical School, recalls as a youngster watching an episode involving automobile accidents and finding it "frightening." When sponsors as well as religious groups grew uncomfortable with *Medic*'s explicitness (an episode about a cesarean birth was especially controversial), NBC canceled the show after two years. Already a trend was set—*too much* realism in television medicine may lead to trouble.

In 1961 the golden era of the television doctor dawned with NBC's *Dr. Kildare*, starring Richard Chamberlain, and ABC's *Ben Casey*, starring Vince Edwards. Both shows spotlighted virile, telegenic actors as young physicians, each with his crusty older mentor (Chamberlain, a resident in internal medicine, was under the aegis of Raymond Massey as Dr. Leonard Gillespie; Casey, a neurosurgeon, was kept in line by Sam Jaffe's Dr. David Zorba.)

In the beginning years of the series, Kildare (originally a character played by Lew Ayres in a series of movies between 1938 and 1943) was new, and the show's main theme was whether he would survive his training. The scripts stressed medicine's emotional aspects over its technical ones—largely, perhaps, because its handsome yet unproven hero was, as *TV Guide* put it at the time, "liable to inspire women with an ardent desire to mend his socks." By 1963, Kildare had been promoted to resident physician and the show was being watched by 80 million viewers in 31 countries.

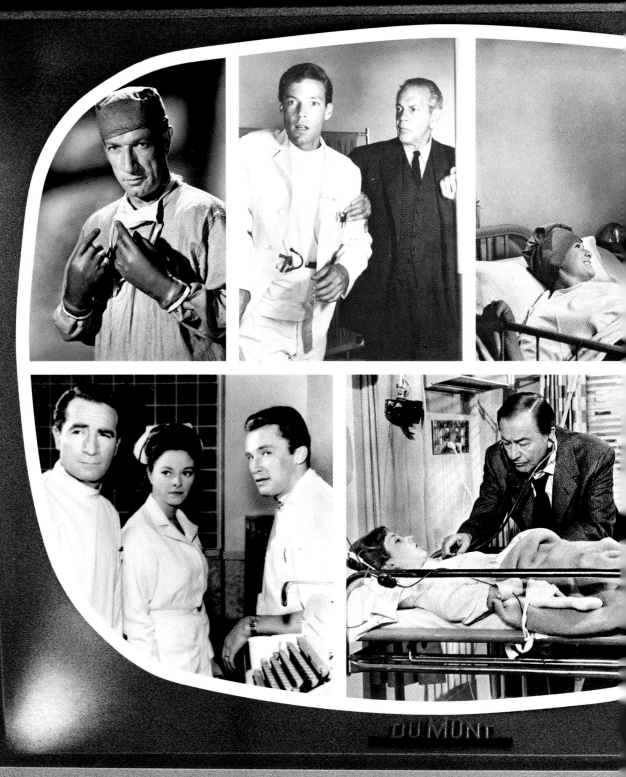

Top left: Richard Boone as Dr. Konrad Styner in Medic.

Top center: Richard Chamberlain (left) as Dr. Kildare was kept in tow by Raymond Massey's Dr. Gillespie.

Bottom left: Nurse Jessie Brewer (center) was played by Emily McLaughlin, who starred on General Hospital with Joe Bernadino (left) and Roy Thinnes.

Bottom center: The wise (and always available) Marcus Welby M.D., as portrayed by Robert Young.

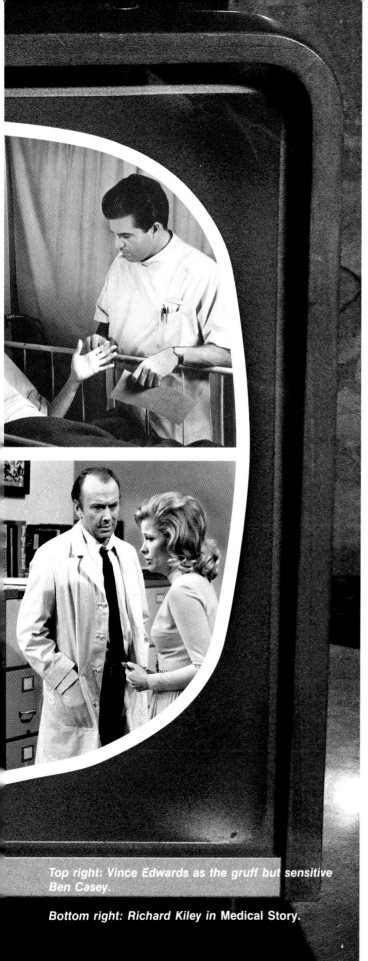

Top right: Vince Edwards as the gruff but sensitive Ben Casey.

Bottom right: Richard Kiley in Medical Story.

Dark, broad-shouldered, brooding, and combative, Edwards's Ben Casey was different. In his hospital, medicine was truly a battle, not only with disease, but, as *Look* magazine described it in 1962, "with the hospital board, patients' relations, other doctors, and most of the human race." The same article said that Casey, "as portrayed by Edwards . . ., runs the gamut from snapping to snarling." Nevertheless, *Variety* called Casey "the most spectacular success of the 1961-62 television season," and it was so popular it spawned a fad in women's blouses patterned after Casey's white, high-necked jacket.

Dissimilar as they were, Kildare and Casey shared a sense of idealism and justice. Casey would gripe about the higher incomes enjoyed by doctors in private practice but remain committed to his own less-lucrative job as a hospital staff physician. During the optimistic Kennedy years at the beginning of the 1960s, such dedication struck a chord with the young. Dr. Yogman recalls being "fascinated" by these two physicians; indeed, they remain a paradigm for what a television doctor is. The networks were now on the right track—a successful medical show needs a likable doctor.

In true television fashion, success brought imitation, and ten medical shows were prepped for the 1962-1963 season. Most were forgettable, but the genre was indestructible, and 1969 brought *Marcus Welby, M.D.*, with the avuncular Robert Young as the gray-haired family physician. *Welby* was produced by David Victor, who had produced *Dr. Kildare*, and he once pointed out that Welby "takes up a Dr. Kildare figure in the later years." Welby is often cynically remembered today as a doctor who actually made house calls, but his wise bedside manner can also be seen as a fantasy wish, in an age of increasingly technical medicine, for a doctor who cared about the whole patient. On the other hand, Welby's saintliness provoked criticism at the time for being a deification of physicians—a mode of thought, it was felt, that could too easily absolve patients of the primary responsibility for maintaining their own health.

Breaking Taboos

Medical Center, which went on in the same year as *Welby*, showed that, although Welby harkened back to a vanishing breed, a new generation was on the

Joseph Gustaitis is a staff editor and writer.

way. Dr. Joe Gannon (played by Chad Everett) was "hip," a character for the times—which is why the show was a hit with younger viewers. More than that, the program revealed how television was beginning to treat more adult, more controversial material. For example, a 1963 *Ben Casey* episode dealt with impotence, but since censors would not permit the word itself to be used, the problem was cloaked in euphemism, such as the patient's lament, "I am not a real man." By the 1970s, however, Joe Gannon could be seen defending the decision of a patient desiring a sex-change operation and the rights of a young woman who wanted an abortion in defiance of her parents' wishes. This increasing frankness, of course, was true of television across the board, but it is arguable that medical shows were leaders of the trend. In a 1975 interview the producers of *Medical Center* acknowledged that one of the express purposes of the show was to explore subjects previously taboo.

One of the more interesting medical programs of the period was *Medical Story* of 1975, which tried to take an investigative approach and explore medicine's failures as well as its successes, while also tackling controversial issues. One episode concerned a doctor (portrayed, interestingly, by the post-*Casey* Vince Edwards) who was arrested for performing an illegal abortion. A reviewer in *TV Guide* said, "Imagine a doctor show without a pat or a happy ending. We tell you it's a medical millennium." The series, however, was a ratings failure and lasted a bare four months. One could argue that, like *Medic, Medical Story* prescribed a pill that was a bit too strong for the audience.

Television's next prominent medical show was NBC's *St. Elsewhere*, which premiered in 1982. With its hand-held cameras, running plots, hard-edged realism, and tight ensemble acting, the program, while never a smash, captured critical acclaim and a loyal following—even among medical personnel. Dr. Yogman recalls it as "one show that really tried to grapple with reality," and Dr. Michael Koren, now clinical assistant professor of medicine at the University of Florida, remembers as a medical student being part of a small fan club that gathered every week to catch it. Toward the end of its six-year run, *St. Elsewhere* tended to slide toward sensationalism, and later scripts dealt heavily in such attention-getting topics as drug addiction, rape, amnesia, artificial insemination, and the physicians' sex lives.

More recent television fare has seen no reason to forgo uncommon subject matter, yet in some ways there has been a drift not only away from reality, but from strictly medical themes. *Northern Exposure* is nominally about a doctor, but the practice of medicine has little to do with the show, as its creators acknowledge. *Doogie Howser, M.D.*, is based on a wholly untenable premise—a 16-year-old physician. As James F. Jekel, M.D., of the Yale University School of Medicine points out, no medical school in the United States would admit a 12-year-old: "Becoming a doctor takes more than intelligence. Emotional maturity and the ability to 'hang in there' are just as important." Even so, *Doogie* is not often about medicine, either, but about the problems—and especially dating habits—of a superbright teen. *The Cosby Show*, of course, is about a doctor, too, but medicine plays virtually no role in the program.

Dr. Perri Klass, a Boston pediatrician writing in the New York *Times*, noted that many of the newer medical shows (*Doogie Howser, Northern Exposure, STAT,* and *Doctor, Doctor*) played for laughs in a way the older ones did not. Being comedies, these were a new wrinkle in the genre. Perhaps this represents a trend—audiences may now want their TV doctors to be not only understanding, but amusing as well (the long-running *M*A*S*H*, though not strictly a medical show, can be seen as a harbinger of the drift and Alan Alda's Hawkeye Pierce as the original wisecracking, lovable—though quite competent—doctor). As a physician, incidentally, Klass did not find the same things funny that the audience was supposed to—to her, it was amusing when the doctors on *STAT* performed an unnecessary barium enema. For those who missed it, *STAT* was a sitcom about life in a New York City emergency room which had a brief run in the 1990-1991 season. A physician reviewing it in the *Medical Tribune*, a professional newspaper, dismissed it with the remark that "its scripts seem to be left over from 13 years ago." (He may not have known how right he was; *STAT*'s scripts were in fact recycled from an earlier show, *A.E.S. Hudson Street*, which went on the air in 1978.)

What Price Reality?

"Since the human body has only two sides—front and back," says Dr. Koren, "you'd think that TV medical shows would get a chest X ray right at least half the time. But it seems to me that nine times out of ten they X-ray the patient from the wrong angle." Dr. Koren raises an interesting issue—just how accurate is the medical information viewers get from these programs?

The question is more than a matter of idle curiosity. In 1982 researchers at the University of Pennsylvania's Annenberg School of Communications reported the results of a survey of daytime soap operas. They found that nearly half of all the characters on these shows became, at one time or another, deeply involved in health matters and that health was the most frequent topic of conversation. They concluded that "it may well be that daytime serials provide the most prolific single source of medical advice in America."

Many television medical shows (as opposed to soaps) have employed technical or medical advisers, sometimes both. The technical adviser is often a nurse who ensures that machines and equipment are being used correctly. The medical adviser is usually a physician who supplies information and helps writers with terminology and procedure. For soap operas and other shows that are not exclusively medical and do not have full-time advisers, the American Medical Association has set up the Physician Advisory Panel on Radio, Television, and Motion Pictures—a group of medical specialists who volunteer to answer technical questions from scriptwriters via a toll-free number. One panel member, Dr. Bates Noble, recalls having to disappoint a writer who wanted to have his surgeon call for a "scalpel," when in reality surgeons use the term "knife."

While accuracy in technical matters such as this can save programs from embarrassment, in the larger picture drama comes first. As Tom Fontana, the co-producer of *St. Elsewhere* once put it, "Medicine is the by-product. We want to make good stories about human beings who happen to be doctors and nurses and patients." Real-life doctors concede that liberties have to be taken. As Dr. Iris Boettcher, assistant professor in the Department of Medicine at Michigan State, explains, "These are *not* information programs, but dramas. If you want information, you can find good documentaries on cable." Dr. Koren points out that TV emergency room scenes can never capture the frenzy and complexity of the real thing and probably shouldn't try: "On television [the treatment to restart a patient's heart] takes about 20 seconds. They shock somebody, and that's it. If they showed the whole pro-

cedure, it would take up the entire program." Dr. Jekel says, "While medicine can involve moments of tension and drama, these shows make it look like a doctor goes from one excitement to another. Most medicine is tedious, ordinary work."

Medical professionals tend to agree that there is one area, however, in which viewers should exercise caution. Dr. Boettcher often feels that her patients, inspired by the omniscience of the Welby type, expect that she, too, can always give them clear-cut answers and "a step-by-step account of what to do." Or, as Dr. Yogman puts it, "Decision-making can be tough. These shows err when they reduce a scientific controversy to something simplistic. You can't act as if the answers were all in." Dr. William A. Nolen, the medical essayist and author of *Making of a Surgeon*, recalled a woman who came into his office certain that she needed a hysterectomy because she had the same symptoms as a woman on television. Actually, his patient needed only hormones. He went on to point out, "Because these shows run for only 51 minutes (9 minutes being devoted to commercials) there isn't enough time to deal in depth with any disease. There is no time, for example, to explain in detail what each symptom means; nor is there time for a discussion of all possible means of therapy. You see one interpretation of symptoms and one method of therapy per patient, when in actual medical practice dozens of alternatives of diagnosis and therapy may be considered before the proper one is chosen."

The Physician's Image

Over 40 years ago the British medical journal *The Lancet* surveyed the ways in which physicians were portrayed in motion pictures and found the portrayals overwhelmingly favorable. For the years 1949 and 1950 it counted 448 doctors in 839 movies and found that only 25 of these doctors were "bad."

In general, this favorable view has continued, although as television became increasingly candid, flawed physicians came to be more prominent. A 1975 episode of *Doctors' Hospital*, for example, was about a surgeon who performed unnecessary surgery—badly—in order to meet his alimony payments. In the same year *Medical Story* dealt with such topics as malpractice and unauthorized experimentation on patients. One of the juiciest characters on *St. Elsewhere* was heart surgeon Dr. Mark Craig (played by William Daniels), who was dis-

27

liked by just about everyone, including his wife. More recently, a *STAT* episode concerned the attempts of a rich uptown Manhattan doctor, obviously in the profession for the money, to lure away the dedicated head of the beleaguered emergency room with a $300,000 yearly salary (the offer, of course, was refused). Yet programs of this sort do not attack the medical profession as a whole, but instead set up the dishonest/incompetent/greedy physician as a foil for the idealistic/dedicated/proficient one, who is really the hero of the show.

Dr. Yogman, however, has noted that there has been a progression from the omnipotent saint-like figure (Welby) to a doctor who is more realistic, which, he says, is all to the good. "Shows that reveal that doctors have crises in their own lives and difficulty making decisions," he says, "can help patients understand that they have to join the treatment process by asking questions and participating in the decision making."

An Enduring Popularity

For today's patient, modern medicine, with its esoteric language, fast-arriving new developments, and forbidding technology, can seem a bewildering place. One reason for the appeal of television medical shows is that they purport to remove some of that mystery. Commenting on the advent of the new medical comedies, Dr. Klass wrote, "Maybe this humor defuses the public's anxiety about doctors and their hocus-pocus, the terror of illness and the strangeness of hospitals. . . ."

Yet while medical programs have been steadily popular, it has been pointed out that there have never been that many successful ones on the air at one time (unlike, say, westerns or police dramas, which have been, at one time or another, all over the dial). Also, fans of one medical show are not necessarily fans of another—viewers tend to have their favorite doctor and watch that one only.

The most compelling explanation for this is that the Kildares, Welbys, and Trapper Johns become for viewers models of what a doctor should be. As people would like their real doctors to do—and which they don't always—the TV doctors form a firm one-to-one relationship with the patient, and, by extension, the viewer, who is the vicarious patient. A television medical show may X-ray a patient incorrectly, but in the wider picture, the message is reassuring. □

28

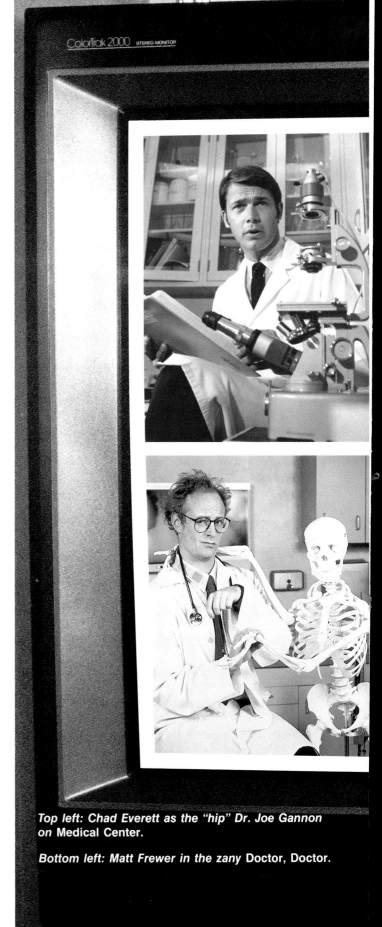

Top left: Chad Everett as the "hip" Dr. Joe Gannon on Medical Center.

Bottom left: Matt Frewer in the zany Doctor, Doctor.

times out of ten they X-ray the patient from the wrong angle." Dr. Koren raises an interesting issue—just how accurate is the medical information viewers get from these programs?

The question is more than a matter of idle curiosity. In 1982 researchers at the University of Pennsylvania's Annenberg School of Communications reported the results of a survey of daytime soap operas. They found that nearly half of all the characters on these shows became, at one time or another, deeply involved in health matters and that health was the most frequent topic of conversation. They concluded that "it may well be that daytime serials provide the most prolific single source of medical advice in America."

Many television medical shows (as opposed to soaps) have employed technical or medical advisers, sometimes both. The technical adviser is often a nurse who ensures that machines and equipment are being used correctly. The medical adviser is usually a physician who supplies information and helps writers with terminology and procedure. For soap operas and other shows that are not exclusively medical and do not have full-time advisers, the American Medical Association has set up the Physician Advisory Panel on Radio, Television, and Motion Pictures—a group of medical specialists who volunteer to answer technical questions from scriptwriters via a toll-free number. One panel member, Dr. Bates Noble, recalls having to disappoint a writer who wanted to have his surgeon call for a "scalpel," when in reality surgeons use the term "knife."

While accuracy in technical matters such as this can save programs from embarrassment, in the larger picture drama comes first. As Tom Fontana, the co-producer of *St. Elsewhere* once put it, "Medicine is the by-product. We want to make good stories about human beings who happen to be doctors and nurses and patients." Real-life doctors concede that liberties have to be taken. As Dr. Iris Boettcher, assistant professor in the Department of Medicine at Michigan State, explains, "These are *not* information programs, but dramas. If you want information, you can find good documentaries on cable." Dr. Koren points out that TV emergency room scenes can never capture the frenzy and complexity of the real thing and probably shouldn't try: "On television [the treatment to restart a patient's heart] takes about 20 seconds. They shock somebody, and that's it. If they showed the whole pro-

cedure, it would take up the entire program." Dr. Jekel says, "While medicine can involve moments of tension and drama, these shows make it look like a doctor goes from one excitement to another. Most medicine is tedious, ordinary work."

Medical professionals tend to agree that there is one area, however, in which viewers should exercise caution. Dr. Boettcher often feels that her patients, inspired by the omniscience of the Welby type, expect that she, too, can always give them clear-cut answers and "a step-by-step account of what to do." Or, as Dr. Yogman puts it, "Decision-making can be tough. These shows err when they reduce a scientific controversy to something simplistic. You can't act as if the answers were all in." Dr. William A. Nolen, the medical essayist and author of *Making of a Surgeon*, recalled a woman who came into his office certain that she needed a hysterectomy because she had the same symptoms as a woman on television. Actually, his patient needed only hormones. He went on to point out, "Because these shows run for only 51 minutes (9 minutes being devoted to commercials) there isn't enough time to deal in depth with any disease. There is no time, for example, to explain in detail what each symptom means; nor is there time for a discussion of all possible means of therapy. You see one interpretation of symptoms and one method of therapy per patient, when in actual medical practice dozens of alternatives of diagnosis and therapy may be considered before the proper one is chosen."

The Physician's Image

Over 40 years ago the British medical journal *The Lancet* surveyed the ways in which physicians were portrayed in motion pictures and found the portrayals overwhelmingly favorable. For the years 1949 and 1950 it counted 448 doctors in 839 movies and found that only 25 of these doctors were "bad."

In general, this favorable view has continued, although as television became increasingly candid, flawed physicians came to be more prominent. A 1975 episode of *Doctors' Hospital*, for example, was about a surgeon who performed unnecessary surgery—badly—in order to meet his alimony payments. In the same year *Medical Story* dealt with such topics as malpractice and unauthorized experimentation on patients. One of the juiciest characters on *St. Elsewhere* was heart surgeon Dr. Mark Craig (played by William Daniels), who was disliked by just about everyone, including his wife. More recently, a *STAT* episode concerned the attempts of a rich uptown Manhattan doctor, obviously in the profession for the money, to lure away the dedicated head of the beleaguered emergency room with a $300,000 yearly salary (the offer, of course, was refused). Yet programs of this sort do not attack the medical profession as a whole, but instead set up the dishonest/incompetent/greedy physician as a foil for the idealistic/dedicated/proficient one, who is really the hero of the show.

Dr. Yogman, however, has noted that there has been a progression from the omnipotent saint-like figure (Welby) to a doctor who is more realistic, which, he says, is all to the good. "Shows that reveal that doctors have crises in their own lives and difficulty making decisions," he says, "can help patients understand that they have to join the treatment process by asking questions and participating in the decision making."

An Enduring Popularity

For today's patient, modern medicine, with its esoteric language, fast-arriving new developments, and forbidding technology, can seem a bewildering place. One reason for the appeal of television medical shows is that they purport to remove some of that mystery. Commenting on the advent of the new medical comedies, Dr. Klass wrote, "Maybe this humor defuses the public's anxiety about doctors and their hocus-pocus, the terror of illness and the strangeness of hospitals. . . ."

Yet while medical programs have been steadily popular, it has been pointed out that there have never been that many successful ones on the air at one time (unlike, say, westerns or police dramas, which have been, at one time or another, all over the dial). Also, fans of one medical show are not necessarily fans of another—viewers tend to have their favorite doctor and watch that one only.

The most compelling explanation for this is that the Kildares, Welbys, and Trapper Johns become for viewers models of what a doctor should be. As people would like their real doctors to do—and which they don't always—the TV doctors form a firm one-to-one relationship with the patient, and, by extension, the viewer, who is the vicarious patient. A television medical show may X-ray a patient incorrectly, but in the wider picture, the message is reassuring. □

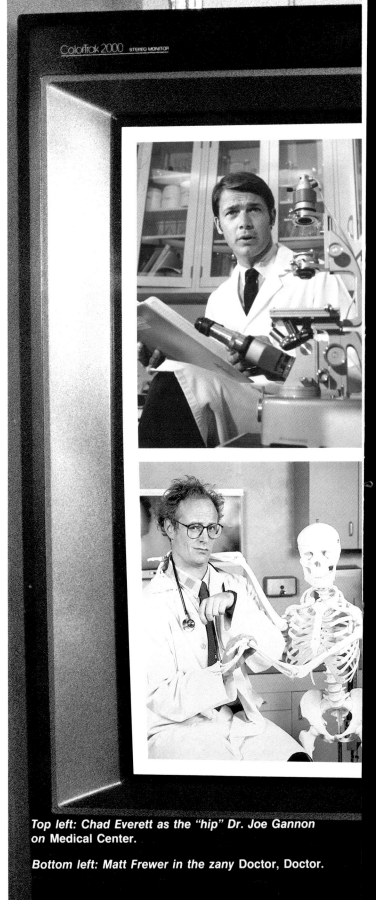

Top left: Chad Everett as the "hip" Dr. Joe Gannon on **Medical Center.**

Bottom left: Matt Frewer in the zany **Doctor, Doctor.**

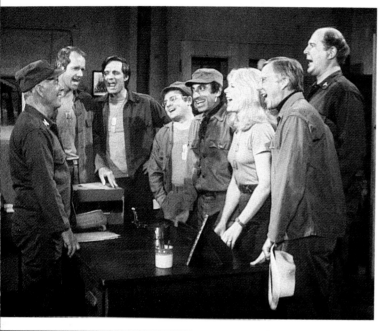

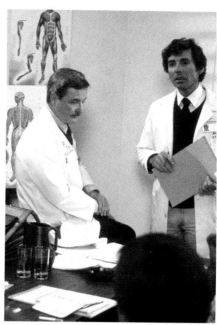

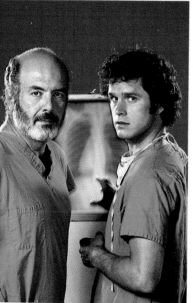

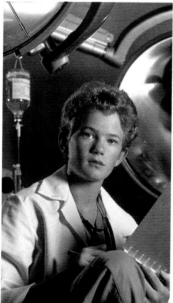

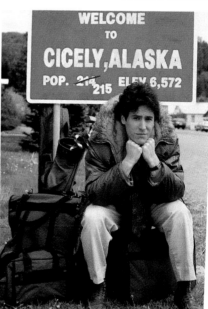

Top center: The gang from M*A*S*H showed that medicine and mirth could mix.

Bottom left center: Pernell Roberts (left, with Gregory Harrison) played the title role in Trapper John, M.D.

Bottom right center: Neil Patrick Harris as the improbable Doogie Howser, M.D.

Top right: William Daniels (left) and David Birney, two of the cast of St. Elsewhere.

Bottom right: The bemused and befuddled Dr. Joel Fleischman, as played by Rob Morrow, in Northern Exposure.

WATER

FIT TO

DRINK

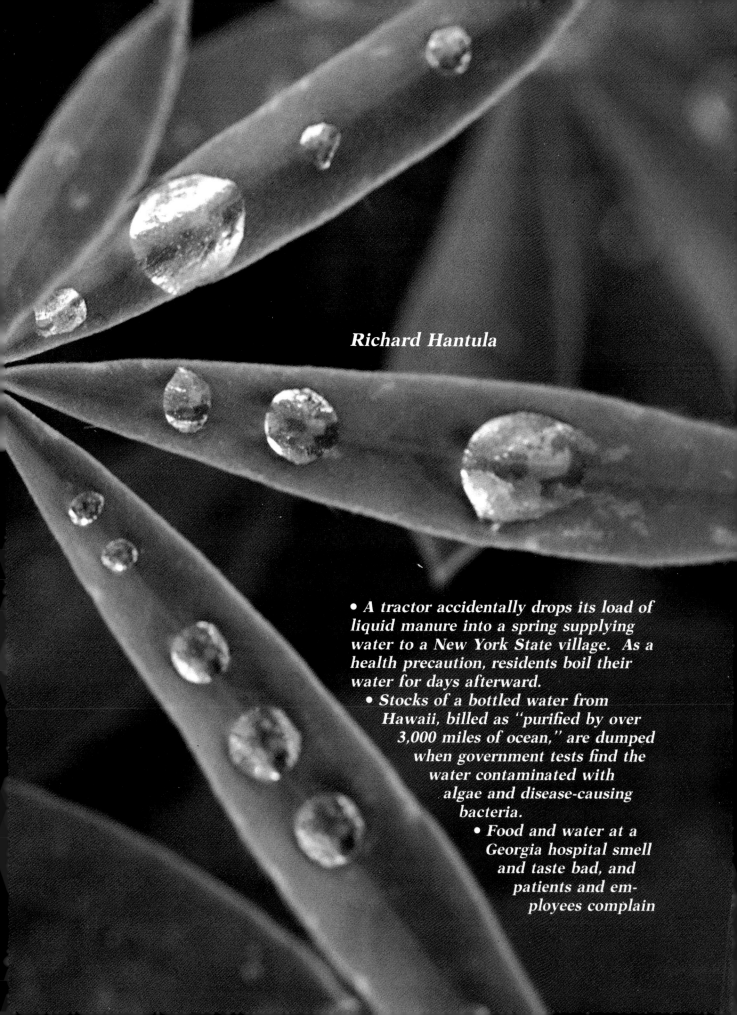

Richard Hantula

• *A tractor accidentally drops its load of liquid manure into a spring supplying water to a New York State village. As a health precaution, residents boil their water for days afterward.*
  • *Stocks of a bottled water from Hawaii, billed as "purified by over 3,000 miles of ocean," are dumped when government tests find the water contaminated with algae and disease-causing bacteria.*
    • *Food and water at a Georgia hospital smell and taste bad, and patients and employees complain*

of nausea, vomiting, and diarrhea, after phenol enters the hospital water from a water storage tank coated with an improperly cured phenol resin.
• For decades the federal nuclear installation at Hanford, Wash., discharges billions of gallons of liquids containing radioactive materials into the Columbia River.

Everyone needs water, and the United States is endowed with immense quantities of it. But, as the above news items from recent years remind us, this resource is fragile. Its quality is easily damaged. Water tainted with more than tiny amounts of certain microbes or chemicals can be hazardous for drinking, or even bathing, or can have a repellent taste, odor, or appearance.

Perfectly pure water is exceedingly hard to find in nature. (Actually, perfectly pure water would be utterly tasteless, and most people would find it unappetizing.) Even the clearest mountain stream may contain germs and minerals or other substances. Thanks to government clean-water programs, the water supplied to American homes today is generally safe. Especially likely to receive good water are people served by large, well-funded public water-supply systems equipped with powerful treatment and filtration technology and up-to-date distribution networks. Some households, however, have chosen to install special purification devices to ensure the wholesomeness of their water.

Groundwater and Surface Water

About half the drinking water in the United States comes from surface sources, such as lakes and rivers. The other half is groundwater, from underground aquifers. Many major U.S. cities use mostly groundwater, and the majority of rural homes have wells.

Both surface water and groundwater can fall prey to contamination. Sewage and industrial waste may be discharged into rivers and lakes. Water filtering into the ground from polluted streams and lakes can poison an aquifer, as can liquids leaking from underground storage tanks, landfills, hazardous waste sites, and the like. In farming areas runoff, the water that drains from the land into rivers and streams and into the soil, can carry pesticides, herbicides, and fertilizer chemicals, and irrigation water may pick up salts from the soil. Runoff from mining operations can carry toxic chemicals. Runoff from streets and roads may contain petrochemicals and metals, as well as salt from road deicing. The quality of a water supply depends also on natural factors like drought, which can cause water quality to deteriorate as pollutants become more concentrated.

The threat from pollution has probably lessened since the 1960s, which saw Cleveland's oil-contaminated Cuyahoga River erupt in flames 200 feet high. Largely because of a massive pollution-control effort that began in the following decade, a major 1987 study found widespread decreases in levels of fecal bacteria and lead in U.S. rivers. Pollution from factories has been declining, according to the U.S. Environmental Protection Agency's annual Toxics Release Inventory, a sur-

Some Water Words

hardness and softness

Hard water contains high amounts of calcium and magnesium (and perhaps other minerals), which cause it to reduce the sudsing power of soap and to produce "scale" in boilers, hot water heaters, and hot water pipes. Hard water is less corrosive than soft and so is less likely to pick up lead from plumbing. Some research suggests a possible link between soft water and an increased risk of heart disease.

pH

A measure of water's acidity or alkalinity (the opposite of acidity). On a scale from 0 to 14, 7 is neutral. The lower the pH falls below 7, the higher the acidity. Acidic water is more corrosive and more likely to leach harmful substances like lead from plumbing.

turbidity

Water becomes cloudy, or turbid, when particles of material are suspended in it. The U.S. Environmental Protection Agency sets standards for turbidity because the particles can shield microorganisms against disinfection. Also, the particles may affect the results of some tests for bacteria and may readily combine with toxic substances or themselves be toxic.

Richard Hantula is a staff editor and writer.

vey of hundreds of hazardous substances discharged into the air, water, and ground by manufacturers.

Still, pollution problems remain. Many toxic chemicals are not monitored in the Toxics Release Inventory. The 1987 study of river water quality found widespread *increases* in concentrations of such substances as nitrates, chlorides, and arsenic. Moreover, while lakes and streams can be cleaned up, groundwater is much less accessible. Once poisoned, the water lying in an aquifer may be difficult or impossible to clean. Seemingly slight leaks of chemicals into an aquifer can be disastrous. A pea-sized hole in a pipe at a gasoline storage terminal on Long Island, N.Y., allowed a million gallons of gasoline to escape over more than a decade before it was detected in 1987. The gasoline spread over 30 acres and threatened the aquifer supplying the heavily populated region with drinking water.

Some studies put at 1-2 percent the proportion of underground water sources near the surface that are contaminated by "point" sources, such as leaking landfills. This may seem a small amount, but the contamination often occurs near thickly populated areas, whose use of groundwater is increasing. About a third of American homes use septic tanks, which can contaminate adjacent groundwater—a problem particularly for those with private wells.

Of course, a polluted water supply is not necessarily dangerous, since, as a government water official pointed out, "you can purify just about any water." But this can be expensive. And even when a utility adequately purifies its water, the water may become contaminated on the way to the tap. It may pick up lead from old lead pipes or from solder in home copper plumbing. Newer plastic pipes can be penetrated by toxic chemicals and may themselves contain hazardous substances. A break in any kind of pipe may allow disease-causing microorganisms—bacteria, viruses, and parasites—or toxic chemicals to enter the water.

Germs in Water

Many decades ago, bad drinking water was a major cause of epidemics of diseases like cholera and typhoid fever. Although government standards and treatment systems in place today protect most developed nations against such epidemics, microorganisms are still responsible for most reported cases of illness caused by water.

Between 1986 and 1988, 50 outbreaks of illness caused by drinking water from public or private supplies were reported to the U.S. Centers for Disease Control; over 25,000 people were affected. Also, there were 26 outbreaks, involving nearly 1,400 people, caused by recreational water use (such as swimming, or bathing in hot tubs or whirlpools). The actual extent of waterborne illness must have been much higher. Many cases were undoubtedly not reported, and the reporting system would not pick up illnesses that develop only after years of exposure to contaminated water.

The overwhelming majority of reported cases were known, or suspected, to be caused by microorganisms. As might be expected, most of the illnesses were digestive system disorders. The parasite *Giardia*

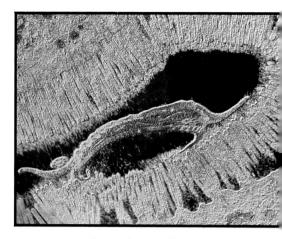

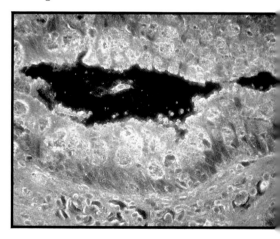

Many cases of waterborne illnesses are caused by the parasite Giardia lamblia, *the orange organism (above) adhering to the inner surface of the small intestine. A major outbreak of gastrointestinal illness in Georgia in 1987 was caused by the parasite* Cryptosporidium *(below), the tiny pinkish globes seen in the photo's center attached to a part of the large intestine.*

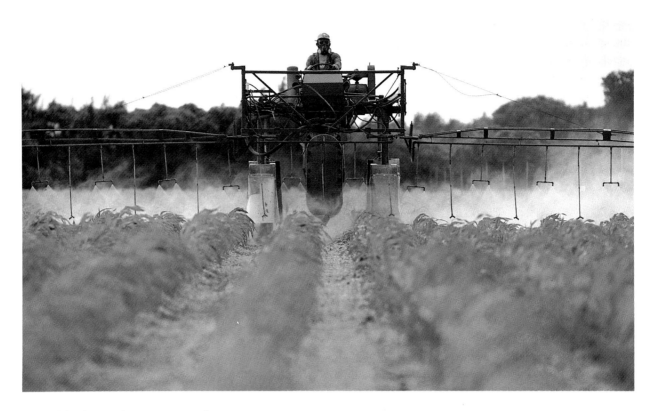

Harmful chemicals can enter the water supply in many ways. Two common ones are the agricultural use of pesticides (above) and the discharge of wastes from industry.

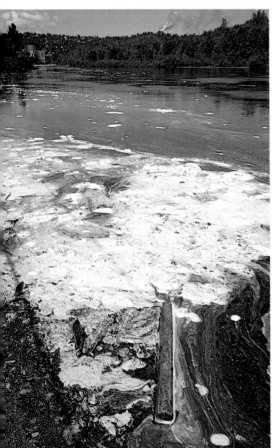

lamblia was responsible for the greatest number of outbreaks. Often found in seemingly clear mountain streams, as well as other water sources, it causes an intestinal infection called giardiasis, familiarly known as backpacker's lament, that may cause gas, diarrhea, vomiting, and weight loss.

Safeguards designed to protect public water supplies against scourges of the past like cholera may not be effective against trouble from an unexpected source. In a major outbreak in 1987, 13,000 people in western Georgia developed gastrointestinal problems after the parasite *Cryptosporidium* appeared in their drinking water, even though the water had been chlorinated (disinfected) and filtered in accordance with government standards. Roughly a fifth of outbreaks of waterborne disease occur in areas that are regarded as having full water treatment facilities.

Troublesome Chemicals

Thousands of chemical compounds have been detected in U.S. drinking water; some are known or suspected to be harmful to health, but they are generally present in what is regarded as insignificant amounts. Very rarely do hazardous chemicals occur in large enough amounts to cause illness to develop immediately. Of the 50 outbreaks of disease caused by drinking water in 1986-1988, only five, affecting about 100 people, were attributed to chemical contamination.

Scientists are still seeking to determine the risks, if any, of long-term exposure to drinking water containing very low levels of various toxic chemicals. A health problem might conceivably arise after years of using the water for drinking or for swimming or bathing (some pollutants are readily absorbed through the skin). There already is enough evidence to raise concern about a few potentially hazardous substances that may occur in water over wide areas of the United States, including radon, lead, and nitrates.

Radon. A radioactive gas, radon has in recent years emerged as a major health concern for residents of some areas, where it has been found to seep into buildings from certain underlying rock formations. When inhaled, the gas can lead to the development of lung cancer. Seepage from the ground is not the only way radon can enter the air in a house, since the gas may also be dissolved in groundwater. When such water is used for showering, laundering, or dish washing, the radon can escape into the air. The Environmental Protection Agency estimates that radon in water causes 200 cancer deaths a year. (This includes a few cases of stomach cancer caused by drinking such water.)

Water from major public water systems has usually undergone aeration, which allows radon to dissipate in the atmosphere. In any event, household water coming from rivers or lakes or from storage reservoirs will probably have released any radon in it harmlessly into the atmosphere. Those who should be concerned that their water may be exposing them to excessive quantities of radon are people in high-radon areas who get their water from private wells or small community water systems that use groundwater. Levels of radon in groundwater are generally highest in certain areas of the Northeast and lowest in the Midwest.

Lead and Other Metals. Some metals that occur in drinking water can be good for us, at least in small doses. Examples are calcium, copper, iron, magnesium, manganese, and zinc. But these may be dangerous in large amounts. Other metals, which are not necessary for good health, may also be harmful if they accumulate in the body. Both groundwater and surface water, for example, may be contaminated by metals like arsenic, barium, cadmium, lead, mercury, and silver from landfills or inadequately treated industrial waste water. (Also, in many cases, much of the lead that may be found in tap water has leached from household plumbing.) Some metals may cause birth defects or damage various organs. Research so far indicates that drinking water that meets current federal standards for metal content poses very little risk to health. People generally take in more metals from food, smoking, and polluted air than from water.

Lead, however, is a particularly insidious threat. In large doses it can harm the nervous system, brain, kidneys, and circulatory system. Water with lead levels too low to poison adults can present a significant risk to young children and fetuses, whose nervous systems are still developing. The lead can cause low birth weight, developmental and learning disabilities, and hyperactive behavior.

Nitrates. The nitrogen-containing chemicals called nitrates can enter groundwater from septic tanks or from the soil, where they arise out of nitrogen compounds from fertilizers, feedlots, and manure. The level of nitrates in U.S. water has been rising. A five-year national study of drinking-water wells released by the Environmental Protection

Lead found in tap water often comes from the plumbing.

35

Agency in 1990 found that over half of the wells contained nitrates. In most cases the amounts were very small, reaching potentially harmful levels in 1.2 percent of community wells and 2.4 percent of private rural wells. In the digestive system nitrates are converted to nitrites, which in infants can cause methemoglobinemia, a blood disorder that deprives organs of oxygen. Extreme cases can produce brain damage or death.

Organic Chemicals. Hundreds of different "organic" chemicals— chemicals whose components include carbon and hydrogen—have been detected in U.S. water, especially in industrial areas. They include trichloroethylene, which comes from industrial discharges and hazardous waste sites, and trihalomethanes, such as chloroform, which may result from chlorination of water. In agricultural regions water may be contaminated by organic pesticides. Little is known about the possible risks to health, if any, of these chemicals in the low concentrations at which they generally appear in water. Exposure to large quantities of some of them can be harmful. Trichloroethylene, for example, has been linked to cancer, as have some organic pesticides.

Salt, Chlorine, Fluoride. Common salt is a combination of the metal sodium and chlorine. High levels of sodium in food and drinking water are associated with high blood pressure in some people. For that reason, the American Heart Association recommends that drinking water have less than 20 parts of sodium per million. Ways in which sodium can enter groundwater include intrusion by seawater and contamination from natural salt deposits. Municipal sewage discharge may raise the sodium content of surface water. Runoff in northern states will carry salt used on icy roads in the winter. A water softener will increase the sodium content of water in the home.

Many water supply systems treat their water with chemicals containing chlorine in order to disinfect it. Some studies have suggested a link between chlorination by-products like trihalomethanes and a slightly increased risk of disorders such as heart disease and cancer. The evidence so far, however, suggests that the benefits of chlorination far outweigh the possible increased risk.

Fluoride is widely added to water supplies to reduce tooth decay. Although critics have for years argued that this fluoride can harm the body, there is no solid evidence that the small amount used can be dangerous to health. A 1990 study did suggest a weak link between sodium fluoride and a rare bone cancer in male rats. The researchers had given the fluoride in drinking water to over 1,000 male and female mice and rats. Only 4 male rats (out of 130) developed the cancer, and they had received dozens of times more fluoride than the dose recommended for human drinking water.

While fluoride levels are carefully monitored in public water systems, they generally are not for private wells. A 1991 study pointed out that in certain areas (including parts of Arizona, Colorado, Illinois, Iowa, New Mexico, Ohio, Oklahoma, and Texas) groundwater may be very high in fluoride, and people who drink it run an increased risk of eventually developing fluorosis, which in extreme cases can produce bone abnormalities. The researchers recommended that fluoride levels be measured at least when a well is drilled.

The fluoride added to water to reduce tooth decay is not dangerous to one's health.

BOTTLED WATER

Anxiety in recent years over water quality helped drive a boom in the U.S. bottled water market. Sales grew 400 percent in the 1980s, reaching $2.6 billion by 1990, and hundreds of brands are now marketed.

Bottled water, however, is not necessarily more wholesome than tap water that meets federal standards. Some brands take their water from public supplies (albeit perhaps specially treated); others use water from springs or more exotic sources—which does not necessarily guarantee purity. A 1991 Food and Drug Administration study discovered bacteria in 31 percent of the 52 brands surveyed. It is unclear whether so-called mineral water truly provides any health benefits.

That is not to say there are no valid reasons for buying bottled water. Some people just don't like the flavor of the stuff that flows from their taps. If a household's water supply becomes contaminated, a trustworthy bottled brand can provide a safe alternative.

Federal standards for bottled water are more limited than those for tap water. Some states, such as California, New Jersey, and New York, have their own, more strict regulations. The Food and Drug Administration regulates bottled waters (at least those that cross state lines), requiring that they meet the safety standards set by the Environmental Protection Agency for public water supplies. In addition, the FDA conducts occasional inspections to ensure that federal standards for cleanliness of food-handling plants are observed. Also, most companies belong to the International Bottled Water Association, which encourages them to have their plants inspected regularly by the National Sanitation Foundation to verify that the association's treatment and bottling standards are being observed.

Still, problems may arise. The Food and Drug Administration's enforcement activity is less extensive than the Environmental Protection Agency's supervision of public water supplies, and the FDA has not set quality standards for mineral waters. In a famous 1990 incident, France's Perrier company recalled 170 million bottles worldwide after tiny amounts of benzene, a suspected carcinogen, were found in its water. Benzene occurs as a contaminant in the gas used to carbonate Perrier water, and the company had failed to change the filters used to screen it out.

Sodium and fluoride are particular concerns. Some bottled waters have very high sodium levels, and some do not contain enough fluoride to provide the protection against cavities that is expected from water supplied by public utilities.

Terms used to characterize bottled water include the following:

- distilled water—all minerals have been removed through vaporization and condensation. Many people find that distilled water tastes "flat" or "lifeless."

- mineral water—water that, according to the International Bottled Water Association, "contains not less than 500 parts per million total dissolved solids," although some experts use this name for any nondistilled water.

- natural water—this comes from a "natural" source, such as a well or a spring, not from a community water supply, and should have had no minerals added or removed.

- sparkling water—carbonated water; it contains dissolved carbon dioxide, which may have been present at the source or may have been added during bottling.

- spring water—groundwater that flows naturally from a surface opening. If the bottler follows the guidelines of the International Bottled Water Association, no minerals have been added or removed. The law requires that water labeled "spring water" actually come from a spring. If the word "spring" merely appears in the bottler's name, the bottle may contain just repackaged tap water.

- still water—noncarbonated water.

Club soda and seltzer are carbonated waters classed for regulatory purposes as soft drinks rather than bottled waters. Club soda, but not seltzer, contains added salts and minerals.

Regulation

A number of laws in the United States protect the quality of drinking water, notably, for public water systems, the Safe Drinking Water Act. This legislation, enacted in 1974 and amended in 1986, mandates certain standards and requires that the public be notified when these standards are violated, such as by accidental contamination of a water supply. The details of the standards are established by the Environmental Protection Agency. Individual states sometimes impose stricter requirements. In addition to mandatory "primary" standards, which are based on health considerations, the Environmental Protection Agency sets secondary standards, which concern water's taste, odor, or color and are guidelines only (although states may choose to enforce them). For some contaminants, primary standards define a maximum allowable level. For contaminants that are difficult or expensive to measure, primary standards require the use of specific water treatment techniques, like filtration or corrosion control.

The U.S. government issued its first water quality standards back in 1914.

The earliest federal efforts at controlling the quality of drinking water focused on disease-causing microorganisms. Standards introduced in 1914 were aimed against interstate transmission of communicable diseases. About five decades later, interstate water supplies were subjected to limits on hazardous chemical as well as biological contaminants. The Safe Drinking Water Act was enacted after a 1970 study found that 5,000 public water supplies were providing potentially harmful water to 8 million Americans. Applying to all public water supplies, the act mandated standards for ten inorganic chemicals, six pesticides, and radioactive materials, as well as for "coliform" bacteria. Even though they do not themselves necessarily cause disease, coliform bacteria have long been used in testing water as an indicator that disease-causing microorganisms may be present, since coliforms are easy to detect and occur in large numbers in human and animal fecal matter, which is the most common source of disease-causing microorganisms in water.

The amendments to the Safe Drinking Water Act adopted in 1986 required that standards be set for 83 contaminants, with more to be added in groups of 25 at regular intervals. (Issuance of the 83 standards is not expected to be completed until at least 1992.) The microorganisms specified included *Legionella*, the cause of Legionnaires' disease; *Giardia*; and enteric viruses (viruses of the intestine). The amendments virtually (but not completely) banned the use of lead materials in new pipes and plumbing and required water suppliers to inform customers of the existence of excess lead levels. The maximum acceptable lead content in plumbing components was put at 0.2 percent for solder and flux. A limit of 8 percent lead, however, was set for pipes and fittings, thereby allowing the continued use of popular brass faucets and fittings containing some lead.

In 1991 the Environmental Protection Agency lowered its limit for lead in drinking water to an average level of 5 parts per billion, down from 50, and water utilities were ordered to begin monitoring lead levels in water at customers' faucets. (Previously, monitoring could be done anywhere in the distribution system.) The regulation required that lead levels at the tap not exceed 15 parts per billion in at least 90 percent of households from which samples are taken. This corresponds to an average of 5 parts per billion for the water system. Utilities would have to eventually replace their lead pipes if high lead levels could not be sufficiently reduced by chemically treating their water. (Water from lead pipes may not contain high levels of lead if, say, lime salts have covered the inner surfaces of the pipes, thereby shielding the water from the lead, or if the water is not corrosive enough to dissolve significant amounts of lead.)

Laws and regulations, however, are effective only if they are implemented. Lead is a case in point. Seeking to lower lead levels in the drinking water used in schools, Congress a few years ago ordered school districts to check their water for lead and required government agencies to establish guidelines for the testing; it also prohibited the interstate sale of water coolers releasing too much lead and required that faulty school coolers be repaired or removed by 1990. But for budgetary and other reasons, comprehensive guidelines were not issued, and many school systems failed to meet the legislation's requirements. A 1990 federal study found that because of inadequate implementation of the legislation, some water coolers and water fountains in schools and other public buildings still had lead-containing pipes that were capable of raising lead levels above the then federal limit of 50 parts per billion.

Public water systems generally test their water at regular intervals, and the results are made available to the public.

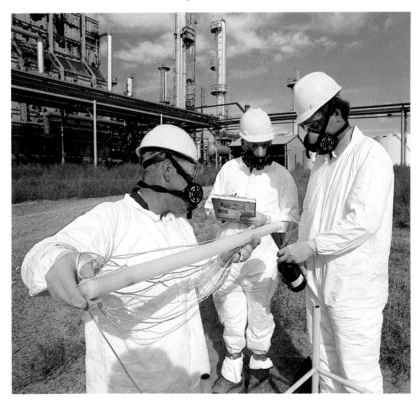

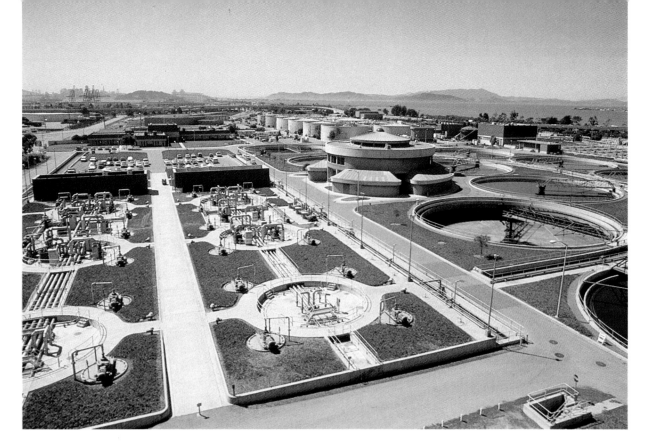

Modern water treatment plants, such as this one in Oakland, Calif., go a long way toward ensuring the safety of a community's water supply.

Water Testing

The only way to be truly sure about the quality of water is to have it analyzed. Water that tastes good and looks clean may harbor harmful contaminants such as lead or *Giardia lamblia*, while water that tastes or looks a little strange may be fit to drink. Water from private wells, for example, may contain enough manganese or iron to affect its smell and taste or to leave a rust stain, but the levels of these metals are typically not high enough to be harmful to health.

Public water systems generally must test their water for certain contaminants at regular intervals, with the results made available to the public. People considering whether to have their own testing done on their household water should, at least at first, focus on contaminants suspected to possibly be present. Checking for a wide variety of contaminants can be expensive. A simple test just for lead or radon will not cost much, but some substances are hard to identify even with sophisticated equipment.

A lead test is a good idea where the plumbing contains lead pipe or lead solder, especially if the household has small children or a pregnant woman. Samples should be taken from every tap used for drinking water, and they should be obtained early in the morning, before any water has been used. The water will have been in the pipes all night and so will be more likely to have dissolved lead from the plumbing (if it contains any).

People living in areas known to be high in radon ought to have the air in their home tested. If it is found to contain potentially harmful levels of radon and the household uses groundwater, the water should be tested for the gas. There is controversy over what levels of radon in water are safe, but in mid-1991 the Environmental Protection Agency proposed setting the maximum allowable level for public water systems at 300 picocuries per liter (about 1 quart) of water. Some experts had previously recommended specially purifying household water if the radon level is at least 10,000 picocuries per liter, arguing that at lower levels it might be more practical for a home owner to simply try to reduce the amount of radon entering the house from the ground.

People getting their drinking water from private wells are not protected by the safeguards governing public water systems. Local health officials may be able to advise regarding specific threats to water quality. Groundwater may be contaminated, for example, if a hazardous waste site, landfill, chemical plant, military base, or munitions factory is in the vicinity. Well water should certainly be checked at least once a year for bacteria. In farming areas a periodic test for nitrates is recommended, especially if there are infants or pregnant women in the household. It is also a good idea to test the water for lead, petrochemicals (particularly if a gasoline station or refinery is nearby), and pesticides and herbicides known to be used in the area.

Some local water companies or health departments will check a household's water for certain contaminants for a moderate fee, and some states offer radon testing of water at a small charge. But government laboratories generally offer only a few tests, and they may be slow to provide the results. For a more comprehensive analysis a private laboratory will probably be needed. Local labs can be found in the Yellow Pages under headings like "Laboratories-Testing," "Water Analysis," or "Water Testing." It is best to look for a lab that is certified by the state and by the Environmental Protection Agency. The EPA's Safe Drinking Water Hotline (800-426-4791) can provide the telephone number for the state agency responsible for certifying. The lab used should be independent, not connected with any water treatment equipment company, which has an interest in selling its products. An appropriate bottle for collecting the sample should be obtained from the lab doing the analysis. If the test report indicates high levels of hazardous contaminants that would require an expensive treatment system, the results should be confirmed by a second test done by another lab.

Home Treatment Devices

A variety of water purification and treatment equipment is available. No single device can remove all possible contaminants. So-called point-of-entry systems, which handle all the water entering the household, can be very costly, but they may be justified in situations where all water, not just drinking water, should be purified. According to one study, a 50-pound child who spent an hour in a swimming pool polluted with certain toxic chemicals would absorb far more of the substances than would be ingested by drinking a quart of the same water. In some cases, such as nitrate contamination, people who use well water may have the option of digging a deeper well to reach uncontaminated water instead of installing purification equipment.

The most popular purification devices treat only the water at, say, a particular tap. The most widely sold of these "point-of-use" devices

No single water purification device can remove all possible contaminants.

41

WATER WISDOM

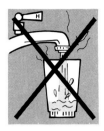

1 Don't use water from the hot water tap for drinking or cooking. Use water from the cold water tap, and let it run until cold.

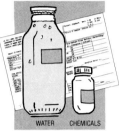

WATER   CHEMICALS

2 Have your water analyzed if you doubt its wholesomeness.

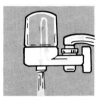

3 Consider purification equipment if testing finds a water problem.

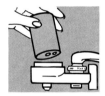

4 Change filters in purification equipment regularly.

have activated carbon (charcoal) filters. Large carbon filters mounted under the sink or on a countertop can significantly reduce levels of chlorine and some organic chemicals, including pesticides and chloroform, and are good at eliminating bad tastes or odors. They generally cannot remove microorganisms, sodium, nitrates, fluoride, or lead or other heavy metals. Small carbon filters that are mounted on a faucet, as well as water pitchers with a built-in carbon filter, are much less effective. While good carbon filters can remove radon, a point-of-entry system is really needed for this, because any water used in the house, not just drinking water, can be a source of the gas.

Carbon filter cartridges have to be changed regularly, since they not only become saturated, and thus ineffective, but can develop into a breeding ground for bacteria. (Also to protect against bacteria, the unit should be flushed after a period of nonuse.) To avoid clogging the filter, water should be made to pass first through a sediment filter.

A different kind of filtering device, based on "reverse osmosis," passes water through high-tech membranes that remove ions and large molecules. Such systems are recommended for water with high levels of inorganic substances like salt, fluoride, or heavy metals such as lead or iron. They may also remove organic chemicals with large molecules, as well as large microorganisms. Reverse osmosis, however, works slowly and is wasteful of water, since most of the water entering the device generally goes down the drain. Systems on the market typically include a sediment filter and an activated carbon filter and are installed under the sink or on the countertop. The reverse-osmosis membrane needs to be replaced once a year or so, depending on use and water quality.

Water softeners improve water's aesthetic qualities by replacing calcium and magnesium with sodium, from salt. This helps to reduce scaly rings around the bathtub as well as sediments ("scale") that can clog the water heater, hot water pipes, and boiler; it can also help solve the problem of low suds in the dishwasher. Softeners may also remove a little lead, as well as iron, which can leave brown stains. The increased sodium content of water from a softener may pose a health problem for some individuals. Also, it should be kept in mind that softening makes water more corrosive and more likely to leach out lead from pipes or solder if any is present.

A third type of treatment device is the distillation unit, which boils water to form steam and then condenses it back into water. This procedure will not protect against toxic chemicals that have a boiling point similar to, or lower than, that of water, but it can remove salts, nitrates, fluoride, sediment, and heavy metals (for metals it is better than reverse osmosis). The distillation process is very slow and consumes a great deal of electricity, and it softens the water.

Other types of equipment are also on the market. In home aerators, which can reduce radon levels, water held in an aeration tank is agitated by pumped-in air; the radon bubbles out and is piped outside, where it dissipates. There are filters specifically designed to trap lead that are cheaper than reverse-osmosis systems. There are also devices that disinfect water by using ultraviolet light, ozone, or chlorine to kill any germs that are present.

If, after testing your water, you decide to buy a water treatment system, get one that meets your needs and has a good track record. Some machines have been known to release harmful chemicals into the water. Look for units certified by the National Sanitation Foundation and manufacturers that belong to the Water Quality Association. It's a good idea to have your water tested again after the unit is installed. That way you can find out if the water treatment system is doing what it is supposed to do.

Playing It Safe

Whether you buy treatment equipment or not, a few simple precautions can make your water safer. Before drawing water from the tap for drinking or cooking, let the water run until it turns cold. At the beginning of the day this may take as long as three minutes. Unlike the warmer water that first appears, the cold water will not have been lying in the pipes for a long time, and thus will be less likely to have absorbed lead or other contaminants from them. Also, warm water is more corrosive, and more readily takes lead from pipes. (This is also one reason why warm or hot water from the tap should not be used for cooking or drinking.) If a lab test shows that letting the water run to flush the pipes does not reduce the lead level enough, a water purification system may need to be installed.

Flushing the pipes need not be wasteful of water. The warm water that comes out first can be collected and used for nondrinking purposes like washing. (Also, cold water for drinking can be stored in a refrigerator, so the pipes don't have to be flushed as often.) The flushing procedure is not practical with water fountains of the type found in schools, which may contain as much as several quarts of water.

The water heater is another possible source of water contamination, since sediments accumulate in it. Experts recommend flushing it out on a regular basis, such as every six months. □

SOURCES OF FURTHER INFORMATION

National Sanitation Foundation. P.O. Box 1468, Ann Arbor, MI 48106. This nonprofit organization tests water treatment systems for certification and verifies manufacturers' claims.
Safe Drinking Water Hotline. Tel.: (800) 426-4791. Sponsored by the U.S. Environmental Protection Agency.
State departments of public health or environmental engineering.
U.S. Environmental Protection Agency regional offices.
Water Quality Association. 4151 Naperville Road, Lisle, IL 60532. A water-treatment industry group.

SUGGESTIONS FOR FURTHER READING

COFFEL, STEVE. *But Not a Drop to Drink! The Lifesaving Guide to Good Water.* New York, Rawson, 1989.
STEWART, JOHN CARY. *Drinking Water Hazards: How to Know If There Are Toxic Chemicals in Your Water and What to Do If There Are.* Hiram, Ohio, Envirographics, 1990.

UPS AND DOWNS OF AIR TRAVEL

Ingrid J. Strauch

ir travel, once considered an adventure in itself, has become almost as commonplace as driving a car for many people worldwide. In today's modern jets very few people experience motion sickness or severe ill effects, but it's no secret that a long flight can present problems. Luckily there are a number of things passengers can do to counterbalance the fact that the human body objects to sitting for hours in cramped quarters miles above the earth.

The Importance of Exercise

Even before the plane takes off, it's hard to ignore how small the seats are and how little leg room there is between rows. Sitting in such conditions for long periods of time can leave passengers feeling stiff and can also cause swelling of the legs and feet as circulation slows and blood pools in the lower extremities. To alleviate these symptoms, passengers on long flights should exercise periodically. Doctors recommend an hourly walk in the aisle, provided the airplane isn't experiencing turbulence and the flight attendants aren't serving food. When walking isn't possible (or in addition to it), occasionally tensing and relaxing the muscles of the abdomen, buttocks, and legs for several repetitions while seated and extending the legs will help blood circulate. Loose, comfortable clothing and shoes are also advised. Exercises that can help relax a stiff neck and shoulders (and that can be performed in cramped quarters) include gently rolling the head forward and to the sides (dropping the head back can create too much pressure on the spine), stretching the arms forward and overhead, and rolling the shoulders forward, up, and back, then going in the reverse direction.

In rare instances the near-claustrophobic accommodations in economy class are not just uncomfortable; they can be dangerous. When blood pools in the legs, there is risk of a blood clot developing in the deep veins of the legs or pelvis. Such a clot may break free, circulate through the bloodstream, and block an artery leading to the lungs. This potentially fatal condition is called a pulmonary embolism. A single, large clot can cause instant death, but fortunately, most clots are small. They can cause shortness of breath or sharp chest pain during deep breathing. Sometimes clots that form in the legs during a long flight will break off and circulate to the lungs days or weeks later.

Blood clots can develop even in people with no previous history of circulatory disorders, but some people are at higher risk than others. These include pregnant women, women who use birth control pills, and people with varicose veins or a history of thrombophlebitis (inflammation of the veins). Such people may want to ask their doctors if it is appropriate for them to wear elastic support hose, in addition to exercising during the flight.

Easing Ear Discomfort

Although modern jets have come a long way in minimizing the discomfort of flying at high altitude by maintaining acceptable air pressure in the cabin, the changes in air pressure as the airplane takes off

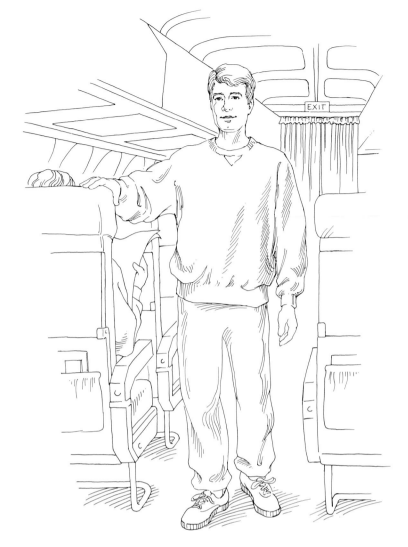

Walking periodically in the aisle wards off stiffness and circulation problems.

or lands can cause pain in the ears and sinuses for some people, especially infants and small children. Giving a young child a bottle or pacifier during ascent and descent will, in most cases, alleviate the problem. For older children and adults, remedies include chewing gum, swallowing, or performing the Valsalva maneuver—pinching the nose shut, closing the mouth, and exhaling, thus forcing air into the ears. (An individual with a cold or sinus infection or a heart condition should not perform the Valsalva maneuver.) If those fail, flight attendants sometimes recommend holding over the ears paper cups stuffed with paper towels that have been soaked in hot water and wrung out. The warmth from the towels relieves the pressure.

Cabin pressure changes are also likely to cause discomfort for those flying with a cold or respiratory infection. If the trip cannot be postponed for a few days, a passenger with such a problem may want to take an over-the-counter decongestant an hour before boarding and, if the flight is very long, again before the plane lands. Infants and young children with colds or with a history of easily-blocked eustachian tubes should be given a decongestant that is specially formulated for their age and weight. Parents may need to consult their pediatricians for a safe medication.

Ingrid J. Strauch is a staff editor and writer.

Eating

Although many airlines have made efforts to improve their food service in recent years, most high-altitude cuisine is still notoriously unappetizing and high in sodium and fat. Aesthetics aside, such fare can pose real problems for people whose diets are restricted for medical reasons as well as for people observing religious dietary laws. However, most airlines will provide special meals—for example, vegetarian, kosher, low-fat, or low-sodium—at no extra charge if such meals are requested in advance. Ideally, a special meal should be ordered when the ticket is reserved, but some can be ordered as little as 6 hours before takeoff; kosher meals may require as long as 12 hours. Travelers who change their flight reservations must remember to reorder their special meals.

To ensure that a meal is on board, a passenger should mention to the gate attendant before boarding that a special meal has been ordered. In addition, a flight attendant should be notified so that the meal is delivered to the right person.

Drinking

For many people, alcoholic beverages provide an easy way to relieve the tedium of flying. Drinks are readily available on most airlines and sometimes even offered free when there is a long delay or other inconvenience to passengers. However, for health and safety reasons, it is not advisable to drink when flying. In an emergency, alcohol can in-

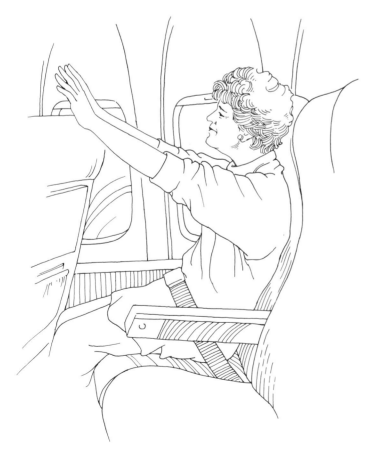

Stretching exercises relieve the discomfort of sitting for long periods.

hibit the ability to think and act quickly, possibly delaying a quick exit from the plane and endangering many lives. In addition, the air inside an airplane is very dry (relative humidity is typically 5 to 10 percent, comparable to a desert), and alcohol tends to dehydrate the body. For this reason, the wise choice of beverage during a flight is plenty of water. Caffeinated drinks—coffee, tea, and colas—also cause dehydration and should be avoided in favor of water, fruit juice, or milk.

Traveling With Young Children

Even a five-minute car ride with an infant or young child seems to require a bagful of equipment, and a trip on an airplane is no exception. Parents will need all the usual paraphernalia—diapers, moistened wipes, extra bottles, pacifier, baby blanket, diaper rash ointment, baby food (airlines do not provide this), snacks, toys, coloring books, and plenty of time to settle into their seats. Most airlines offer an early boarding call for persons traveling with young children; parents should take advantage of it to get all family members settled and bottles and pacifiers ready for takeoff.

Although infant car seats are not required by law on airplanes, they are considered the safest way for small children to fly. The drawback, however, is that on most airlines parents wanting to bring an infant car seat on board must purchase a ticket for the infant (normally, children under two ride free but are not guaranteed a seat and must ride

Milk is a better choice than alcohol, for both health and safety reasons.

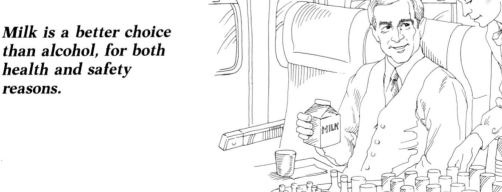

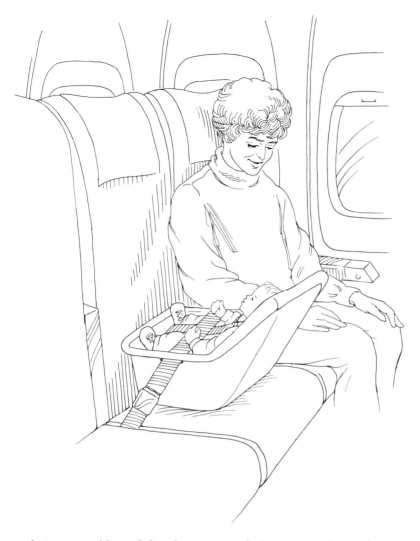

The safest way for an infant to fly is securely buckled into a car seat.

on their parents' laps if the plane is crowded). Since airline policies differ, before buying tickets parents should inform the airline that they want to bring along a car seat and should get a clear answer on whether a ticket must be purchased to guarantee the child a seat. Parents who keep their children on their laps should not fasten the children into their safety belts. If the adult is thrown forward, the child could be crushed.

Traveling While Pregnant

Before flying, a pregnant woman should discuss her travel plans with her doctor and should also check with the airline on its policy or recommendation. Most discourage flying after the 32nd week of pregnancy, and U.S. airlines generally do not allow air travel after 36 weeks; most international airlines have a cutoff of 35 weeks. Some airlines may require a note from a woman's physician stating her expected delivery date. Such regulations exist not because flying poses any particular danger to a healthy mother and fetus, but because flight crews are unable to cope with labor or delivery on board.

The lowered air pressure in a jet flying at high altitude can cause

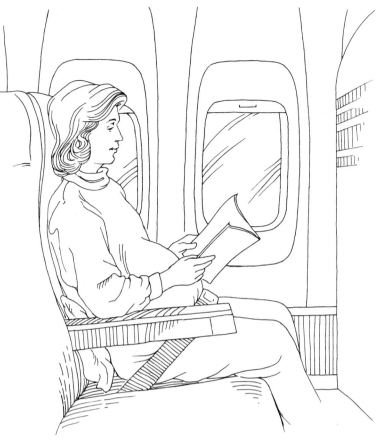

A pregnant passenger should request a bulkhead seat, fasten the seat belt low on her abdomen, and support her back with a pillow.

significant complications in pregnant women with anemia, sickle cell anemia, or the sickle cell trait. Women with any of these conditions should follow their doctor's recommendations. Because problems and complications are more likely during a multiple pregnancy, air travel should be avoided if multiple births are expected. It should also be avoided if a woman has a history of pregnancy-induced high blood pressure or bleeding.

If a pregnant woman does decide to fly, she should request a bulkhead, aisle seat for maximum leg room and ease in getting in and out of the seat. Exercising periodically—ideally, walking 15 minutes every hour—to prevent the legs and feet from swelling and to lower the risk of developing blood clots is especially important during pregnancy. So is drinking plenty of water to avoid dehydration. Comfortable clothes and shoes and a small pillow to support the back will also make the ride easier. Some women prefer to bring their own meals and snacks so they can eat when they need to. This may be of particular concern if morning sickness is a problem.

The proper placement of a seat belt for a pregnant woman is low across the hips, under the bulge of the abdomen. Some women may hesitate to use their seat belts for fear of injuring the fetus, but studies of car crashes have shown that the cushioning provided by the amniotic sac protects the fetus from injury when pressure is exerted by a seat belt. A pregnant woman should never forgo using a seat belt because of discomfort; this would jeopardize both mother and fetus.

Safety Aloft

Flying is one of the safest ways to travel, as borne out by statistics, but in-flight injuries—including fractures, sprains, cuts, and bruises—do occur almost daily as a result of ordinary turbulence. In rough weather improperly stowed luggage or unattended beverage carts can be pitched about, hitting or falling on passengers and attendants. A bumpy ride can also cause people to lose their balance and fall when walking in the aisle or using the lavatory. To avoid in-flight injuries, it is important to listen to the flight attendants' safety instructions and read the printed safety information provided by the airline.

Jet Lag

Circadian dyschronism, more commonly known as jet lag, is the fatigue and disorientation that result when a person travels east or west across more than three time zones. The body's biological rhythms continue to operate on "home" time, and it can take several days to adjust to the new clock setting. Symptoms of jet lag include daytime fatigue and nighttime insomnia, confusion, poor concentration, slowed reflexes, headache, loss of appetite, and constipation or diarrhea. Generally, flying east causes more severe jet lag than traveling west because it drastically shortens the day, and the human body seems more able to adapt to a lengthened day. Jet lag can be a serious problem for military personnel responding to an emergency or people who must conduct business soon after arrival; it is a serious annoyance to vacationers whose week abroad may well be nearly over by the time their bodies have adjusted to local time.

Theories abound on how to minimize the effects of jet lag. Research on the body's circadian rhythm—or inner clock—-suggests that exposure to sunlight at certain times of the day may be key to getting the body back in sync. While sunlight is not the only factor affecting body rhythms, scientists studying circadian rhythms advise doing the following to the extent one's schedule permits:

1. After traveling east through one to six time zones, spend several hours outdoors in the early morning for the first few days following the flight to help the body reset its clock.

2. After traveling east through 6 to 12 time zones, avoid morning sunlight but spend time outside at midday.

3. After traveling west through one to six time zones, go outside in the late afternoon.

4. After traveling west through 6 to 12 zones, go outside at midday but avoid sunlight in the late afternoon.

Even in inclement weather, being outside in natural light is important so that ambient light is absorbed through the eyes. In very sunny weather it is not necessary to be in direct sunlight; sitting in the shade is fine. At no time should a person look directly into the sun.

Another remedy that has gained much popularity in the United States, although it has not been scientifically proven effective, is called the Anti-Jet-Lag Diet. Developed at the Argonne National Laboratory, the diet consists of three days of alternately feasting and fasting and drinking caffeinated beverages only at prescribed times. The diet also calls for abstaining from alcohol on the plane. Argonne cautions people already on special diets to consult with their doctors before trying this diet. Although some people swear by the Anti-Jet-Lag Diet, a recent test conducted by the U.S. Army showed that those who followed the diet had no fewer symptoms of jet lag than anyone else.

Even with no surefire method of avoiding jet lag, experts say there are still a few things travelers can do to adjust as quickly as possible.

• Several days before departure, try to shift eating and sleeping schedules, to the extent possible, to correspond with time at the destination.

• Before the flight, avoid overeating or drinking.

• If possible, break up long flights in one direction with layovers of at least a day.

• Adopt local time for eating, sleeping, and other routines immediately upon arrival.

• If your schedule permits, allow plenty of time for relaxation the first day in a new location.

Sleeping pills or sedatives to induce sleep during the flight are not

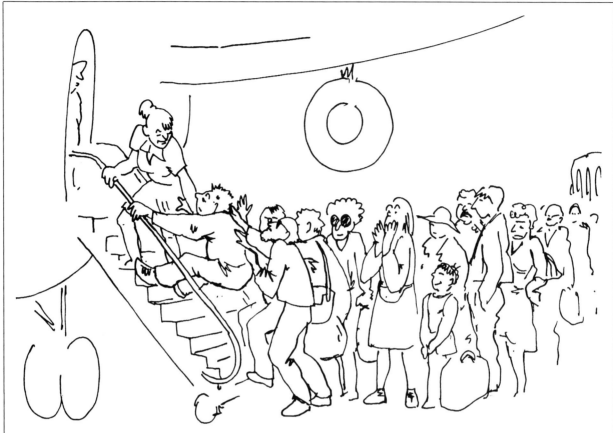

Fear of Flying

Despite statistical evidence that flying is much safer than traveling by car, as many as 44 percent of Americans report that they are sometimes afraid to board an airplane. No doubt many are influenced by the media coverage of plane crashes with high death tolls; car accidents, which cumulatively kill tens of thousands of people each year, receive relatively little attention. For some the fear of flying takes the form of a little uneasiness, but for others it can turn into a full-blown panic attack.

Many fearful flyers seek to overcome their anxiety—or at least numb it—by drinking large quantities of alcohol before and during a flight. Not only is this practice unhealthy, but the disorientation that alcohol causes can exacerbate anxiety, making the ride even worse. Others turn to tranquilizers to calm them down, but depending on a pill only reinforces the message that a person can't cope with flying; it doesn't solve the problem.

A potentially more helpful approach is to enroll in one of the many programs or clinics designed to help people overcome their fears about flying. Programs may last anywhere from a weekend to several months. In addition, there are therapists who specialize in treating fear of flying, although long-term psychotherapy for this problem is rarely needed. Generally, fear of flying programs provide information on the actual dangers of flying, teach relaxation techniques, and schedule short plane trips for participants in the company of a counselor. People who are unable to take part in a suitable program may find it helpful to list their fears, then research the probability of those fears actually coming true by talking with flight attendants or pilots. There are also many books you can read and courses you can take that teach relaxation techniques, which usually include deep breathing, relaxing the muscles, and visualizing pleasant scenes.

recommended. Some of them can actually cause a type of short-term amnesia that can last for hours after the pill is taken. While a person may continue to function normally during this time, nothing that takes place will be remembered.

Special Problems

For people with certain medical conditions, air travel can pose special problems. For example, doctors recommend that patients recovering from a heart attack wait several weeks before traveling by airplane. This is also recommended for patients recovering from gastrointestinal surgery, because gases in the stomach and intestines expand at high altitudes. (For the same reason, people with colostomies require larger bags during flight.) Some doctors advise people with certain lung disorders, such as emphysema, to avoid air travel, and people with severe anemia may require oxygen because of difficulty adapting to changes in oxygen concentration at high altitudes.

Because airport security systems can interfere with older model cardiac pacemakers, anyone wearing one should contact the airport security agency to make other arrangements for passing through security gates. (The airlines themselves are usually not in charge of airport functions.) People with disabilities who are traveling with guide dogs can bring the dogs on board at no extra charge, but they must inform the airline beforehand of their intention to do so. Some airlines may require some form of written documentation for a guide dog.

People who are taking prescription drugs need to adjust their dosage schedules when crossing time zones; they should consult their doctor about this before flying. People with diabetes who take insulin must also remember to carry on board any necessary equipment such as syringes and testing materials (as well as pack a complete backup set of supplies in their luggage). It is wise to bring along a doctor's note explaining why this equipment is necessary.

Anyone using a prescription medication should carry it on board in its original package, especially if going through customs. It is also a good idea to bring along a doctor's written prescription. Within the United States a prescription written in one state can generally be filled in any other. If a traveler must visit a local doctor, the prescription serves to inform the doctor of exactly what the patient is currently using. People with conditions that could potentially necessitate emergency treatment should wear some form of medical identification, such as a bracelet, and carry a card with emergency information, including the phone numbers of physicians or relatives to be contacted.

Since individual cases and needs differ, anyone who is unsure about whether to fly because of a health condition should consult a physician before boarding a plane. In the United States flight attendants are not allowed to diagnose or administer medications in flight; they are trained only in basic first aid, and passengers cannot count on there being a doctor on board. No one likes to cancel a vacation, but it's wise to remember that while Honolulu will still be there next year, someone who denies the symptoms of an impending medical problem or ignores the doctor's orders may not be. ☐

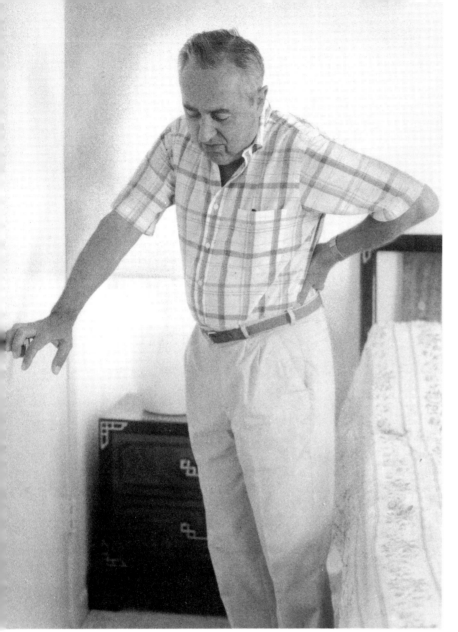

The Challenge of Relieving PAIN

Dori Stehlin

The lucky among us have only an occasional headache. For others, pain is a constant, though unwelcome, companion. Relieving pain is sometimes simple, sometimes impossible. It depends on the source of the pain and it may also depend on the person.

There are three main nonprescription choices for pain relief—aspirin, acetaminophen (brand names, Datril, Tylenol, and others), and ibuprofen (Motrin IB, Advil, Nuprin, and others). All three block the production of chemicals called prostaglandins, which the body usually releases when cells are injured. Prostaglandins are believed to play an important role in the pain, heat, redness, and swelling that occur following tissue damage.

So what's the best choice for your headache, pulled muscle, or menstrual cramps? When it comes to mild, nonspecific pain, headaches, or menstrual discomfort, "all three [nonprescription pain relievers] are quite useful," says Dr. Patricia Love, a rheumatologist with the Center

54

for Drug Evaluation and Research of the U.S. Food and Drug Administration. "There are probably persons who are not able to detect a difference in the effectiveness of the over-the-counter products."

It has been suggested, Love says, that aspirin or ibuprofen may be more effective than acetaminophen for pain caused by inflammation or mild menstrual discomfort because they have more prostaglandin-blocking effects. "Our best advice at present is that, for mild pain, individuals may use what works best and is safe for them," says Love. In other words, what doesn't cause them problems.

Because prostaglandins play a role in protecting the stomach lining from being attacked by the acid of digestive fluid, aspirin, ibuprofen, and, apparently to a lesser extent, according to Love, acetaminophen may cause stomach irritation, ulcers or bleeding. "If you have a history of stomach disorders, first talk to your doctor [before taking a nonprescription pain reliever]," says Love.

For some people who take aspirin, stomach irritation may be decreased by taking either enteric-coated aspirin, buffered aspirin, or other modified aspirin derivatives such as choline salicylate or magnesium salicylate.

Buffered aspirin contains an ingredient that neutralizes some of the digestive system's acid and, therefore, may produce less irritation than plain aspirin.

Coated aspirin dissolves mainly in the intestine. (Uncoated aspirin dissolves in the stomach.) In theory, that difference may mean less stomach irritation, says Love. But, she adds, it still depends on an individual's metabolism. For example, some people can't digest the coating, so while they don't get any stomach irritation, they don't get any benefit either. The aspirin passes out of the body undigested and unabsorbed.

People who can't take aspirin because of allergic reactions (e.g., rash, asthma, anaphylaxis) generally can't take ibuprofen either. For them, acetaminophen may be the only nonprescription choice.

"Persons with medication allergies should discuss the use of any nonprescription medication with their doctor," Love says.

She adds that all three drugs have the potential to cause liver damage, although liver toxicity is much less common than gastric ulcers or bleeding.

The FDA is reviewing recent studies that suggest an association between use of all three nonprescription pain relievers and kidney disease. But the agency says that not enough is known yet about these possible associations to make any changes in current recommendations for use for healthy individuals.

"I think one of the important safety issues in choosing a medication is it's not just whether or not you have minor pain, but what is your medical history on top of the minor pain," says Love. "People who have specific disorders—kidney disease, heart disease, bleeding problems, liver disorders, medication allergies, and the like—should talk to their physicians."

Dori Stehlin is a staff writer for the FDA Consumer.

When it comes to nonprescription pain relievers, the consumer has basically three choices—ibuprofen, acetaminophen, and aspirin.

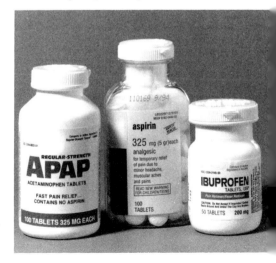

Acute Pain from Injury or Surgery

When the pain becomes too much to bear or is the result of a serious injury or surgery, relief requires stronger medicine and a doctor's prescription. One class of frequently prescribed pain relievers is nonsteroidal anti-inflammatory drugs, often abbreviated NSAIDs. (The three nonprescription pain relievers are also NSAIDs, according to Love, although acetaminophen is not commonly referred to by that term.) Pre-

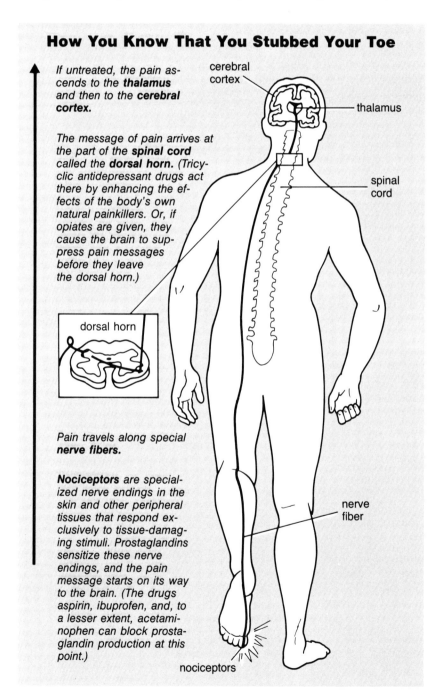

How You Know That You Stubbed Your Toe

*If untreated, the pain ascends to the **thalamus** and then to the **cerebral cortex**.*

*The message of pain arrives at the part of the **spinal cord** called the **dorsal horn**. (Tricyclic antidepressant drugs act there by enhancing the effects of the body's own natural painkillers. Or, if opiates are given, they cause the brain to suppress pain messages before they leave the dorsal horn.)*

dorsal horn

*Pain travels along special **nerve fibers**.*

Nociceptors *are specialized nerve endings in the skin and other peripheral tissues that respond exclusively to tissue-damaging stimuli. Prostaglandins sensitize these nerve endings, and the pain message starts on its way to the brain. (The drugs aspirin, ibuprofen, and, to a lesser extent, acetaminophen can block prostaglandin production at this point.)*

cerebral cortex

thalamus

spinal cord

nerve fiber

nociceptors

scription NSAIDs are given at higher doses than the nonprescription types, but the mechanism for pain relief is the same—blocking the production of prostaglandins.

Opiate drugs are another class of pain-relieving prescription drugs. Commonly prescribed opiates include morphine, codeine, hydromorphone (brand name, Dilaudid), and meperidine (Demerol). (In some states, some forms of codeine are sold without a prescription in limited amounts.) Most of these drugs are derived from opium, the juice of the poppy flower.

Opiate drugs work by altering the transmission of pain messages in the brain and spinal cord, blocking pain messages or altering their character. The pain-blocking action of the opiates can be enhanced by taking aspirin, ibuprofen, or acetaminophen at the same time as the opiate. This hits pain with a "double-whammy." The NSAIDs block the pain at the site of injury, while the opiates suppress in the brain any remaining pain.

Unfortunately, the effect of opiates on the brain isn't limited to pain control. Opiates can cause drowsiness, nausea, constipation, and even unpleasant mood changes in some people. However, sometimes simply trying a different opiate may be all that's needed to reduce these side effects.

Tolerance and Addiction

Because doctors are afraid patients may become dependent on opiate drugs, they sometimes hold back on the amount or number of doses, even if this means the patient doesn't get sufficient pain relief.

Ronald Dubner, D.D.S., chief of the Neurobiology and Anesthesiology Branch of the U.S. National Institute of Dental Research, says those fears are unfounded. But, he explains, "One needs to be very clear about making the distinction between tolerance and addiction." Tolerance occurs when the body no longer responds as well to the opiate's pain-relieving properties at the current dose. For example, some cancer patients with severe pain may need increasing amounts of morphine to maintain the same level of pain relief.

Addiction, on the other hand, is an overwhelming compulsion to continue use of the drug even when pain relief is no longer needed. While some of the addiction is physical, it is mainly considered a psychological dependence that has a detrimental effect not only on the individual but also on society, because the addicted individual may have to obtain the drug illegally.

Addiction is "really a red herring in the field of pain control," says Dubner. The fear that giving patients opiates will turn them into addicts craving the drugs long after the pain has ended is unfounded, says Dubner. "People who are truly seeking help for their pain and who are in good hands do not have addiction problems," he explains.

In any case, Dubner says, it is very rare for a patient to reach a point where no amount of an opiate will relieve pain and that should never be used as a reason for not increasing the drug's dose.

Anesthesiologist Francis Balestrieri agrees. "There's no reason to hold back the drug dose for people in acute pain," says Balestrieri,

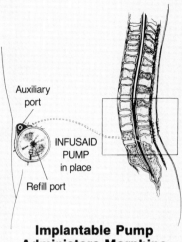

Implantable Pump Administers Morphine

A concentrated form of morphine specially developed for administration by implantable pump is now available for people in severe pain, such as terminal cancer patients.

The small pump provides a steady stream of the drug to nerves along the spine, giving more constant relief, without the "peaks and valleys" of pain sometimes associated with capsules, pills, and intravenous injections. The FDA approved the drug in 1991. It will be marketed under the trade name Infumorph.

The pumps, called microinfusion devices, can be implanted under the skin of the abdomen or worn outside the body. A specially concentrated morphine was needed because the pumps are so small (about 3 inches in diameter). At the FDA's request the drug was developed by Elkins-Sinn Inc. of Cherry Hill, N.J., under the agency's orphan products program, which encourages the development of needed therapies for diseases or conditions affecting fewer than 200,000 people.

The pump is programmed with dosing information before being filled with concentrated morphine and is thus able to constantly administer fractional doses of the drug. If the pump is implanted, the dose can be changed by beaming information through skin and tissues.

Misjudgment in the starting dose can result in severe side effects, such as seizures and respiratory problems. Therefore, patients must be monitored in a fully equipped and staffed facility for at least 24 hours after the initial dose. After this first "test" dose, however, patients may go home and return periodically—sometimes only once a month—for the physician to refill the pump reservoir with the medication.

who is the director of the Woodburn Surgery Center at Fairfax Hospital in Falls Church, Va.

However, the FDA's Dr. Curtis Wright warns that the pain relief from higher doses of opiates must be weighed against the side effects these drugs can cause. "It's a balancing act," says Wright, who is a medical review officer for the agency's center for drug evaluation and research. "The amount of pain relief must be weighed against the effects of adverse reactions such as agitation, nausea, confusion, and potentially lethal respiratory depression."

Patients in Control

Frequently, however, the doses of narcotics physicians prescribe are too low, not too high, and the time between doses is too long, according to a book by Dr. Barry Stimmel, *Pain, Analgesia, and Addiction: The Pharmacologic Treatment of Pain.* Stimmel writes that, "Analgesic medications should be prescribed regularly around the clock in the presence of acute pain. The intervals between administration should be sufficiently close together to avoid swings in pain levels. Both laboratory and clinical studies have shown that the presence of anxiety will result in an increased need for narcotics, thus setting up a vicious cycle whereby escalating doses of analgesics are needed, without adequate pain relief being obtained."

Pain itself can be considered a disease that needs treatment.

The use of analgesics provides more benefits to the patient than just relieving pain. "Evidence from laboratory experiments has begun to accumulate showing that pain can accelerate the growth of tumors and increase mortality after tumor challenge," writes John C. Liebeskind in an editorial in the January 1991 issue of *Pain*. "It appears that the dictum 'pain does not kill,' sometimes invoked to justify ignoring pain complaints, may be dangerously wrong."

Dubner agrees. "Pain is not a passive symptom. We consider pain, in many instances, an aggressive disease in itself. Therefore it becomes very, very critical to control pain as rapidly and as completely as possible."

One solution to inadequate doses of analgesics is patient-controlled intravenous analgesia (PCA), which is usually used in hospitals for acute pain following surgery. In PCA, the patient is connected to a machine called a PCA pump. When the patient pushes a control button, the machine delivers a dose of narcotic or other pain reliever intravenously. The doses are smaller than what would be given by injection, but because the drug goes directly into the bloodstream, relief can occur within seconds. A patient receiving traditional administration with an injection in the muscle or under the skin may have to wait anywhere from 5 to 30 minutes for pain relief.

Although the pain relief with PCA's small doses may only last for 10 to 15 minutes, the patient can get another dose the second pain begins to return. Injections, on the other hand, may last up to two hours, but since the usual dosage schedule is three to four hours, the pain returns long before the nurse does. "PCA matches the patients' relief to their pain," says Balestrieri. "It also relieves patients of the worry over their pain relief in the majority of cases."

It also helps patients deal with the side effects opiates can cause, says the FDA's Wright. "A substantial portion of patients don't want complete pain relief," says Wright. "They want as much pain relief as they can get without bad side effects." Wright says that when the first studies were done on the effectiveness of PCA, "We thought that the pain scores [the patients gave] would be zero." (Patients generally rated pain on a four-point scale with four being the greatest amount of pain and zero, no pain.) "What we found was that patients didn't titrate down to zero, but instead brought the pain down to one or two," he says.

The undesirable side effects of narcotics can be avoided completely with another form of continuous administration—epidural therapy. Epidurals, which inject the narcotics into the membrane surrounding the spinal cord, have been used for many years to block the pain of labor. Now this is being adapted to control pain after some major surgery, especially abdominal.

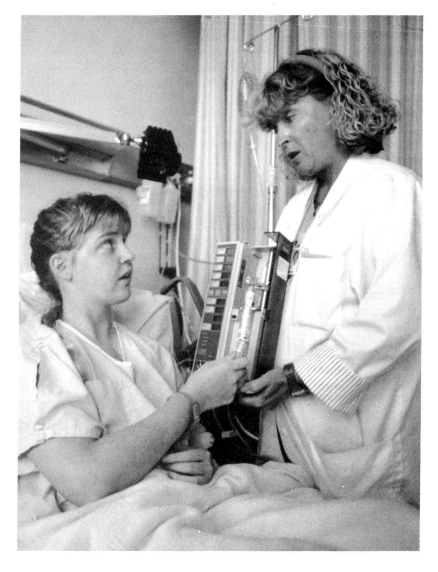

A device called a PCA pump allows hospital patients to choose their own levels of pain relief.

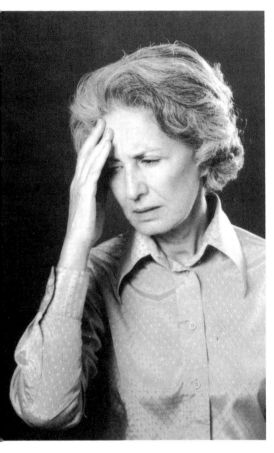

Chronic pain, such as that from migraine headaches, can be difficult to control.

Drugs injected into the epidural space don't travel to the brain like other types of injections, explains Sherry Fisher, R.N., pain management coordinator at Fairfax Hospital. Therefore, complications such as nausea and respiratory depression don't occur.

With epidurals "patients can talk to me, take deep breaths, cough, and even be up and walking around, sometimes 24 hours after surgery," says Fisher. Normally, after the type of major surgery that requires the kind of pain control epidural therapy provides, "the patient would still be on a ventilator after 24 hours," she says.

However, epidurals aren't effective for every type of pain. Besides pain from abdominal surgeries, epidurals are best used for pain following major chest and urologic surgery, according to Fisher.

No matter what the form of administration, "I don't think people should be exposed to any more pain than they're willing to tolerate," says Dubner.

Chronic Pain

Unfortunately, "When it comes to chronic pain, there are situations where pain cannot be controlled as well with the approaches that are available to us today," says Dubner. Opiate drugs are usually avoided in chronic pain management because of the potential for tolerance. The following are some of the types of chronic pain that are difficult to control:
• pain from nerve damage caused by diabetes or shingles
• lower back pain that continues long after the initial injury has healed
• arthritis
• migraine and other chronic headaches.
There is some hope though. Tricyclic antidepressants, especially amitriptyline, have been found to relieve pain in patients with nerve damage. These drugs aid the body's own defenses by trapping serotonin, a pain-blocking chemical, at its point of production in the nerve endings in the dorsal horn of the spinal cord. An excess of serotonin builds up and suppresses pain signals longer than usual.

Although the FDA has not approved tricyclic antidepressants for pain control, these drugs are gaining wide acceptance for this purpose. (The practice of medicine may include the prescribing of approved drugs for unapproved uses supported by research and not otherwise contraindicated.)

Treatment of chronic and migraine headache pain may include two drugs approved for heart problems—calcium channel blockers and beta blockers.

Treatment for mild arthritis pain, on the other hand, often begins with aspirin. If the patient can't tolerate aspirin, ibuprofen is a reasonable substitute, says Love. She warns, however, that even though people can buy aspirin and ibuprofen without a prescription, the doses required to treat arthritis pain are too high to be taken without a physician's care. "The treatment of chronic arthritis, regardless of severity, requires an adequate diagnosis and possible use of many different types of medications, physical therapy, or surgery," says Love.

TENS

Another potential source of relief for chronic pain is transcutaneous electrical nerve stimulation (TENS). Through the use of the TENS device—a battery-powered generator that could be mistaken for a Walkman portable radio or a beeper—electrical impulses are transmitted to the site of pain through electrodes placed on the skin.

With the most common course of treatment, the physician or physical therapist sets the TENS device to deliver 80 to 100 impulses a second for 45 minutes, three times a day. But there are a wide variety of parameter ranges, and what works for one person may have no effect on another. Determining the most effective settings "is a real art," says Stephen M. Hinckley, a physiologist with the FDA's Center for Devices and Radiological Health. Pain can be very subjective, explains Hinckley. Two people whose pain is caused by the same problem may need very different settings to achieve relief.

If a patient doesn't require hospital care, the patient can use the TENS device, preset to the proper level, at home. The device does not interfere with most normal activities.

A study published in the *New England Journal of Medicine* in June 1990 questioned the effectiveness of TENS. The study concluded "that for patients with chronic low back pain, treatment with TENS is no more effective than treatment with a placebo, and TENS adds no apparent benefit to that of exercise alone." But, because a number of previous studies support the use of TENS, the FDA still considers TENS to be effective for pain relief for some people.

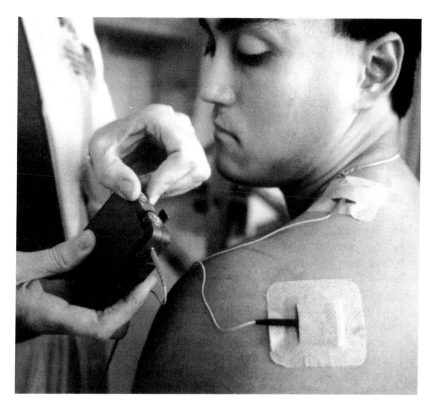

Some patients find that they get relief from the TENS device, which transmits electrical impulses to the painful area through electrodes placed on the skin.

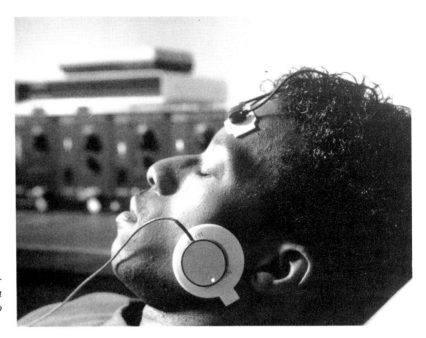

Biofeedback is one of several behavior modification techniques that can bring relief when other therapies do not completely succeed.

Although it isn't clear why TENS works, there are two plausible theories, according to the *Harvard Medical School Health Letter*. The first holds that nerves can easily carry only one message at a time. The electrical pulses from TENS overload the nerves, and the pain message shuts down. A second theory hypothesizes that the electrical pulses stimulate the body to release its own painkilling molecules, called endorphins, into the fluid bathing the spinal cord.

Pain researchers are studying how to stimulate production of the brain's own opiates, such as endorphins and enkephalins, since they may act as natural painkillers, according to NIH's Dubner. "There are clear indications that stimulation in certain parts of the brain can be helpful in some patients," he says.

Focus on Life

Sometimes, though, none of these therapies will completely relieve the pain for chronic sufferers. They don't have to give up hope, though. For many in chronic pain, behavior modification techniques such as biofeedback, meditation, and relaxation training may offer some relief. These treatment approaches are designed to alter a patient's reactions and behavior in response to pain.

"They learn that they can deal with their pain effectively if they focus on improving their quality of life instead of focusing on their pain," says Dubner.

Seymour Rubin, 67, who has suffered with chronic back pain for 40 years, agrees. "If I focus on the pain, it just gets worse," he says. Instead, Rubin keeps busy with walking, reading, and running errands with his wife. "Singing helps, talking helps," adds Rubin. "And I've just learned to accept the fact that I have pain."

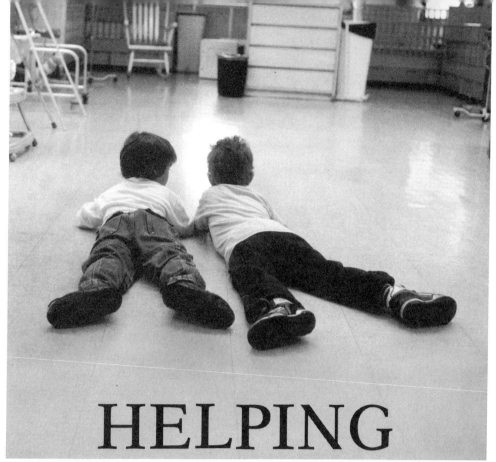

HELPING
THE SMALLEST VICTIMS

Dennis Sanders

"As with many things in life, if it's going to happen, you're going to have to make it happen yourself." Dr. Margaret Heagarty, chief of pediatrics at Harlem Hospital and professor at Columbia's College of Physicians and Surgeons (P&S), was talking to Dr. Stephen Nicholas, a young pediatrician on her staff. It was 1987, and Heagarty and her colleague were trying to find solutions for one of the biggest crises urban medical and social services had faced in decades: the boarder-baby boom.

Like many of their colleagues in urban hospitals around the nation, Heagarty and Nicholas, an assistant professor of pediatrics at P&S, had to find a way of dealing with an immediate and critical problem: the overwhelming number of infants crowding their wards who were born to families that could not take care of them. Virtually all of the boarder babies, so called because they became "boarders" in hospital pediatric wards, were born to drug-addicted mothers. Most were black or Hispanic. Many had serious medical problems, such as birth defects, prematurity, low birth weight, cerebral palsy, or prenatal drug addiction. As the 1980s progressed, more and more were born infected with the human immunodeficiency virus (HIV) that causes AIDS, contracted in utero from their mothers.

More than anywhere else, these infants were being born in urban hospitals like Harlem; older children, who had developed AIDS symptoms after leaving the hospital, were coming back with acute and chronic AIDS-related illnesses. They, too, often stayed indefinitely in pediatric wards because their parents were addicts, many of them dying of AIDS.

In the days before crack and AIDS, according to Heagarty, the problem of newborn children without homes or stable families had been more or less manageable. "Almost any department of pediatrics that I have known about over the years would typically have one or two children who could be termed boarder babies," Heagarty recalls. "These were usually children with serious chronic diseases whose parents couldn't take care of them and whose medical problems made them essentially unplaceable in foster homes."

That changed in the 1980s. The problem—urban hospitals having to provide long-term care for newborns whose parents were unable to take them—was the same. The difference was in the numbers.

"Within what seemed like weeks, we were overwhelmed," Heagarty remembers. "We found our nurseries crowded with significant numbers of newborn infants whose families could not take care of them. Thirty to fifty at a time. There was a point at which we literally ran out of bassinets." According to Heagarty, by 1987 about 10 to 15 percent of her department's 60 beds were at any one time filled with children suffering from AIDS-related or cocaine-related illnesses.

Because of Harlem's intense involvement in the AIDS and boarder-baby crises, Heagarty became a frequent spokesperson for the plight of urban hospitals and their youngest patients. When Diana, the Princess of Wales, came to New York, she toured a children's AIDS ward with Dr. Heagarty. In one of the early editions of *AIDS Quarterly* on public television, host Peter Jennings interviewed Heagarty at length on the problems of infants born to HIV-positive and AIDS-afflicted mothers. In 1989, First Lady Barbara Bush met with Heagarty to learn about the hospital's programs in pediatric AIDS treatment.

National media attention on Harlem Hospital and its struggle with pediatric AIDS and boarder babies was helping to educate the public about the scope of the problem. According to Nicholas, televised footage of figures such as Princess Diana holding a child with AIDS contributed to the public's lessening fear of contact with infected children. Still, in spite of progress in public awareness, hospitals were faced with the immediate problem of caring long-term for children with nowhere to go.

Harlem's boarder-baby boom was repeated at hospitals nationwide, in every city with acute healthcare problems. It hit hardest and earli-

Dennis Sanders is director of academic services publications at the University of Colorado at Boulder.

est in places like New York, Newark, and Chicago. Los Angeles saw a 1,000 percent increase in drug-addicted infants in the four years between 1985 and 1989. Many of these infants were also at high risk for HIV infection. In New York City, the impact of crack and AIDS on social services was staggering. As long ago as 1986, Special Services for Children, the city agency responsible for monitoring the foster care system, recognized that two-thirds of all boarder babies, at that time numbering in the hundreds, were born to mothers who used crack, cocaine, or heroin. The agency also acknowledged that the inadequacies of the foster care system allowed for hospital stays averaging two months for the city's boarder-baby population.

The city-managed foster care system was reeling under the burden of an overload of these hard-to-place infants and children. By 1989, New York City had an estimated 25,000 children in foster homes—what Heagarty describes as "a small city of foster children."

The costs of maintaining boarder babies in hospitals were, and still are, enormous, ranging from $12,000 to $27,000 a month per child. For infants requiring neonatal intensive care, costs can soar to $1,800 per day. The burden of this expense is borne by hospitals, mainly from their bad-debt pools, with some help coming from federal, state, and city funds.

The Challenge of Caring

The boarder problem, of course, is not only financial. At the height of the New York City crisis, healthy babies without homes to go to were occupying beds desperately needed by seriously ill infants and children. Doctors and nurses, already busy providing medical care to crowded neonatal and pediatric units, found themselves trying to give at least some of the nurturing care and personal attention that are so crucial to child development.

"We're trying to be mothers, grandmothers, aunts," said one stressed neonatal nurse as she held a drug-addicted newborn in a rocking chair that had been brought into the nurses' station. "At the same time, we've got our medical duties, too." Staffs in many of New York's hospitals set up programs for volunteers to come to wards to hold and play with their boarder babies. Hospitals are, as one doctor put it, "legally and morally bound" to care for infants and children who have no home to go to. Yet hospitals have traditionally had little or no influence over the social service systems responsible for placing boarder babies in foster care.

Hospitals like Harlem could not stand up indefinitely under the burden of the boarder-baby boom. The question for administrators, and physicians like Heagarty and Nicholas was, what could be done? In the middle of the crisis, a big increase in the number of foster homes willing to take in AIDS babies seemed unlikely. Programs to help drug-addicted parents get in shape to care for their families were minimal, and, when available, had long waiting lists and took more time than pediatric wards could afford to wait.

To Heagarty and other pediatric experts, the only alternative seemed to be halfway houses, or transitional group care homes as they are

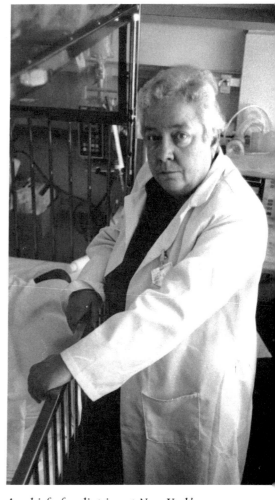

As chief of pediatrics at New York's Harlem Hospital, Dr. Margaret Heagarty was in the front lines of the boarder-baby crisis and was one of the first to see group homes as the solution.

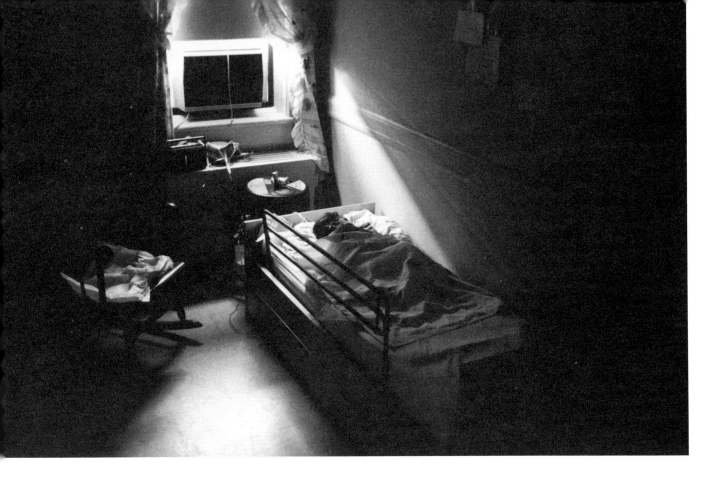

The rooms at the Incarnation Children's Center are designed to provide a cozy atmosphere as unlike the traditional concept of the orphanage as possible.

known among foster care professionals, where infants who were being boarded in hospitals could be moved once they were well enough.

"We're having to look at group homes as solutions to the problem," Heagarty commented at the time. "Yet this flies in the face of conventional child-care wisdom. Repeated studies have shown that children reared for any length of time in group homes lag behind their counterparts in foster care. They are more likely to suffer long-term emotional and socialization problems."

The alternatives, such as extended stays in hospital environments, or roughing it on the streets and in the slums with addicted or AIDS-infected parents, were simply not acceptable long-term solutions. "The challenge," Heagarty knew, "is to make sure the group care these little ones get is of the quality that the best group situations can provide. If we warehouse them someplace, putting them in group homes just to achieve economies of scale, we are running the real risk of reinventing Dickens's orphanage, especially given the scope of the problem in New York City and other urban centers. We've got to rethink the whole process."

A few good group-care situations were already in place. One of the best-known was Hale House, founded by "Mother" Clara Hale and headed by her daughter, Dr. Lorraine Hale, which had pioneered group care for drug-addicted infants. Another was the St. Clare's group home for AIDS babies in Newark. These homes had already paved the way for high-quality group care for infants and children. However, they were filled to capacity. And they were not able to provide on-site medical care, which Nicholas and Heagarty saw as a real need for HIV-positive children.

The catalyst for the creation of what was to become Incarnation Children's Center came in 1986, when Nicholas went to Children's Hospital in Philadelphia on a fellowship. While there, he helped to organize the U.S. Surgeon General's workshop on HIV children and their families. At the workshop, healthcare and social service experts from around the nation discussed problems of HIV-positive and AIDS boarder babies, including alternatives to housing these infants in hospitals. By the time he returned to Harlem, Nicholas had a clearer idea of what kind of group-care home would work for AIDS boarder babies. The model addressed the concerns that Heagarty had raised about the Dickensian orphanage aspect of group care at its worst. Nicholas believed that a well run transitional group care home could provide both effective nurturing and high-quality medical care in a nonhospital, noninstitutional environment.

Finding a Home

Faced with the tremendous overload of HIV-positive boarders filling Harlem's pediatric wards, the big question was how and when this kind of care would become available. At this point, Heagarty challenged Nicholas to take on the task of helping to make it happen. The final concept for the transitional group home was simple, but a site would have to be found and the project would require a level of cooperation between the public and private sectors, and between healthcare and social service agencies, that had seldom been attempted.

Group homes provide both love and medical care.

By a stroke of luck, Dr. John Nicholson, associate professor of pediatrics at P&S, after spending a month as an attending physician at Harlem Hospital, learned that there was an empty convent in northern Manhattan, belonging to the Church of the Incarnation. Nicholson, Heagarty, Nicholas, and Dr. Michael Katz, Carpentier Professor of Pediatrics at Columbia, met with Monsignor Thomas Leonard, pastor, and Sister Una McCormack, executive director of the Catholic Home Bureau, a foster care agency, to explore the possibility of using the convent as a residence for HIV-positive boarder babies. Nicholas recalls, "Our expertise was in healthcare, and, clearly, we didn't know much about foster care so we really needed help in that area." To fund the medical portion of the program, Katz, who is also chief of pediatrics at Presbyterian Hospital, approached the Samuel and May Rudin Foundation, which has supported many Columbia programs over the years.

As the plans drew closer to completion, Nicholas and his team presented it to New York City's Child Welfare Administration and the New York State Division of Social Services, the other essential partners in the project. According to these plans, the center would provide loving, homelike shelter and nurturing for boarder babies currently in pediatric wards. The center's medical staff, under Dr. Nicholas's direction, would provide all nonacute medical care. If a child experienced one of the serious opportunistic infections associated with AIDS, such as pneumocystis pneumonia, he or she would be taken to a hospital equipped to provide care and returned to the center when well enough.

By early 1988, the coalition of public and private agencies and insti-

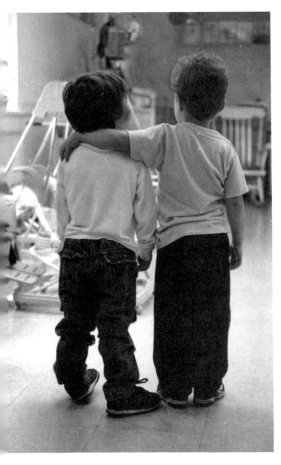

A tyke can always find a friend in one of the Incarnation Children's Center's two playrooms.

tutions had come to an agreement, an administrative staff was hired, and renovations on the convent began. The Incarnation Children's Center, or ICC, opened on March 21, 1989, with space for 24 HIV-infected or AIDS infants and children.

"This must be a speed record of sorts," says Nicholas. "To have a public hospital, a private hospital, city and state social services agencies, a church, a university, and a private foundation all sitting in one room and agreeing on something—well, it's so unlikely. In retrospect, it's hard to believe it happened in such a short time."

Because the center was charting new territory, Nicholas and his staff weren't sure how things would go. "It was conceivable," Nicholas recalls, "that we would get 24 kids, and that they would simply live at the center and never move. And that would have been okay. They would have been better off than living in a hospital."

But the outcome was very different. Instead of becoming a permanent residence for children from Harlem, Presbyterian, and other metropolitan-area hospitals with large boarder-baby populations, ICC became a true halfway house, providing a stopping-off point while foster homes were found for the children.

What contributed to this, according to Nicholas, was the Child Welfare Administration's efforts to increase the number of foster care agencies with placement programs for HIV-positive and AIDS children, and an increase in the number of foster parents willing to care for them. "Clearly, during the height of the boarder crisis in the 1980s," says Nicholas, "foster parents were afraid of AIDS in their homes. And the foster care agencies knew this, and felt that efforts to place these kids were pretty much futile. In 1985, for example, only one agency in the New York area had a placement program for HIV-infected babies."

By the time ICC opened, more agencies were working with HIV and AIDS placement, and the Catholic Home Bureau developed its own program as an outgrowth of its involvement in the center. The response to these active placement programs was so strong that within six months eight agencies were working with ICC.

"Education had a lot to do with it, of course," observes Nicholas. "Families who were interested in fostering had learned that having a child with AIDS in their care was not dangerous to them or to their children. They discovered that there were even special satisfactions in caring for these kids."

The unexpected success that foster care agencies have had in placing HIV-positive and AIDS children has had a profound impact on the boarder-baby crisis. It has allowed ICC to provide care for numbers of infants and children far beyond original expectations. According to Nicholas, by March 1991 the center had taken in about 158 children. Of these, 140 were placed in foster homes.

"Before ICC opened," Nicholas recalls, "most HIV-positive boarder babies stayed in Harlem Hospital for almost a year, just because there was no place for them to go. Now, at the center, the average stay is about a month or, if a child is a little sicker than most, two or three months."

Nicholas adds, "The boarder-baby problem for HIV-positive infants is, for all intents and purposes, fixed, because we're never filled to ca-

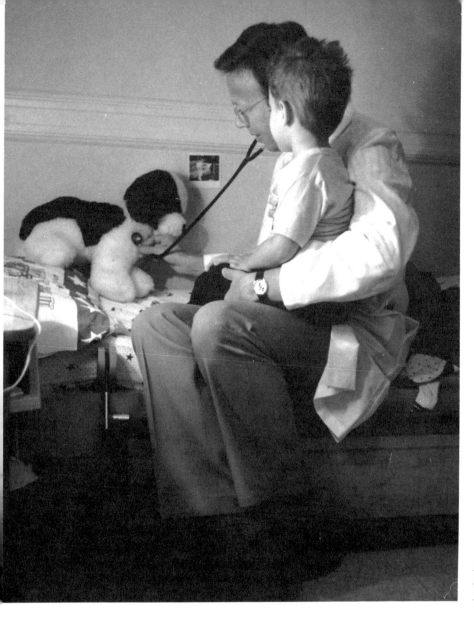

*Every resident gets medical checkups
at the Incarnation Children's Center.
Left, Dr. Stephen Nicholas at work.*

pacity. We always have beds available, so that the minute a kid who
needs foster care is ready to leave the hospital, and a home is not
available, they can come here. And now that foster parents are easier
to find, many kids are going directly to homes from the hospital."

When the center was conceived, a decision was made to focus on
HIV-positive and AIDS children only because, as Nicholas puts it,
"This was the hardest end of the boarder-baby spectrum to deal with.
We felt that if we could find a solution for these kids, we could find a
solution for the others."

The Incarnation Children's Center has been designed to avoid the
aura of a "pediatric warehouse" or of the Dickensian orphanage that
so concerned Heagarty. Common rooms at the center include a living
room, two playrooms, and a roof garden. Two children share each of
the homey bedrooms, and one child-care worker is assigned to each
room, with only those two children to look after. The center also provides a setting in which students in several of Columbia's divisions—
P&S, Nursing, Teachers College, and Social Work, for instance—can
gain valuable and fulfilling experience.

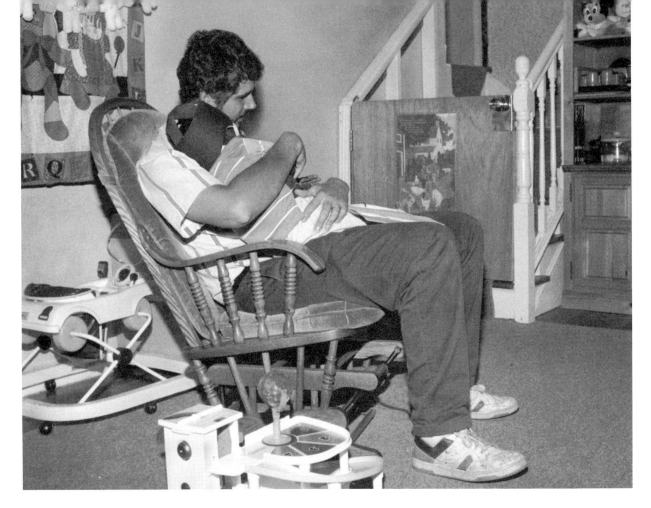

Caregivers are often called upon to give a loving cuddle at the St. Clare's group home for AIDS babies in Newark, N.J., one of the pioneers of the group home idea.

The Bigger Picture

In spite of improvements in the treatment available to AIDS patients, both children and adults, in the last few years, the disease is still fatal. The homelike, familial atmosphere at ICC, although it may only be a stopping place between hospital and a foster family, provides infants and children with a warm, caring environment for part—perhaps a big part—of their brief lives.

As Nicholas points out, the center has also become a place where parents and extended families of these children can come to spend some time with the children for whom, sadly, they are incapable of caring themselves.

"One of the biggest myths about boarder babies is that they are all abandoned," says Nicholas. "Almost all the kids we see have some family involved with them. There are some instances where the mother will have the child in a hospital and simply leave. But these are the exceptions. For the most part, we find that the mothers just don't have it together. They can't possibly take care of their kids." However, Nicholas emphasizes, "This doesn't mean that they don't love them."

At ICC, the staff has found that only about one-third of their children have no contact from family members. Another third of the children are visited occasionally—once every two or three weeks—by their mothers, fathers, or members of their extended families, especially their grandmothers.

"What's interesting," according to Nicholas, "is that fully a third of the children at the center have frequent visits from someone in their families. Many mothers come often to the center to see their children. The tragedy is that these women care, but they still are not always capable of providing care for their children. In almost 100 percent of the cases, drugs are the problem. But there are the other realities of inner-city life: homelessness, maternal AIDS, physical abuse or neglect within the family." In many cases, the only able person may be a grandmother, often very young herself—30 or so—who bears the burden of trying to keep these families together.

The effectiveness of halfway houses and foster-care services in caring for boarder babies and children with AIDS is working wonders to alleviate what was a crisis in healthcare and social services just a few years ago. But, as Nicholas points out, this "good news" is only one paragraph in a long and troubling story.

"When you're talking inner-city poverty, the list of problems is much longer—drugs, housing, education, isolation, weakened family fabric, lack of social support and political clout. Those of us in healthcare and social services do as much as we can. Sometimes we achieve a degree of success, as we have with the center. Even so, we can work on only one small piece of the bigger problem. Our inner-city poor are struggling to deal with problems that the rest of us take for granted being able to solve." ☐

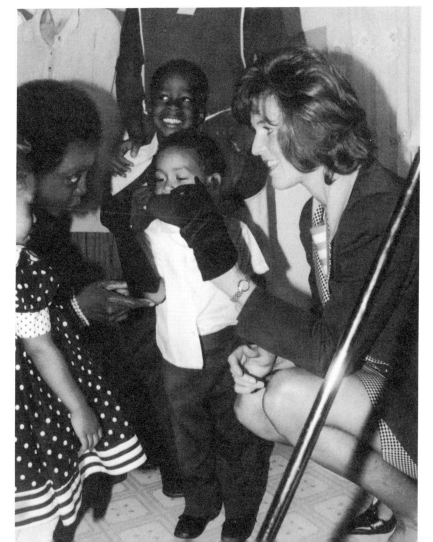

The willingness of high-profile personalities to reach out to young AIDS victims did much to allay the public's fears of contact with infected children. Left, Sarah, the Duchess of York, visits the well-known group home, Hale House.

71

Focus on Women

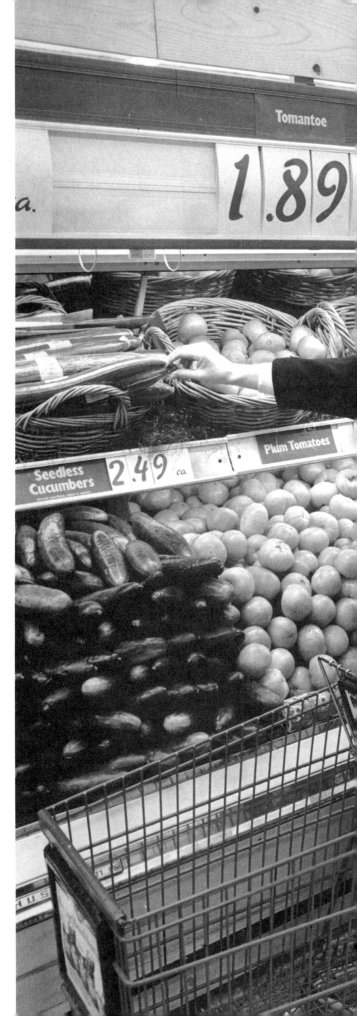

The evidence is mounting: developing and maintaining strength is essential to a healthy life. This is especially important for women, who are less strong than men to begin with. Women have special dietary needs, too, to help them avoid conditions unique to or more prevalent among women. The first of the two articles that follow looks at what women need to eat to stay healthy. The second explores how strength, or lack of it, affects women's health and the benefits of weight training—at any age.

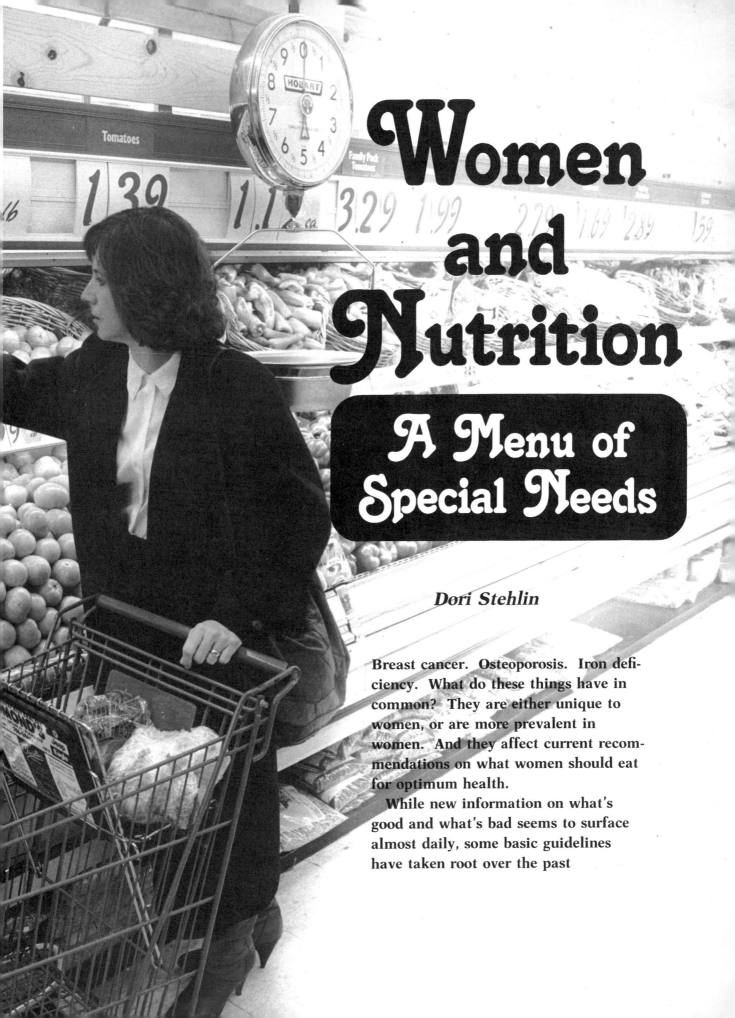

Women and Nutrition

A Menu of Special Needs

Dori Stehlin

Breast cancer. Osteoporosis. Iron deficiency. What do these things have in common? They are either unique to women, or are more prevalent in women. And they affect current recommendations on what women should eat for optimum health.

While new information on what's good and what's bad seems to surface almost daily, some basic guidelines have taken root over the past

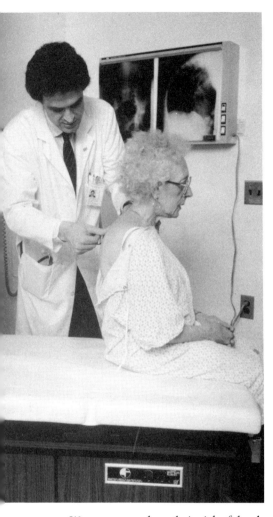

Women can reduce their risk of developing osteoporosis—a thinning of the bones that tends to occur in later life—by getting enough calcium, especially during the years in which bones are growing.

several years. The bottom line (also known as the Dietary Guidelines for Americans, from the federal departments of Health and Human Services and Agriculture) is:
- eat a variety of foods
- maintain healthy weight
- choose a diet low in fat, saturated fat, and cholesterol
- choose a diet with plenty of vegetables, fruits, and grain products
- use sugar and salt/sodium only in moderation
- if you drink alcoholic beverages, do so in moderation.

That sounds simple enough. Except, what exactly is variety? Cake one day, cookies the next? What is a diet low in fat, saturated fat, and cholesterol? And, finally, what parts of a healthy diet have special importance for women?

Vitamins and Minerals

There are several vitamins and minerals essential to a healthy diet. A well-balanced diet will usually meet women's allowances for them. However, for good health, women need to pay special attention to two minerals, calcium and iron.

Calcium

Both women and men need enough calcium to build peak (maximum) bone mass during their early years of life. Low calcium intake appears to be one important factor in the development of osteoporosis. Women have a greater risk than men of developing osteoporosis.

A condition in which progressive loss of bone mass occurs with aging, osteoporosis causes the bones to be more susceptible to fracture. If a woman has a high level of bone mass when her skeleton matures, this may modify her risk of developing osteoporosis. Therefore, particularly during adolescence and early adulthood, women should increase their food sources of calcium. "The most important time to get a sufficient amount of calcium is while bone growth and consolidation are occurring, a period that continues until approximately age 30 to 35," says Marilyn Stephenson, a registered dietitian with the Center for Food Safety and Applied Nutrition of the U.S. Food and Drug Administration. "The idea is, if you can build a maximum peak of calcium deposits early on, this may delay fractures that occur later in life."

The recommended dietary allowance (RDA) for calcium for woman 19 to 24 is 1,200 milligrams per day. For women 25 and older, the allowance drops to 800 milligrams, but that is still a significant amount, says Stephenson. "The need for good dietary sources of calcium continues throughout life," she says. How do you get enough calcium without too many calories and fat? After all, the foods that top the calcium charts—milk, cheese, ice cream—aren't calorie and fat lightweights. "There are lots of lower fat choices," says Stephenson.

Dori Stehlin is a staff writer for the FDA Consumer.

"There's 1 percent or skim milk instead of whole milk. There's a good variety of lower fat cheeses, yogurts, and frozen yogurts, and there's a whole flock of substitutes for ice cream."

In addition to dairy foods, other good sources of calcium include salmon, tofu (soybean curd), certain vegetables (for example, broccoli), legumes (peas and beans), calcium-enriched grain products, lime-processed tortillas, seeds, and nuts.

Iron

For women, the RDA for iron is 15 milligrams per day, 5 milligrams more than the RDA for men. Women need more of this mineral because they lose an average of 15 to 20 milligrams of iron each month during menstruation. Without enough iron, iron deficiency anemia can develop and cause symptoms that include pallor, fatigue, and headaches. After menopause, body iron stores generally begin to increase. Therefore, iron deficiency in women over 50 may indicate that they are losing blood from another source and they should be checked by a physician.

Animal products—meat, fish, and poultry—are good and important sources of iron. In addition, the type of iron, known as heme iron, in these foods is well absorbed in the human intestine. Dietary iron from plant sources, called nonheme, are found in peas and beans, spinach and other green leafy vegetables, potatoes, and whole-grain and iron-fortified cereal products. Although nonheme iron is not as well absorbed as heme iron, the amount of nonheme iron absorbed from a meal is influenced by other constituents in the diet. The addition of even relatively small amounts of meat or foods containing vitamin C substantially increases the total amount of iron absorbed from the entire meal.

Calories and Weight Control

The Food and Nutrition Board of the U.S. National Research Council recommends that the average woman between 23 and 50 eat about 2,200 calories a day to maintain weight. The best way for a woman to determine whether she's eating the right number of calories is to "keep stepping on the scale," says the FDA's Stephenson. She cautions, however, that cutting back on calories isn't always the answer to losing weight. "You don't really want to cut back any more [calories] if you're down around that [1,500 calories] range," says Stephenson. She explains that the fewer the calories you have to work with, the harder it is to meet all your daily requirements for a healthy diet. "If you find you are gaining weight, you need to think of not only cutting calories, but also about increasing exercise," she says. "Calories are only half the equation for weight control. Physical activity burns calories, increases the proportion of lean to fat body mass, and raises your metabolism. So, a combination of both calorie control and increased physical activity is important for attaining healthy weight. On the other hand, if you've been pigging out—well, you know what you have to do."

Suggested Weights for Adults

Height[1]	Weight (in pounds)[2]	
	19 to 34	35 and over
5'0"	97-128[3]	108-138
5'1"	101-132	111-143
5'2"	104-137	115-148
5'3"	107-141	119-152
5'4"	111-146	122-157
5'5"	114-150	126-162
5'6"	118-155	130-167
5'7"	121-160	134-172
5'8"	125-164	138-178
5'9"	129-169	142-183
5'10"	132-174	146-188
5'11"	136-179	151-194
6'0"	140-184	155-199
6'1"	144-189	159-205
6'2"	148-195	165-210
6'3"	152-200	168-216
6'4"	156-205	173-222
6'5"	160-211	177-228
6'6"	164-216	182-234

[1]Without shoes
[2]Without clothes
[3]The higher weights in the range generally apply to men, who tend to have larger body frames and more muscle; the lower weights more often apply to women, who have smaller body frames and less muscle. Weights even below the range may be appropriate for some small-boned people.

Source: National Research Council, 1989

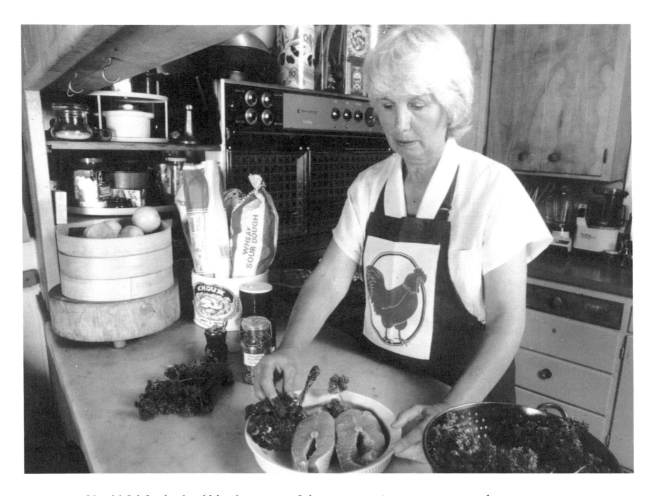

A variety of healthful foods should be the source of the many nutrients a woman needs.

Cholesterol

Women tend to have higher levels than men of a desirable type of cholesterol called HDLs (high-density lipoproteins) until menopause, leading some researchers to believe there is a link between HDLs and estrogen levels. But this doesn't let women off the hook—a diet high in saturated fat and cholesterol can still mean trouble.

For both women and men, blood cholesterol levels of below 200 milligrams are desirable. Levels between 200 and 239 milligrams are considered borderline, and anything over 240 milligrams is high. High levels of blood cholesterol increase the risk of coronary heart disease. To keep levels in the good range, the National Cholesterol Education Program of the U.S. National Heart, Lung, and Blood Institute recommends eating no more than 300 milligrams of cholesterol a day. Cholesterol is found only in food from animal sources, such as egg yolks, dairy products, meat, poultry, shellfish, and—in smaller amounts—fish and some processed products containing animal foods.

Even more important than limiting cholesterol to under 300 milligrams is keeping saturated fat to under 10 percent of total calories, says Nancy Ernst, the nutrition coordinator for the National Heart, Lung, and Blood Institute. "Don't even think about cholesterol in your diet," says Ernst. "Focus on reducing saturated fat."

Fat

In the United States, out of every 100,000 women, approximately 27 die from breast cancer each year. In Japan breast cancer deaths are fewer than 7 per 100,000. Some scientists think that the difference in death rates may be related to the different amounts of fat in the average diet in each country—40 percent for American women versus 20 percent in Japan. "We believe pretty strongly in the link [between high-fat diets and breast cancer]," says Jeffrey McKenna, director of the U.S. Cancer Awareness Program. Population studies have also linked high-fat diets to other cancers, particularly colorectal cancer.

Fat does, however, serve a purpose in the diet. Fats in foods provide energy and help the body absorb certain vitamins. But it is as easy as pie (and doughnuts, ice cream, and sirloin steaks) to eat too much.

For a healthy diet, the diet and health report of the National Research Council recommends reducing fat to no more than 30 percent of total calories (see box to figure out how). But that's not all. In terms

Figure Out Your Fat

The recommendation is that no more than 30 percent of total calories come from fat. Food labels list fat in grams. To find out what your total intake of fats in grams should be limited to, multiply your daily calories by 0.30 (30 percent) and divide by 9 (the number of calories in a gram of fat).

Example: 2,200 calories × 0.30 = 660 calories from fat

660 calories ÷ 9 = 73 grams of fat

A blood test can provide a woman with important information about her cholesterol level.

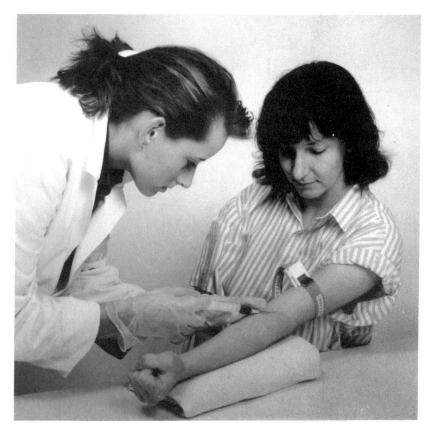

of heart disease, the kinds of fat you eat are as important as how much of it you eat.

There are three kinds of fat—saturated, polyunsaturated, and monounsaturated. All three are equal when it comes to calories—9 per gram (compared to 4 calories per gram for protein or carbohydrate). But they aren't equal when it comes to how they affect your health.

More than anything else in the diet, saturated fat can raise your blood cholesterol level. Because of this risk, less than one-third of your daily fat intake (less than 10 percent of total calories) should come from saturated fats. That's the bad news. The good news is that polyunsaturated and monounsaturated may actually lower blood cholesterol levels. The diet and health report recommends that not more than 10 percent of total calories should be from polyunsaturated fat, and monounsaturated fat should make up the remaining 10 percent.

The foods with the highest amounts of saturated fat come from animals—meat, of course, and foods derived from animals, such as butter, cream, ice cream, and cheese. In addition to animal products, coconut and palm kernel oils are very high in saturated fat—over 90 percent. The best sources for polyunsaturated fats are plant-based oils—sunflower, corn, soybean, cottonseed, and safflower. Monounsaturated fats are found in the largest amounts in olive, canola, and peanut oils.

Fiber

An apple a day—that is, a whole apple with the skin—will give you approximately 3.6 grams of fiber. That's a good start, but you still need a lot more fruits, vegetables, and whole grains to meet the daily level of 20 to 30 grams of fiber recommended by the National Cancer Institute.

Eating foods with plenty of complex carbohydrates and fiber (vegetables, fruits, and grain products) is part of a healthy diet for several reasons. A fiber-rich diet is helpful in the management of constipation and may be related to lower rates of colon cancer. These types of foods are generally low in fat and can be substitutes for fatty foods.

Fiber comes in two forms—insoluble and soluble. Insoluble fiber, mostly found in whole-grain products, vegetables, and fruit, provides bulk for stool formation and helps move wastes more quickly through the colon. Another benefit is the full feeling fiber may create in the stomach, a possible deterrent to overeating.

Soluble fiber has been linked to lowering blood cholesterol levels, but that's still a research area according to the *Surgeon General's Report on Nutrition and Health*. There are many sources of soluble fiber, including peas and beans, many vegetables and fruits, and rice, corn, and oat bran. There are even small amounts in pasta, crackers, and other bakery products.

Although foods containing fiber seem to exert a protective effect against some cancers, the diet and health report points out there is no conclusive evidence that dietary fiber itself, rather than other components, exerts this effect. Therefore, the report does not recommend the use of fiber supplements.

As important as fiber is to good health, it can be overdone. The Na-

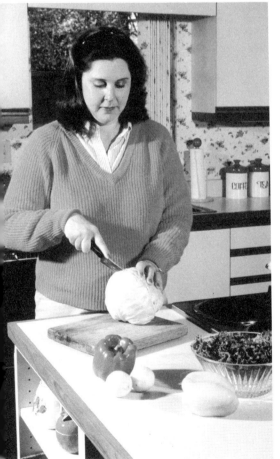

Vegetables are one good source of fiber, which helps prevent constipation and may even protect against some cancers.

tional Cancer Institute recommends an upper limit of 35 grams a day. More probably won't further increase the benefits from fiber and may interfere with the body's ability to absorb iron and other minerals. When increasing the amount of fiber in your diet, do it slowly, so your body can become accustomed to handling it. Adding too much fiber too quickly may lead to uncomfortable side effects, including abdominal discomfort, flatulence, and diarrhea.

Food Preparation

Carefully selecting foods for a well-balanced diet can end up a wasted effort if equal care isn't used in the kitchen. Some important points to help make the most of health food:

• To help reduce fat, broil, bake, or microwave food rather than frying or deep-fat frying.

• Cook vegetables in as little water as possible, or, instead of boiling food, try steaming. The steamer basket keeps the food above the water so the nutrients can't be washed away. Also, heat can destroy some nutrients, so don't overcook.

• Use fresh foods as soon as possible to avoid loss of vitamins.

• Season vegetables with herbs and spices instead of high-fat sauces, butter, or margarine. Try lemon juice as a salad dressing.

• Substitute plain low-fat yogurt, blender-whipped low-fat cottage cheese, or buttermilk in recipes that call for sour cream or mayonnaise. Use skim or low-fat milk in place of whole milk in puddings, soups, and baked products.

Getting a Variety of Foods

The Dietary Guidelines say that the many nutrients you need should come from a variety of foods, not from a few highly fortified foods or supplements. A good way to ensure variety is to choose foods each day from the five major food groups. The U.S. Department of Agriculture has developed a daily food guide for a well-balanced diet that suggests the following:

• vegetables—3 to 5 servings
• fruits—2 to 4 servings
• breads, cereals, rice, pasta—6 to 11 servings
• milk, yogurt, cheese—2 to 3 servings
• meat, poultry, fish, dried beans and dried peas, eggs, nuts—2 to 3 servings.

This food guide is "a useful, simple way for women to look at their own diets and see how to improve them," says Stephenson. By choosing different foods from each group daily, the food guide can serve as the basis for the dietary guideline "eat a variety of foods," says Stephenson, and "that's a tenet of nutritional advice for all people."

Finally, the guidelines are meant for the average person, cautions Dr. Walter H. Glinsmann, the FDA's associate director for clinical nutrition. "Almost nobody is average," he says. Lifestyle, genetics, and conditions such as pregnancy or disease can also affect a person's nutritional needs, he explains. ☐

Recommended Dietary Allowances for Women

Vitamins

A	800 micrograms
D	10 micrograms (age 19-24), 5 micrograms (age 25-50)
E	8 milligrams
K	60 micrograms (19-24), 65 micrograms (25-50)
C	60 milligrams
Thiamine	1.1 milligrams
Riboflavin	1.3 milligrams
Niacin	15 milligrams
B_6	1.6 milligrams
Folate	180 milligrams
B_{12}	2 micrograms

Minerals

Calcium	1,200 milligrams (19-24), 800 milligrams (25-50)
Phosphorus	1,200 milligrams (19-24), 800 milligrams (25-50)
Magnesium	280 milligrams
Iron	15 milligrams
Zinc	12 milligrams
Iodine	150 micrograms
Selenium	55 micrograms

Note: RDAs are recommended average daily intakes for women age 19-50.

Source: National Academy of Sciences/National Research Council, 1989

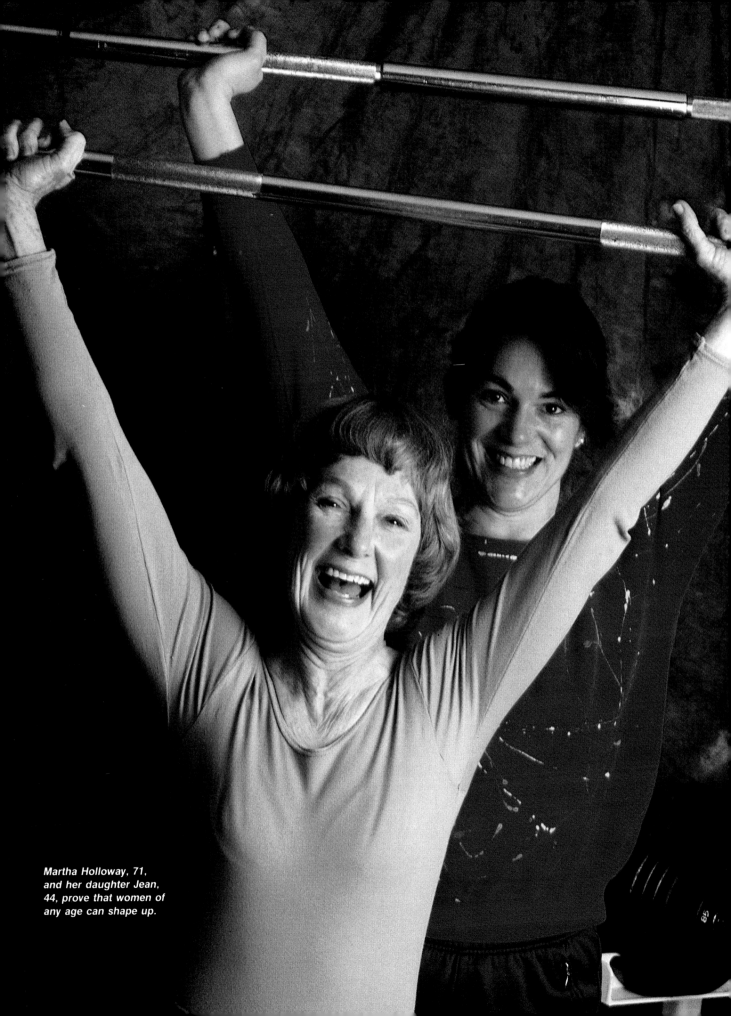

Martha Holloway, 71, and her daughter Jean, 44, prove that women of any age can shape up.

pesticides. For example, it cannot be purchased in Massachusetts or New York, two states where Lyme disease is very common.)

Clothing can also be sprayed with repellents containing diethyl-toluamide (DEET), which is marketed in preparations ranging in concentration from about 5 percent to nearly 100 percent. Stafford, who is an assistant scientist at the Connecticut Agricultural Experiment Station in New Haven, states that products in the range of 30-40 percent DEET should be adequate to protect against ticks. He advises against higher concentrations because the substance is readily absorbed by the skin and may, in sufficient quantity, cause some adverse reactions.

Eliminating ticks in the environment without widespread use of pesticides has proved to be a tough—and perhaps insoluble—problem. But there are some strategies to reduce risk. A basic principle is that deer ticks love woods and hate grass. This suggests that people should cultivate lawns and cut brush back as far as possible from paths and houses. It is also prudent to remove wood piles and other attractive mouse hotels. In warm weather, birds can carry the ticks, so Stafford suggests moving bird feeders away from dwellings during the summer months (although they may be returned in winter).

If a tick bites, the best response is to remove it immediately.

A novel method to rid an area of deer ticks was invented several years ago by the man who originally identified the tick. Andrew Spielman, a professor of tropical public health at the Harvard School of Public Health, and his associates devised a product named Damminix (because it is intended to nix the *I. dammini* tick). It consists of biodegradable cardboard tubes filled with permethrin-saturated cotton balls. Field mice collect soft materials, including the cotton, for their nests. The pesticide in the cotton rubs off on the mice and kills immature ticks feeding on them. If left to grow, these ticks would be ready to feed on humans the following summer.

Generally, improvement occurs the year after initial application, Dr. Spielman says. He and his colleagues have published research supporting the effectiveness of this method, and another group has such an investigation in press. Although no studies to show that the product is ineffective have yet appeared, critics question its usefulness, pointing out that removing the ticks from mice in one's backyard may have little effect if the neighbors' rodents are free to visit.

Damminix is sold in hardware and garden stores in 22 states. Enough tubes to treat an ordinary half-acre house lot cost around $40.00; larger and smaller kits are also available. For best results, tubes should be put out in early spring and again in late summer. Although there is no proof, it stands to reason that Damminix would be more effective the larger the area covered and the more seasons it was treated.

If a tick does get through your defenses, the best response is to remove it immediately, because the likelihood of infection rises the longer the tick is attached. It should be pulled off gently with a pair of tweezers. Trying to smother the critter with nail polish, petroleum jelly, or anything else only prolongs exposure time. Saving the tick in a suitable container, labeled with the date of the bite, could help in making a diagnosis if illness subsequently develops.

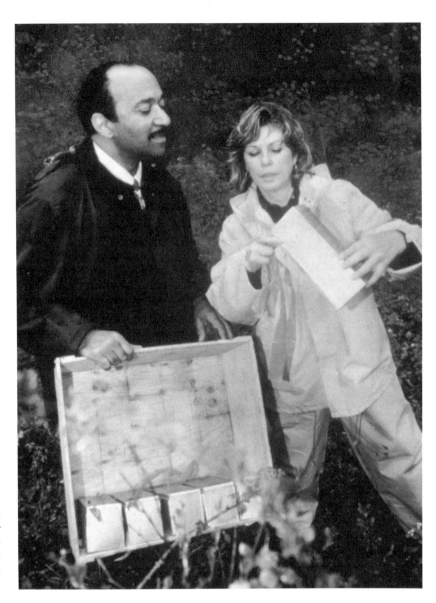

Employees of the Stamford, Conn., health department, trap ticks in the wild for testing to determine whether they carry the bacteria responsible for Lyme disease. Researchers have found that the illness is spreading to more and more states.

Spurious Cures

Public education campaigns aimed at preventing Lyme disease have given this summer scourge a high profile indeed. And scientists studying its distribution say that an increasing number of people are being exposed to this illness each year, in more and more states. As the disease has spread and become better known, it has spawned both an entire subculture and a small flurry of entrepreneurial activity.

Linked by local support groups and newsletters with such names as *the ticked-off tract* and *Lyme Disease Update*, people who call themselves "Lymeys" share experiences, complaints, and beliefs about cures with each other. Whether all Lymeys truly have chronic Lyme disease is not clear. Some of their symptoms, such as fatigue, weakness, and aches, are nonspecific and may be associated with other conditions—

112

chronic fatigue syndrome or fibromyalgia, for example—or may have no clear basis in physical illness.

Lymeys are unified by their belief that infection with the Lyme agent is the cause of their symptoms and by a general mistrust of standard medicine and its limitations. Many of them shun treatment at major medical centers known for research on Lyme disease. Instead, following what they read in the newsletters, some Lymeys travel great distances to consult self-appointed specialists with dubious credentials.

These doctors often prescribe intravenous antibiotic regimens lasting for months or, in extreme cases, years, at a cost of literally hundreds of thousands of dollars. Acting on physicians' orders, private companies will administer intravenous drugs in patients' homes. Some of these companies advertise their services in Lymey newsletters, help pay the publications' costs, and publicize support groups.

The "cure" can, however, be worse than the illness. Long-term dosage with intravenous antibiotics often leads to severe diarrhea, allergic reactions, or colonization by drug-resistant organisms, points out Leonard H. Sigal, who is the director of the Lyme Disease Center at Robert Wood Johnson Medical School in New Brunswick, N.J. Dr. Sigal adds that fibromyalgia may develop after Lyme disease is cured and may be misinterpreted as ongoing Lyme arthritis. Fibromyalgia is not an active infection and does not respond to antibiotics. If it is misdiagnosed as Lyme arthritis, unnecessary and very prolonged antibiotic therapy may be given.

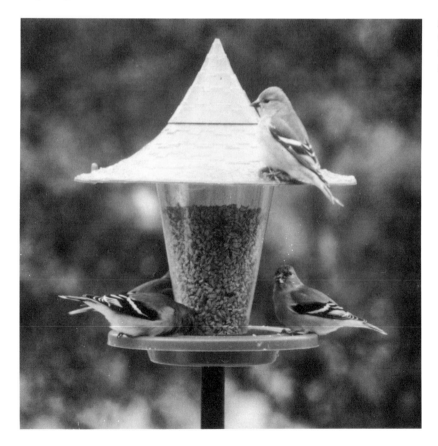

Because birds can carry ticks in warm weather, it is recommended that bird feeders be moved away from dwellings during the summer.

113

Sick as a Person

The good news is that people don't catch Lyme disease from dogs. The bad news is, dogs often get it from ticks.

"Given a choice, a tick would choose a dog over a person every time," says Andrew Spielman of the Harvard School of Public Health. Several years ago his research group compared rates of Lyme infection in humans and dogs sharing 22 coastal Massachusetts households. They found that 74 percent of dogs and 28 percent of people had high levels of antibody to the Lyme bacteria. When dog owners were compared with their dogless neighbors, infection rates were the same. In a letter to the *Journal of Infectious Diseases* published in December 1988, Dr. Spielman interpreted these results to indicate that "dog ownership was not associated with risk of human Lyme disease." He speculated that dogs are more likely to be infected than humans because their owners fail to find and remove ticks before the bacteria are transmitted from tick to pet.

Antibody tests indicate that over half the dogs in veterinarian Steven A. Levy's practice in Durham, Conn., have been exposed to the Lyme agent. By contrast, only about 14 percent of cats in the area test positive. This may be because cats are indoors more than dogs or because they groom themselves more thoroughly, Levy theorizes.

Dogs with Lyme disease are lame, sore all over, lethargic, and uninterested in food. "If they were people, they'd want to get into bed and put pillows over their heads and not move," says Levy, president of the Connecticut Veterinary Medical Association. The same symptoms affect cats. The owner of an affected feline many notice that it makes an uncharacteristically lame landing after a jump.

Animals respond well to treatment with antibiotics. (Some veterinarians may also prescribe a nonsteroidal anti-inflammatory drug such as aspirin.) More than 90 percent of infected dogs improve dramatically one to three days after starting treatment. The remainder have an up-and-down course, improving while treated and relapsing if the drugs are stopped. The majority of treated cats recover within a week.

Prevention is the best strategy for pets as well as people. Kirby Stafford, the Connecticut entomologist, suggests fencing pets out of wooded areas wherever it's feasible. Levy recommends protecting animals with flea and tick collars. They can also be sprayed with permethrin before they are allowed to roam in tick-infested areas. He does not recommend Blockade, a combination insecticide and repellent. This product was once removed from the market because it produced signs of toxicity in dogs and cats, Levy explains, but the same formulation is now being sold again.

In 1990, a Lyme vaccine became available for dogs. Although it appeared to be highly protective in laboratory studies, its effectiveness for pet dogs is still under evaluation. Pet owners should consult their veterinarians for advice on whether their dogs should be immunized.

Levy and Spielman both reject the notion that pets bring in ticks, which then drop off and attach to humans, thus increasing their owners' risk of infection. Research has never shown this to be true, and Levy's own experience argues against it. By day he is in intimate contact with dogs and cats, and at night, he says, obviously speaking as an animal lover and not a scientist, "my dogs all sleep on my bed, and I haven't had Lyme disease."

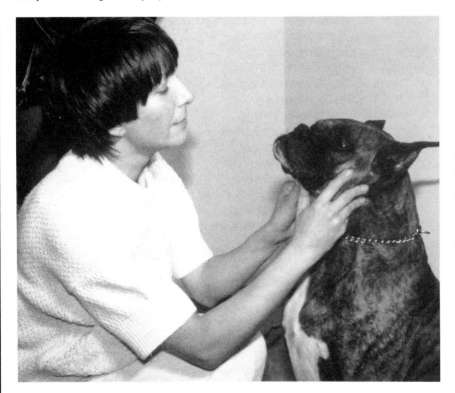

Research has shown that dogs are even more likely than humans to get Lyme disease. There is no evidence, however, that ticks travel from pets to their owners.

Fighting Fire With. . . .

Yet more troubling is malaria therapy for chronic Lyme disease. Some entrepreneurs, among them a few physicians, take groups of Lymeys to Mexico or Panama for injections of human blood containing malaria parasites. The basis for this practice as a treatment for Lyme disease was a thought-provoking but speculative letter to the editor of the *New England Journal of Medicine*, published on April 26, 1990. It was written by Henry J. Heimlich, a physician best known for the antichoking maneuver that bears his name. Dr. Heimlich pointed out that many features of chronic Lyme disease resemble those of late-stage syphilis, an illness caused by a spirochete distantly related to the Lyme organism. As he observed, infection with malaria (made temporary by subsequent antimalaria medication) was used from 1917 to 1975 to treat resistant cases of syphilis affecting the nervous system. He speculated that the same approach might relieve chronic neurological symptoms in patients with Lyme disease. A year later, Dr. Heimlich also made the case for malaria therapy in *Lyme Disease Update*, a newsletter based in Mills Shoals, Illinois.

Did malaria therapy work for syphilis? Dr. Heimlich writes that "tens of thousands of patients with neurosyphilis were cured" and adds that the treatment is still recommended for chronic syphilis affecting the nervous system when repeated courses of antibiotics have failed. But the U.S. Centers for Disease Control has issued a statement that "the effectiveness of malaria therapy for neurosyphilis was variable and unpredictable. Therapeutic trials were not carried out following strict scientific guidelines," and thus the effect of treatment cannot be adequately evaluated. The CDC also terms malaria therapy "obsolete" for neurosyphilis.

Exposure to human blood is required to transmit the malaria parasite—an ironic twist in an era when people store their own blood prior to surgery rather than run the risk of contracting AIDS or hepatitis from even rigorously tested donor blood. According to David T. Dennis, coordinator of the Centers for Disease Control's research program on Lyme disease, "We just don't know how carefully the blood used for malaria therapy outside the United States is screened."

Desperate patients are willing to pay dearly for special trips to places where malaria therapy is legal. For example, at a center in Panama, Lymeys can be injected with malaria-containing blood for $10,000. In addition, the patients must pay for transportation, meals, and hotel accommodations for up to 30 days during the period of treatment.

Two of the first American patients injected with malaria-containing blood at a Mexican "clinic" still harbored malaria parasites when they returned to New Jersey. One of them has since repudiated the treatment, saying that she is just as sick now as she was before she went to Mexico. Last year, an official CDC statement on malaria therapy emphasized that there is no proof that the treatment is safe or effective for Lyme disease, and it warned that "severe illness and death" might result from either runaway malaria or another blood-borne illness, such as hepatitis B or AIDS. □

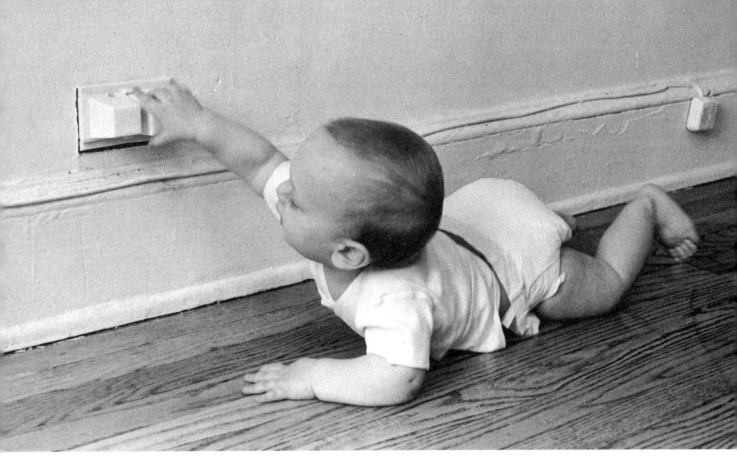

Childproof covers on electrical outlets prevent little fingers from poking where they shouldn't.

Childproofing Your Home

Ingrid J. Strauch

When a baby discovers the world, everything is new—to be touched, tasted, and explored. Infants and toddlers can't yet discriminate between what is safe to handle or put in their mouths and what is not; even preschool children are not fully aware of the dangers lurking in electrical outlets, matches, and furniture polish. Since parents cannot possibly watch their children's every move, accidents do happen, and many of the worst accidents that befall young children occur right in their own homes.

The idea then is to make the child's environment—in other words, the home—as safe as possible. By locking up, placing out of reach, or getting rid of potential dangers, you can actually create an environment where most things can be touched and played with.

116

Staying a Step Ahead

The best time to evaluate household safety and begin making appropriate changes is before your baby is born. Since babies rarely give warning that tomorrow they will be able to do something they couldn't today, parents always need to keep one step ahead of their child's development. Given children's natural curiosity, it is best to assume that they will eventually get their hands on anything that is not locked up or placed high out of reach.

The first two or three months of the infant's life are a kind of breathing spell, since the baby has so little mobility. Safety measures at this age include making sure all baby equipment—seat, swing, crib—is in good repair and has no sharp edges or exposed hardware that can pinch a baby's fingers. Gradually infants become able to interact more actively with their surroundings, waving arms and legs, grabbing at nearby objects, and putting anything and everything in their mouths. At this point anything potentially unsafe—breakable objects, plants, window shade cords—within reaching distance of the crib and play areas must be moved farther away.

Sometime between six months and a year most babies begin to crawl. By this time small or sharp objects should be stowed away, and poisons locked up; dangling cords need to be tied out of reach and electrical outlets covered. Doors and stairways should be blocked off. A good way to identify potential trouble spots is to get down on your hands and knees to see your home from your baby's vantage point.

Babies trying to pull themselves up to stand can knock over unstable furniture or pull drawers out onto their heads. Toddlers pose an additional challenge, since they can get to things faster, sometimes before you even realize they've moved. And toddlers who have learned to climb know no bounds—only extremely high cupboards and closets will be out of reach.

Common Household Dangers

Electrical outlets, to children, look like intriguing little holes in the wall in which to insert fingers, tongues, and playthings, but they can deliver a dangerous shock. This can be prevented by installing dummy plugs or plastic covers on every unused outlet.

Electric cords invite grabbing, which may bring a heavy lamp or appliance crashing down. When not in use, appliances should be unplugged, and the cord placed out of reach. All frayed cords should be replaced in case one does end up in your child's mouth, where it could cause a shock. Cords lying on the floor can trip a toddler, and so should be kept out of the way.

Plastic bags and plastic wrap can suffocate a child and must always be kept out of reach. All plastic packaging should be removed from crib mattresses before use, and plastic bags or large pieces of plastic should be cut into small pieces before being placed in wastebaskets.

Windows are both fascinating and dangerous for young children who don't understand the dangers of leaning out too far. Window bars will keep youngsters safely inside, as will burglar locks, which allow win-

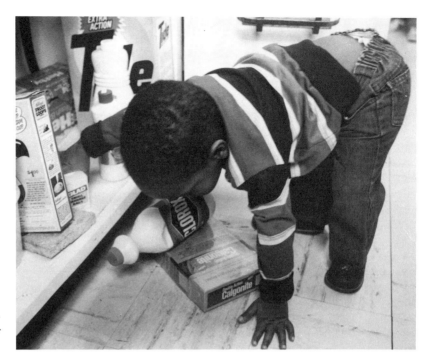

Curiosity can lure toddlers into exploring unlocked cabinets and their often dangerous contents.

dows to be opened only a few inches. Such precautions are especially important for windows above the first floor. Some cities have laws requiring landlords to install window gates in apartments where small children live.

Since radiators and heat ducts get dangerously hot, safety guards should be placed over them to prevent burns. Avoid using kerosene and space heaters. They are impossible to make entirely safe and are easily tipped over.

It takes only a couple of inches of water and a few minutes for a young child to drown, so never leave water standing in bathtubs, sinks, pails, dishpans, or other open containers. Nor should a child be left alone in the tub—even for a minute. The temperature of the hot water coming out of the tap may be hot enough to burn a baby's skin (and hotter than really necessary for household use). In homes which have separate hot water heaters, parents may want to consider turning down the thermostat.

Medicine of all sorts, even vitamins and over-the-counter products, must be kept away from curious children. Some medicines look like candy to young eyes, but sampling such "candy" could be disastrous. For extra insurance, medicine should be bought in childproof containers whenever possible. Be aware that visitors, especially older people, may bring medications with them.

Staircases should have gates at top and bottom until your child is able to climb both up and down stairs. Children often learn to climb up stairs before mastering going back down, and can get stranded at the top of a staircase.

Ingrid J. Strauch is a staff editor and writer.

118

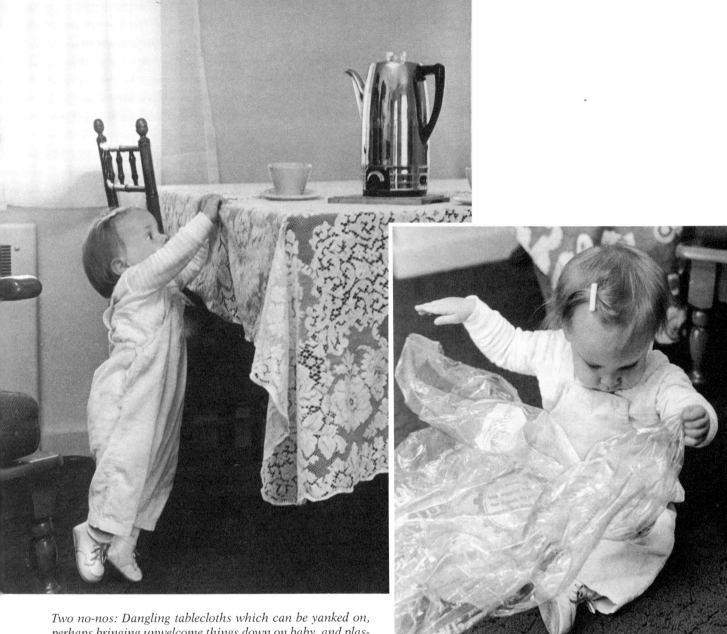

Two no-nos: Dangling tablecloths which can be yanked on, perhaps bringing unwelcome things down on baby, and plastic bags or wrappers, which can cause suffocation.

Some children love to explore wastebaskets, which may contain sharp objects, old food, and other undesirable things. For this reason, wastebaskets should be placed on a high counter out of reach, locked in a closet, or fitted with a lid that is extremely hard to remove.

Some common houseplants are toxic and, if eaten, can make a child sick. These include caladium, dieffenbachia, poinsettia, philodendron, and the castor-oil plant. Parents should make sure any poisonous plants are inaccessible to a child. In general, children should be discouraged from chewing on or eating any houseplant.

Beautifully finished floors are a joy to behold, but they can be slippery—and this can spell danger for a child learning to walk. It's easy for a toddler to slip and fall, especially when wearing just socks. Bare feet or shoes will provide more traction. Throw rugs should be anchored or put away until walking has been mastered.

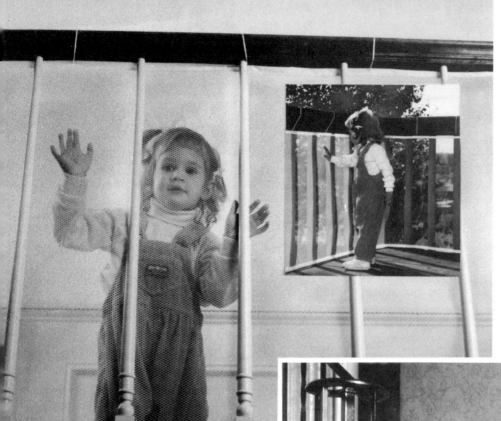

To the Barricades

Nasty falls can be prevented with the use of barrier devices, such as the netting (above) that can be used on a staircase landing or outdoors on a deck or balcony (inset). A baby gate (right) will prevent a youngster from attempting to scale a flight of stairs.

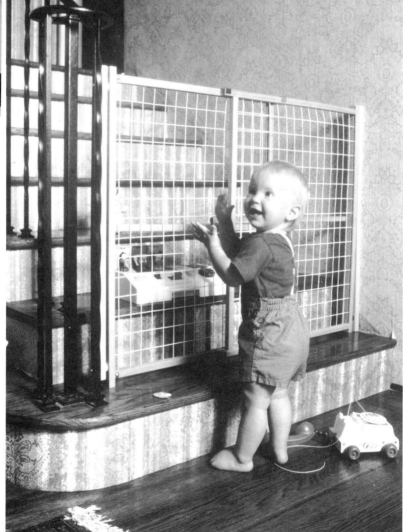

120

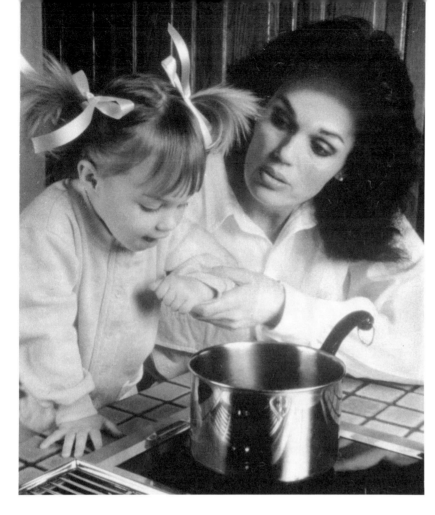

Kitchens are full of hazards for young children, but close supervision and instruction, such as that being practiced by this mother, can help prevent accidents.

Kitchen and Dining Room

The kitchen is a minefield of dangers for a young child. It has sharp knives, breakable crockery, and the stove. When a toddler's every move cannot be watched because the only adult home is busy cooking, the safest place for the child is in a high chair (securely strapped) or in a playpen. But children grow out of high chairs, lose patience with playpens, and wander into the kitchen when they're supposed to be playing in the living room, so the kitchen needs to be made as safe as it possibly can be.

Use just the stove's back burners whenever possible, and keep pot handles pointed inward. Pots with two small handles on either side are more stable and thus safer than those with one long handle, which are more easily grabbed and pulled by curious toddlers. Some ovens are so poorly insulated that a child (or anyone else) can be burned just by touching the outside of the oven door. Ideally such an oven, or at least the door, should be replaced, but this is expensive and not always possible. A fireplace grate placed in front of the door is an awkward alternative, but it may help keep children back. Don't try to insulate the door by placing towels, cardboard, or other materials over it—this creates a fire hazard.

Knives, scissors, forks, and other sharp kitchen items (such as cooking thermometers, skewers, cheese graters, food processor blades, corkscrews, and some can openers) must be stored out of reach or kept in a safety-locked drawer or cabinet. Breakable tableware and cookware

121

should also be stored out of reach. Beware of plastic containers such as those used for yogurt and cottage cheese that are safe while whole but have sharp edges when broken.

Many people use the space under the kitchen sink to store household chemicals like cleansers, insect and rodent poisons, shoe polish, and plant fertilizer. These should be moved to a high cabinet or at least secured with a safety lock.

The lower kitchen cabinets can be used for unbreakable plastic bowls and cups, wooden spoons, metal pots, muffin tins, and bread pans that are safe and fun for a child to play with.

In the dining room, keep knives, forks, glasses and other breakables, and hot cooking and serving dishes away from young children. Some families use tablecloths sparingly until children are old enough to understand that pulling on the cloth can send everything on the table crashing to the floor and possibly on their heads.

Bathroom

A baby should never be left unattended in a bathtub, not even for a minute. Drowning can occur in very little water—and very little time.

The cold, hard surfaces of most bathrooms make them unsafe places for very young children. The bathroom should be kept off-limits until your child has learned to use it independently. Access can be restricted by installing a simple lock, such as a hook and eye, or a childproof doorknob on the outside of the bathroom door. But since you

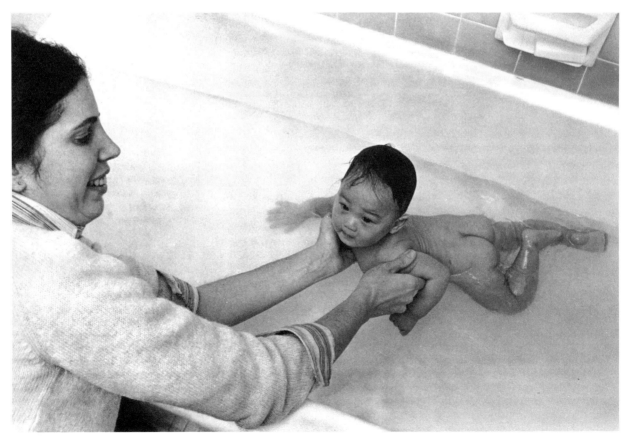

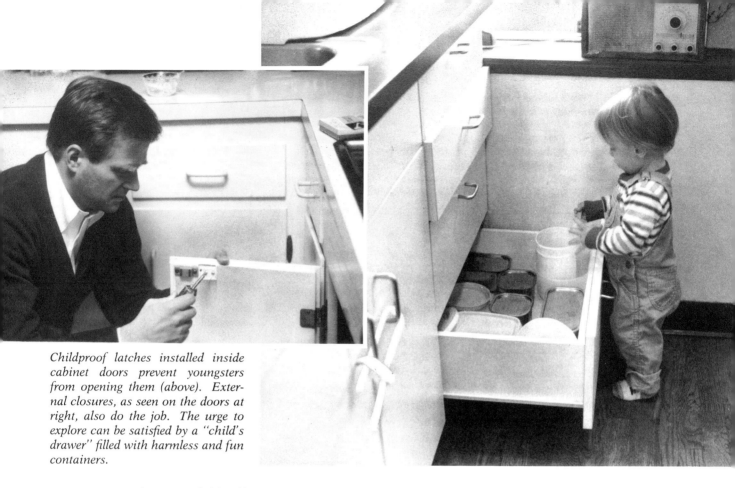

Childproof latches installed inside cabinet doors prevent youngsters from opening them (above). External closures, as seen on the doors at right, also do the job. The urge to explore can be satisfied by a "child's drawer" filled with harmless and fun containers.

cannot assume that your child will never get into the bathroom, you should put a safety lock on the medicine cabinet and keep all cosmetics, beauty and hygiene aids, scissors, razors, and cleaning products high out of reach or in a locked cupboard. Appliances such as hair dryers and hot curlers should be unplugged and put away when not in use. The inside door lock is often best removed, as children frequently learn how to lock themselves in, only to find they can't unlock the door when they want to get out.

Living Room

Before your child begins learning to stand and walk, put away very top-heavy items that are easily knocked over, such as tall, thin planters, and try to repair any furniture that is wobbly because of missing parts or loose joints.

Breakable, valuable, or heavy ornaments are best put in storage until children are older. You can prevent valued books from being pulled onto the floor by using the bottom bookshelves to store old magazines and toys.

When serving hot beverages in the living room, don't put tea and coffee pots and cups on low tables where children can reach them and possibly spill the burning liquid onto themselves. Alcoholic drinks should also be kept out of children's reach so they won't be tempted to sample them.

Plate glass doors can cause horrible injuries if children do not realize they're there and walk through them. One solution is to install safety glass. A less expensive way to avoid accidents is to make the glass more visible by applying decals at a child's eye level.

If you have a working fireplace, put a sturdy grate in front of it. Nothing a young child might want should be kept on the mantle. But these precautions are no substitute for constant supervision. Never leave a young child alone with a fire. And whenever children are present, avoid poking around in the fire with a stick or throwing in bits of trash, since the children will want to imitate you.

Baby's Bedroom

Cribs should meet the safety requirements set by the U.S. Consumer Product Safety Commission: bars no more than $2\frac{3}{8}''$ apart; a latch mechanism that does not allow the dropside rail to release suddenly if jostled from within or without; no exposed sharp edges, screws, or bolts; and a paint or finish that is lead-free and nontoxic. In the United States all newly manufactured cribs are required to meet these standards, but parents may need to inspect a second-hand or handmade crib. The mattress should fit snugly in the crib. If the space between mattress and crib is greater than the width of two fingers, fill it with a rolled blanket. Newborns should never sleep with a pillow or large stuffed animal; these can suffocate a baby who is not strong enough to turn when breathing is obstructed.

Off-limits

For very young children, certain areas of the house should simply be off-limits unless the child is accompanied by an adult. The basement storage area, the toolshed, and the garage may contain too many dangerous things for them to be placed out of reach or secured individually. In many cases a hook and eye installed high up, a childproof doorknob cover, or a safety gate is all that is required.

Remember to put away sharp implements or toxic materials used for sports, collections, or hobbies such as painting, calligraphy, sewing, model building, or darts. Firearms and other weapons should always be kept unloaded and locked up.

Pets

Pets sometimes cause trouble with infants and young children. A dog may be jealous of the attention the newcomer receives and may even attack the baby. A warning sign of jealousy is that the dog demands attention whenever the baby is being held or cared for. Dogs vary in their tolerance for playing with small children—some allow any amount of tail pulling while others get irritated and nip or snap. It is safest never to leave a very young child alone with a dog.

Cats are rarely jealous of a baby, but they often like to jump in the crib and curl up. This should not be allowed, because a cat can suffocate the baby if it lies on top of it. Placing netting over the crib will keep the cat out. Another danger to watch out for is that a cat may scratch a child who treats it roughly or tries to pick it up.

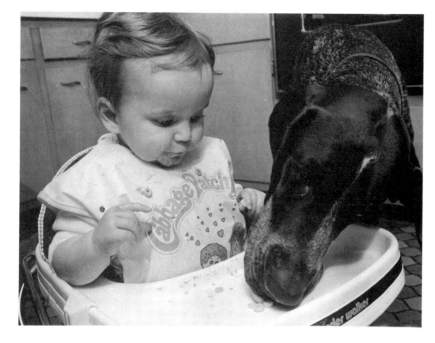

It's fine for babies and pets to be pals, but since pets can carry parasites and diseases, too much togetherness should be avoided.

For the safety of both animal and child, children should not be allowed to hold small animals such as hamsters or guinea pigs. A child who squeezes too hard may be bitten.

Pets may carry parasites and diseases that can be transmitted to children. Dogs and cats should be kept in good health and checked regularly by a veterinarian. Fish tank water is not clean, and children should not be allowed to play with it. Turtles should not be allowed in the house, since some carry *Salmonella* bacteria, which can cause fever, along with diarrhea and a number of other gastrointestinal problems. (The sale of baby turtles for pets has been illegal in the United States since 1975.)

All pet food should be stored where children cannot get to it, and bowls for food and water, pets' beds, and litter boxes should also be placed somewhere inaccessible.

Teaching Safety

As children gain maturity and physical coordination, they should be taught to use some of the items that were previously off-limits. Children who learn to use such objects as scissors, or even simple carpentry tools, safely under adult supervision are less likely to play secretly with them in a dangerous way.

SUGGESTIONS FOR FURTHER READING

FAUCHER, VIVIAN KRAMER. *Safe Kids: A Complete Child Safety Handbook and Resource Guide for Parents.* New York, Wiley, 1991.
LAUSKY, VICKI. *Baby Proofing Basics.* Deephaven, Minn., The Book Peddlers, 1991.

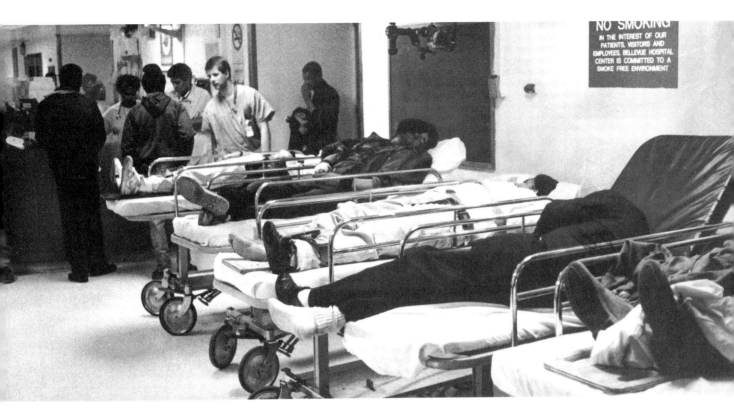

As an emergency physician from the American College of Emergency Physicians (ACEP), I'd like to bring a national perspective on what we consider today's most important crisis in healthcare. We are on the verge—and perhaps over the verge—of a major crisis in healthcare related to overcrowding in hospital emergency departments. Emergency department overcrowding occurs when admitted patients can no longer leave the department because all staffed inpatient and intensive care beds in the hospital are occupied and no beds are available in neighboring facilities for transfer. Patients come to the emergency department requiring inpatient care, and there are no beds, no resources, no intensive care units, and no nurses available to provide that care. Those patients wait in the emergency department, sometimes for hours, sometimes for days, until a bed becomes available.

I am personally familiar with patients who have waited as long as eight days in the emergency department for an inpatient bed. There are emergency departments in New York and in other cities throughout the country in which there have been as many as 50 or 60 patients waiting for inpatient beds that were not available. In large metropolitan areas, emergency department overload can develop despite the availability of staffed beds, because additional patients are being diverted from other overcrowded facilities. When a large percentage of a community's emergency departments simultaneously adopt "ambulance diversion," "standby," or some other limited availability status, emergency departments that remain open may quickly become overwhelmed with patients. This set of circumstances can rapidly lead to

EMERGENCY ROOM GRIDLOCK

Stephan G. Lynn, M.D., FACEP

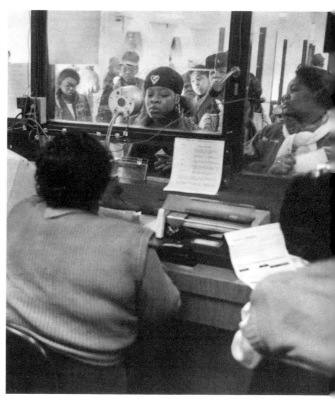

emergency department "gridlock"—a particularly dangerous situation in which no emergency department in the immediate vicinity can safely accommodate additional ambulance patients. In many communities overcrowding is severely limiting the public's right to timely emergency medical care and compromising the quality of that care. The problem in simple terms is that we have too many patients requiring access to healthcare and too few resources available.

As an emergency physician, this significantly limits my ability to provide quality care. Emergency departments were neither designed, planned, nor staffed to provide inpatient services, and when they are asked to provide those services, they have marginal ability to do so.

In overcrowded emergency departments today, we are able to take vital signs, we are able to give medications, we are able to monitor patients, but we cannot provide any of those things that our patients expect when they are admitted to the hospital. We cannot provide privacy, we cannot turn out the lights, we cannot turn off the noise, and we cannot provide access to telephones or visitors. It is difficult, if not impossible, for us to provide three warm meals at appropriate times. It is extremely uncomfortable for our patients to spend days sitting on an emergency department stretcher with a mattress that is two inches thick. When the emergency department is overcrowded, the quality of care suffers, and, far more important, access to care suffers as well.

When 50 percent of an emergency department's staff, space, and equipment are allocated to provide care for patients who require inpatient admission (and have no need for emergency care), what happens to the next patient who walks through the door? The role and mission

Opposite page: The severe overcrowding that is plaguing emergency rooms throughout the United States is painfully apparent in this scene shot at New York City's Bellevue Hospital. Above: For many patients, the tedious process of receiving emergency care begins with a long wait at a swamped intake desk.

of an emergency physician is to be constantly available for that next patient, whoever he or she is, whatever his or her problem is, but when most of an emergency department's resources are allocated to providing inpatient care, we are far less able to do so.

Scope of the Problem

After being attended to, many patients have to spend days—sometimes even a week or more—on an emergency department stretcher while waiting for a regular inpatient bed in the hospital.

How extensive is this problem? A few years ago, emergency department overcrowding was perceived as a problem of the East and West Coasts, with a few scattered areas in between. Unfortunately, over the last few years we have learned that this problem is substantially more extensive. The American College of Emergency Physicians conducted a survey of its chapters in 1989 to assess the extent of emergency depart-

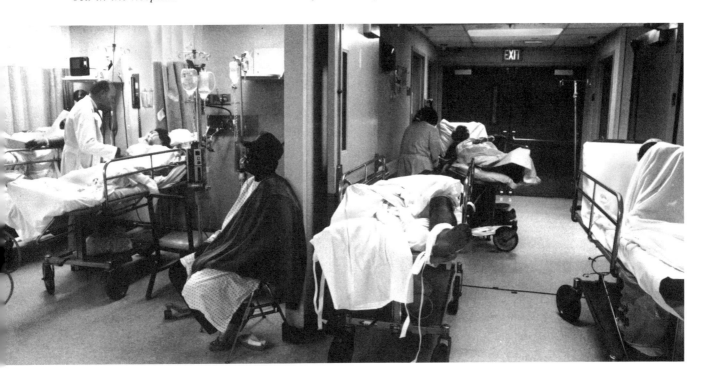

ment and hospital overcrowding nationwide. Each chapter was asked whether its members had experienced emergency department overcrowding, and to what it attributed this problem; all 54 chapters responded. ACEP chapters from 41 states (representing 94 percent of the country's population) reported overcrowding. All four non-state chapters (the District of Columbia, Puerto Rico, Ontario, and Government Services) reported overcrowding as well. Only nine state chapters reported no problem with overcrowding (Idaho, Minnesota, Nebraska,

Stephan G. Lynn, M.D., is Director, Department of Emergency Medicine, St. Luke's-Roosevelt Hospital Center in New York City and Chair of the American College of Emergency Physicians Task Force on Hospital and Emergency Room Overcrowding.

New Hampshire, New Mexico, North Dakota, Oregon, Utah, and Wyoming). Similarly, the Emergency Nurses Association polled its state councilors during its 1989 Scientific Assembly, and all 50 state councilors reported overcrowding.

In the winter of 1990–1991 the entire East Coast, from Atlanta to Toronto, was gridlocked. In 1990, Dallas and Chicago were added to the list of major urban areas that became substantially overcrowded. In 1991–1992 the problem persisted to a significant degree throughout most of the urban centers in the United States. It became substantially worse on the West Coast, although it was beginning to become more sporadic in the Midwest and the East. And when we surveyed ACEP chapters, it was extremely clear that this overcrowding is not simply an urban problem. Our chapters from West Virginia and North

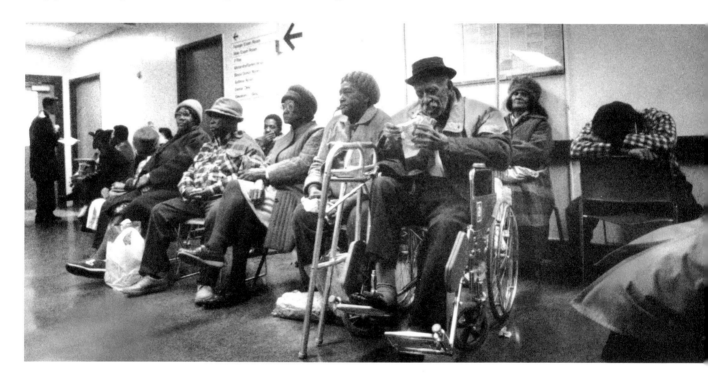

Carolina and Alaska told us that they had substantial overcrowding in areas that were neither urban nor poor.

The National Association of Public Hospitals (NAPH) has issued a report studying overcrowding at all of its member institutions and all the members of the Council of Teaching Hospitals. The study included replies from 277 hospitals in 43 states, among the largest and best hospitals across the country. Based on the preliminary results, the private hospitals experienced the same problems of overcrowding and occupancy as did the public hospitals. Seventy-five percent of those hospitals reported increased emergency department utilization in 1988. (In fact, in 1989 utilization rose to over 90 million visits, the largest annual actual and percentage increase that has ever occurred.) In those hospitals studied, 65 percent reported a substantial effect on quality of care as a result of overcrowding. Forty percent diverted ambulances,

A major cause of emergency room gridlock is the lack of access that many poor people have to primary care. Instead, they must rely on hospital emergency rooms to get treatment for conditions that could be more easily—and more cheaply—handled in a doctor's office.

129

and approximately one-third transferred patients to other institutions during the target month (August 1988), because their hospital and secondarily their emergency department were overwhelmed with patients; there was not room for one additional patient.

Contributing Factors

What contributes to this substantial and increasing problem of emergency department overcrowding? In simple terms, there is inadequate funding and priority for emergency healthcare services during a period of increasing demand. There is increasing demand because more and more people are utilizing the emergency department every year for a large number of reasons. Our population is aging; we have increased drug abuse and poverty; and AIDS patients that we could never have planned for five or ten years ago are utilizing the emergency departments in our hospitals in ever-increasing numbers. And for those 37 million people we constantly hear about that are uninsured or underinsured, the emergency department has became the provider of last (and, frequently, only) resort.

At the same time that demand for services is increasing, the supply of hospital beds is diminishing. Between 1985 and 1990, New York City eliminated 5,000 acute care beds. Emergency departments in California, particularly Southern California, are closing at a rapid rate. In that state, hospitals are allowed to close their emergency departments when they become financially undesirable. There are fewer hospital beds, there are fewer emergency departments available to treat patients. There are not enough nurses; there are particularly not enough skilled nurses in emergency departments and critical care units, and it is these intensive care units that usually become the bottleneck for hospital admissions. There are not enough nursing homes. About 10 percent of the acute care bed capacity in New York City and in the state of Massachusetts in 1989 was occupied by patients who required nursing homes or home healthcare placement. The resources were simply not available in those states.

Solutions

What will bring us to the end of this problem? The first solution is universal access to healthcare and universal access to healthcare reimbursement. The care for about one-third of all patients who come to the emergency department is uncompensated; in a national study by the American College of Emergency Physicians, 31 percent of all emergency care in this country was uncompensated. The emergency department is appropriately mandated to see all patients who seek care there, but society does not provide reimbursement for that care. As a result, our hospitals, our emergency departments, and our patients are suffering.

Another factor that must be addressed is the lack of access to primary care. This is exemplified by a study done in Washington, D.C., for the District of Columbia Hospital Association, which evaluated patients characterized by three very simple factors: the patients (1) had

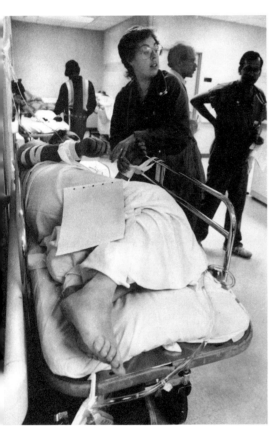

A serious lack of skilled nurses in emergency departments and critical care units is another leading cause of bottlenecks.

no ability to pay, (2) came into the emergency department, and (3) were admitted. Looking at those three characteristics, the study found that about one-quarter of all patients who presented to an emergency department in Washington, D.C., for admission and who had no ability to pay had an "avoidable admission"—avoidable, that is, if that patient had had access to primary care. If one other factor is added to that list—preexisting chronic disease—the percentage of "avoidable admissions" increases from 25 percent to about 45 percent. Lack of access to primary and preventive care is not only injurious, it causes a substantial number of completely avoidable hospital admissions.

Admissions through the emergency department add cost to the system in other ways as well. The Health Care Financing Administration compared patients admitted through the emergency department and patients admitted from all other sources in the same DRG (Diagnosis Related Group—the federal government's method of associating a large number of patients with similar medical problems into a single category. The hospital's reimbursement is the same for all patients classified within the same DRG). The study showed that the length of stay and the cost to the hospital and to the healthcare system are substantially higher for patients with the same diagnosis who are admitted through the emergency department.

Long-term Vision

The problem of emergency department overcrowding is severe and serious today. On one Monday in September 1990 in New York City, 40 of the 55 emergency departments were on total bypass. That means that each of those 40 emergency departments already had 15 patients admitted and waiting for beds, and no inpatient beds were available. This was in the fall, not a season of traditional overcrowding, with winter still to come.

We see little hope for a solution in the short term. Major changes are not occurring to deal with either the causes of this problem— increases in infectious diseases, increases in respiratory emergencies, AIDS, drug-related health crises, and poverty—or to bring about the solutions—universal access to healthcare, more nurses, reweighing of DRGs for patients admitted through the emergency department, implementation of preventive healthcare programs, and a reorganization of healthcare services so that in-hospital treatment is used only for patients with acute health problems. Development of realistic and effective contingency plans may allow emergency physicians and emergency nurses and their colleagues to deal with the immediate consequences of overcrowding. Such management tools, however, while crucial in the face of the immediate problem, will not produce significant long-term changes in the nature of hospital overcrowding.

Emergency departments provide the critically important safety net for our nation's healthcare system, but our capacity to meet the needs of patients is stretched to the breaking point. Long-term resolution of the problem of hospital and emergency department overcrowding will require a substantial commitment of societal resources and vision— and, perhaps, a revolution in our national healthcare priorities. ☐

Our capacity to meet the needs of patients is stretched to the breaking point.

131

LOOKING AFTER YOUR HEART

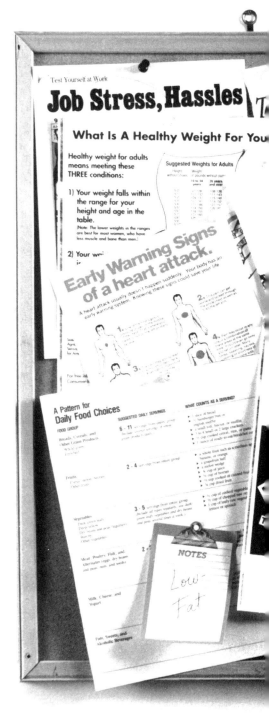

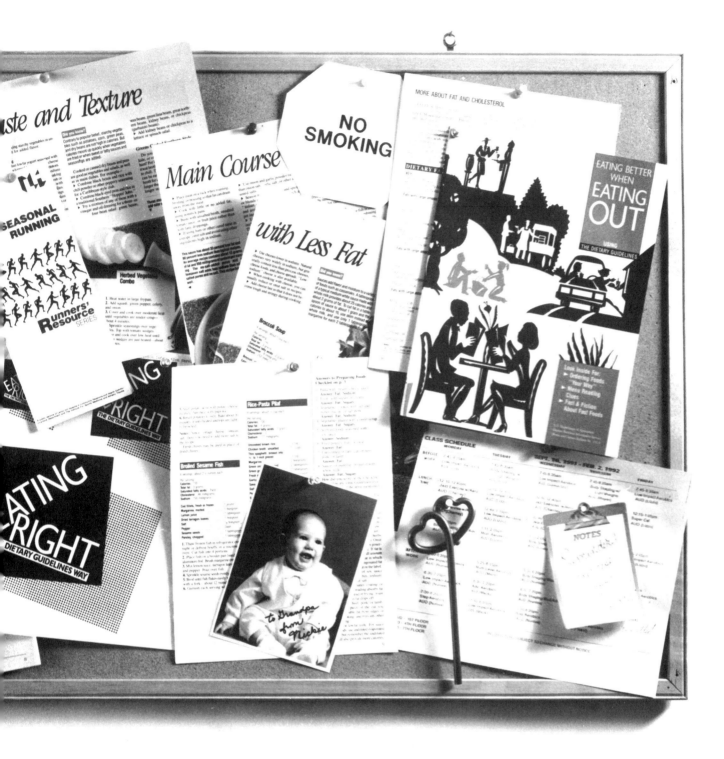

Heart attack—caused by the blockage of one or more arteries supplying blood to the heart—remains a feared and all-too-common killer. But recent advances have given physicians a variety of tools to help prevent heart attacks in high-risk individuals and to help patients survive if they do suffer an attack. The first of the two articles that follow looks at the range of treatments—from diet changes to bypass surgery—that can help people with narrowed arteries avoid life-threatening blockages. The second presents the latest thinking on the best ways for heart attack survivors to resume a full and active life.

Making the Right Treatment Choice

Every year about 300,000 people undergo a coronary artery bypass operation to relieve the pain of angina or to circumvent potentially life-threatening narrowing of the coronary arteries (atherosclerosis). Recently, based on the results of the latest studies of the outcomes of bypass surgery, a joint task force of the American College of Cardiology and the American Heart Association drew up a new set of criteria to guide physicians and patients in deciding just who should—and who should not—have such surgery.

With atherosclerosis, the inner layers of the artery walls become thick due to formation of a plaque, which is made up of cholesterol and other substances. This buildup of plaque narrows the internal circumference (lumen) of the arteries, and that narrowing causes a diminished flow of blood.

When the coronary arteries—those arteries that form a crown of vessels around the heart—become narrowed, they are unable to deliver sufficient blood and, therefore, oxygen to the muscle of the heart itself (the myocardium). This lack of oxygen produces chest pain (angina pectoris), as the heart labors to continue to pump. Some people experience angina only when they increase the work load on the heart—when they climb a flight of stairs, or run to catch a bus, or even walk against a heavy wind. Some, however, may experience angina even when they are resting.

Angina can be mild or so severe as to force people to curtail their activities—and that curtailment can become additionally debilitating. For these reasons alone, angina should be treated. But angina of longer duration or of greater severity is also a warning sign that a person is at risk for a heart attack, since a narrowed coronary artery may eventually be closed off altogether by a buildup of plaque or by a blood clot that forms in the artery (a coronary thrombosis or coronary occlusion). In about two-thirds of people with angina, the pain is associated with at least a 70 percent obstruction of the lumen of two of the three major coronary arteries. If the blood supply is cut off severely, the muscle cells of the heart may suffer irreversible injury or death (myocardial infarction, or heart attack).

The First Step in Treatment

For anyone with angina the first line of treatment is usually cardiac medication. Some drugs, called vasodilators, cause the smooth muscles of the blood vessels to relax so that the lumen opens up and blood flow increases. Nitroglycerin relaxes the veins (which reduces the amount of blood that returns to the heart and so reduces the pumping work load) and also relaxes the coronary arteries (which increases the blood supply to the heart). Other drugs may be used to reduce blood pressure, which in turn reduces the heart's work load and thus its need for oxygen. Still other drugs may slow the action of the heart and reduce its work load.

To inhibit the further progress of atherosclerosis, your physician will also advise you to alter your life-style if indeed you are not already following such health measures as stopping smoking, establishing a nutritious low-fat, low-cholesterol diet, undertaking an exercise regimen,

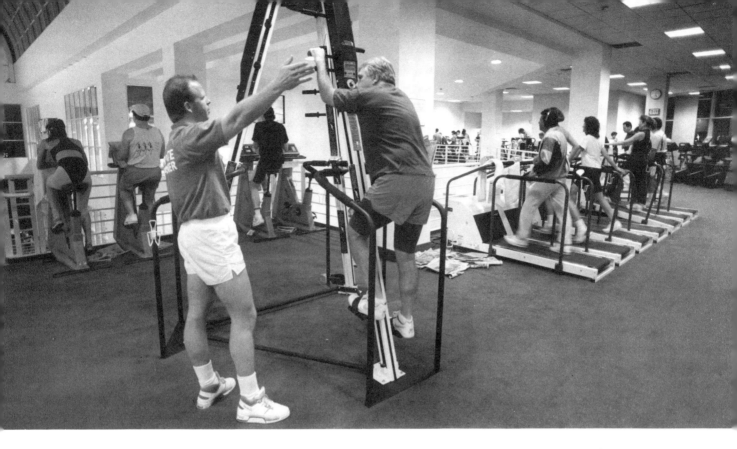

cutting down on weight, bringing blood pressure within the normal range, and reducing stress.

As long as the symptoms of angina are mild, and there is no other overriding reason to perform surgery, "no penalty attaches to a policy of treating angina with life-style changes and medication," as a recent review of treatments in *Patient Care* concludes. In a recent study patients with mild symptoms who were followed for five or ten years had essentially identical mortality rates whether they were treated surgically or medically. There are exceptions to this rule: some patients fall into a group at high risk for a cardiovascular event and are generally well-advised to have bypass surgery at once. This group includes those who have: disease in three or more coronary vessels; impaired function of the left ventricle (the part of the heart responsible for pushing blood out to most of the body); or significant narrowing of the left main coronary artery, which supplies a major part of the left ventricle.

Patients who do not fall into any of these high-risk groups but whose pain is debilitating and is not well controlled by medication are often well-advised to consider angioplasty. In angioplasty a catheter is inserted into a large artery in your arm or leg, and a small, uninflated balloon is fed up into the artery that is narrowed or nearly blocked. The balloon is then inflated to widen the artery. When the balloon is removed, the artery remains open. About 250,000 angioplasties are currently performed each year in the United States. The primary success rate is about 90 percent, although 25 to 35 percent of patients require the procedure again within six months. Moreover, 30 percent of those who have a successful second procedure require a third.

To date, no studies have shown that angioplasty prolongs life expectancy. The procedure is performed only to relieve angina. But it may be useful, too, in helping to postpone the need for bypass surgery.

An important step to take when the first signs of angina occur is the development of sound health habits, such as embarking on an exercise program—as this man has done by joining a health club and consulting with a fitness instructor.

135

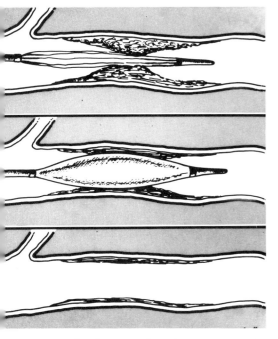

In the procedure known as angioplasty, a small, uninflated balloon on the tip of a catheter is inserted into an artery narrowed by a buildup of plaque (top). When the balloon is inflated (center), the plaque is compressed against the artery wall. The artery remains open after the balloon is removed (bottom).

If you have only one narrowed artery, angioplasty is usually the preferred therapy—though, in some patients, it can be performed on several narrowed arteries. In general, the decision whether to perform angioplasty or opt instead for bypass surgery depends on:
• the number of vessels narrowed or blocked;
• the location of the narrowing or blockage (this determines the relative ease or difficulty of treating the blockage with angioplasty);
• the degree of arterial narrowing;
• and the degree to which the left ventricle may already be damaged.

If these considerations make success with angioplasty unlikely, then bypass surgery is appropriate. It relieves pain and also (in certain risk groups) prolongs life expectancy.

The Bypass Procedure

In a bypass operation a team of surgeons opens the chest and uses a short length of internal mammary artery to create an alternate blood-flow route past a blocked or narrowed artery. (The saphenous vein from the leg is also used if more than one bypass graft is done.) As few as one—or as many as eight or nine—such bypasses can be implanted at one time, though the average is three or four.

Generally speaking, if you are in good health and have normal left ventricular function, you have less than a 1 to 2 percent risk of mortality during the operation and its immediate aftermath, and may expect a successful result—that is, restored blood flow and relief of debilitating pain without other complications. After the surgery, you should expect to spend a week or ten days in the hospital and resume your normal activities within six weeks.

However, while bypass surgery restores blood flow and relieves angina, it does not remove the underlying disease of atherosclerosis. And in time the new bypass arteries may become occluded just like the original arteries before surgery. About 10 to 20 percent of patients who have bypass surgery require a second operation within ten years because of narrowing of the vessels used in the graft. Thus, proper life-style, including strict adherence to a low-fat, low-cholesterol diet, is absolutely crucial after bypass surgery.

Once again, angioplasty may be useful in the first instance to postpone the first bypass and in the second instance—depending on the locations and nature of any new narrowing—as a measure to postpone or avoid a second bypass. Therefore, bypass surgery "can be reserved," as the recent report in *Patient Care* concluded, "for a time when symptoms worsen or no longer respond to medication, or when factors such as deteriorating left ventricular function or an increase in the number of affected vessels provide a more definitive indication for bypass surgery."

If, in this context, you are a candidate for a bypass, how can you maximize the odds for a successful operation? Studies over the years show that a successful outcome depends on:
• the general health of the patient (smoking and being overweight add to the risks);
• the location and number of vessels involved;

• the sex of the patient (women have smaller vessels that are more difficult to operate on);

• the experience of the surgeon (your surgeon should have performed 100 to 150 open-heart operations in the past year, the majority of them bypasses);

• the experience of the surgeon's hospital team, including the nursing and intensive care unit staff (the staff should have handled 200 to 300 open-heart operations in the past year, the majority of them bypasses).

Very recent studies, however, have questioned whether these criteria can accurately predict a good outcome. One of these studies found that mortality rates vary from 1.9 percent to 9.2 percent among surgeons and from 3.1 percent to 6.3 percent among medical centers, and that these outcomes do not vary simply according to the number of operations performed. It has been suggested, not surprisingly, that the skills of individual surgeons—not easily measured by the mere number of operations performed—play a part in the outcome. (You might well ask your surgeon to discuss his or her individual outcomes and look for someone who has a good success rate.) It has also been suggested that the day of the week and the time of the day may affect outcome (with the assumption that surgeons and their teams are at their best early in the week and early in the day). The skills of the anesthesiologist, the anesthesia used, the time spent in intensive care after surgery—all these, and other factors, may affect outcome, too. It may be that drug treatment both before and after surgery affects mortality rates—though more study is needed.

Meanwhile, as further studies are done to sort out all these variables, you are best served by relying on the old commonsense measures of judgment: your health and sex, the complexity of your operation, and the experience and reputation of your surgeon and hospital team. And bear in mind that you ought not to rush into bypass surgery unless you are in a high-risk group. Be sure to give the alternatives a chance. ☐

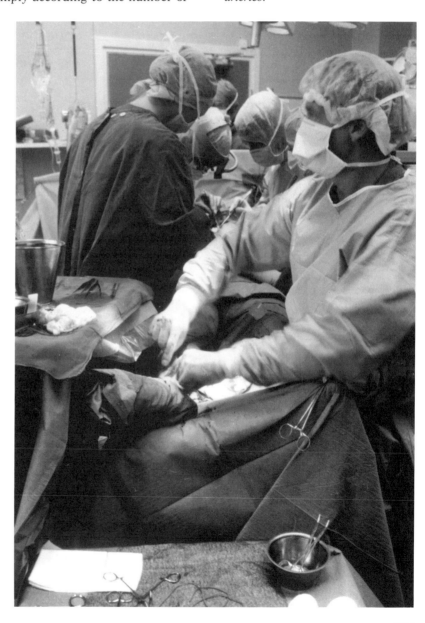

In this bypass operation, a section of vein has been removed from the patient's leg and is being used to construct alternate blood flow routes past blocked or narrowed coronary arteries.

Recovering From a Heart Attack

A heart attack is a frightening "wake-up call"—and for many people, a first confrontation with their own mortality. But thanks to recent treatment advances, most people survive heart attacks. And if they take the right steps, most can resume active lives in just two to three months.

What's more, for many people, life-style changes can actually reverse the process that caused the heart attack in the first place. Dietary fat restriction is now a cornerstone of heart attack care—and it can dramatically lower the risk of a second attack. That provides all the more reason for optimism among patients on the road to recovery.

Getting Back on Your Feet

Perhaps the biggest hurdle in a recovery is getting over the fear and anxiety spawned by a heart attack. A brush with death is a shock, and it's normal to feel like Humpty Dumpty after the fall. A treadmill exercise test usually helps ease those fears. Given before hospital discharge, the test can reassure patients that they're not as fragile or debilitated as they may feel. The doctor will use the results to recommend a safe level of activity to resume at home.

For most heart attack patients, exercise is the key to recovery. Though people with certain conditions, such as heart failure or arrhythmia, may be warned against exercise, regular activity remains the central component of most cardiac rehabilitation programs. The term cardiac rehabilitation is just another way for describing the process of getting back to normal and enjoying life again—often in a healthier way than before. Besides exercise, rehabilitation includes counseling and instruction on how to change risk factors like smoking and a high-fat diet.

Rehabilitation can be accomplished inside or outside a structured program, although a supervised approach, if available, is preferable, says cardiologist Dr. Lance Gould, a professor of medicine at the University of Texas Medical School at Houston. Supervised programs, though more costly and inconvenient, generally are more effective and safer.

Exercise begins in the hospital. Early mobilization, including walking, helps counter the muscle weakening that occurs during bed rest and may speed the return home. Once at home, patients usually can make a gradual return to ordinary household chores. Walking—slowly at first—is an excellent exercise that should be continued for a lifetime to keep a newly healed heart healthy. Cardiologists also prescribe a program of aerobic and muscle-toning exercises to improve physical conditioning. In a cardiac rehabilitation facility, such a program includes treadmill walking and stationary cycling.

The appropriate level of exercise varies from person to person and is determined on the basis of a physical examination, exercise test, and other tests such as an electrocardiogram (ECG). For normally sedentary people, the amount of exercise recommended may well exceed the person's usual level before the heart attack.

Although there's little proof that rehabilitative exercise in the recovery phase prevents another heart attack or lowers the risk of death, it

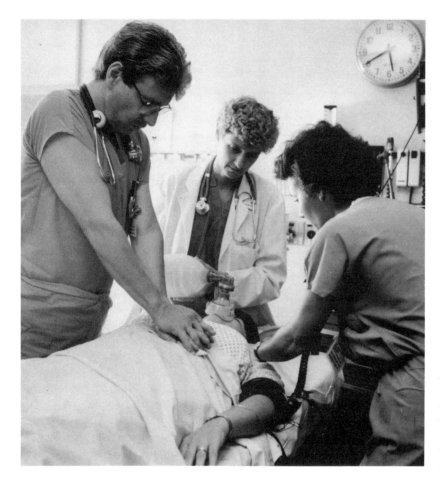

A heart attack victim being revived by a medical emergency team. A heart attack is a frightening "wake-up call," but recent advances in treatment mean that most people can resume active lives in a matter of months.

does confer many immediate benefits. Most important, it enables a quick return to work and other normal daily activities. Exercise improves the efficiency and health of the heart, and by increasing strength, it helps overcome feelings of frailty.

Because a sedentary life-style is a major risk factor for heart disease, it's important to continue regular exercise at home or at a local gym after the recovery phase. Regular exercise also modifies other risk factors: It reduces blood pressure, body fat, and triglyceride levels; increases high-density lipoprotein cholesterol (the "good" cholesterol) and glucose tolerance; and improves mental outlook.

Preventing Another Heart Attack

Whereas exercise gets heart attack patients back on their feet, lowering blood cholesterol can actually prevent future heart attacks. Cholesterol reduction can be accomplished by cutting way back on fats in the diet and, if necessary, by taking cholesterol-lowering drugs.

In collaboration with California investigators, Dr. Gould has produced proof that a very low-fat diet can reverse coronary artery disease, causing regression of plaque—the fatty material that builds up in the arteries supplying the heart. Among patients placed on a diet in

139

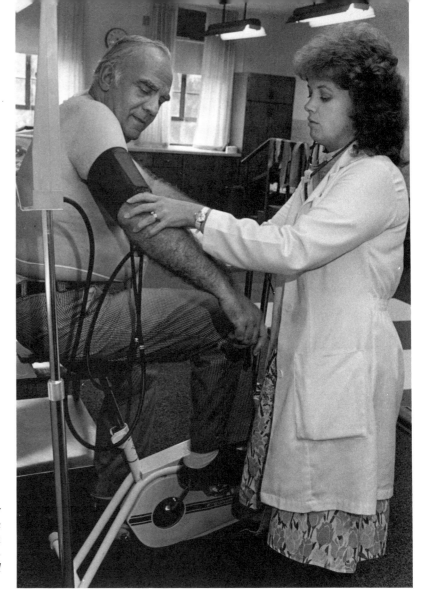

Exercise is the key to recovery for most heart attack survivors, and the use of monitoring devices by a trained healthcare professional enables the patient to find the right level of exercise.

which fat accounted for no more than 10 percent of total calories, 80 percent showed a significant regression of plaque after a year, he says. In contrast, plaque buildup progressed in a comparison group of people who consumed about 30 percent of their total calories as fat—the upper limit of the American Heart Association diet.

Moreover, another study published in 1990 found that lowering high blood cholesterol with the help of drugs also may reverse coronary artery disease. In that study, cholesterol reduction translated into a 73 percent lower incidence of severe coronary artery disease, heart attack, or death over 2½ years.

Aggressively lowering cholesterol also benefits people who've had coronary artery bypass surgery, those who had a heart attack despite having normal cholesterol levels, and anyone else with coronary artery disease, says Dr. Gould.

Other risk factors that heart attack patients must attend to include smoking, high blood pressure, and high levels of stress. All increase the likelihood of another heart attack or death in the years following a heart attack. The so-called Type A behavior pattern—a hard-driving, aggressive or hostile approach to life—also appears to increase the chance of another heart attack. Studies have shown that intervention in all these conditions lowers the risks associated with them.

Overcoming Fears and Depression

Despite all the positive steps a person may take while recuperating from a heart attack, it's normal to feel depressed. Depression may stem from a feeling of being crippled or from worries about not being able to live up to expectations in the role of parent, employee, or mate.

Blue moods may last several months, but they usually dissipate as activities increase. A recent study at the University of California at Los Angeles suggests that participants in a cardiac rehabilitation program that includes group counseling have less anxiety and depression than heart attack patients who go it alone. Another study found that participating in an everyday activity such as walking helps reduce anxiety. If depression or anxiety become difficult to deal with, psychological counseling may help.

What about sex? Although many heart attack patients worry about the safety of resuming sexual activity, few people experience serious heart problems during sex. In general, it's safe to resume sexual activity, just like other forms of moderate exercise, usually within two to four weeks after returning home from the hospital, or as the doctor advises.

Perhaps a more pertinent problem is sexual dysfunction. The fears, depression, and altered body image that may follow a heart attack can cause sexual difficulties in both men and women. It's important to deal with these issues so that sex, or lack of it, doesn't create stress in an important relationship. Beta-blockers, antidepressants, and a number of other drugs may impair sexual performance. The doctor may be able to substitute a different medication or suggest other solutions if sexual difficulties appear to be drug-related.

Despite some of the changes and challenges posed by a heart attack, patients have every reason to be optimistic about the future. According to the American Heart Association, 80 percent to 90 percent of heart attack patients return to work within two to three months, and some are able to return even sooner. Most people can keep the same job as before, although those who perform physically demanding jobs may need to switch to less taxing ones.

For most people, having a heart attack means having to make big life-style changes. Chances are good, however, that those changes will leave the person feeling better and even looking better than before the traumatic event. And, like other people who have had a brush with death, many heart attack patients report a keener appreciation of friends, family, and life itself. □

FOR MORE INFORMATION

After a Heart Attack. This brochure is available free from the American Heart Association, 7320 Greenville Ave., Dallas, TX 75231.

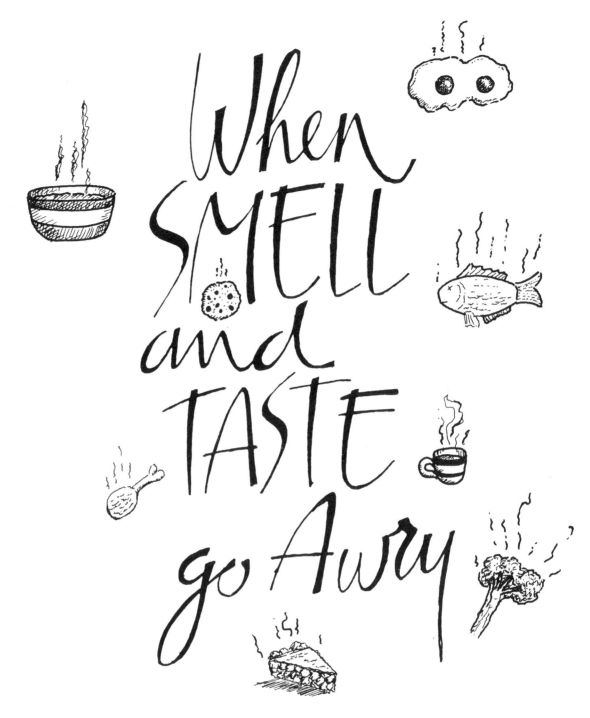

When SMELL and TASTE go Awry

Ricki Lewis, Ph.D.

ILLUSTRATIONS
BY SALEM KRIEGER

Minutes after a sudden April shower, the rich, earthy scent of spring permeates the air. A whiff from a backyard grill evokes cherished images from childhood, and a crisp autumn day has its own aroma.

Imagine a spicy slice of pizza, or freshly brewed coffee, and your mouth waters in anticipation. But for 2 million people in the United States, the senses of smell and taste are dulled, distorted, or gone altogether. Many more of us get some idea of their plight when these senses are temporarily stifled by the sniffles.

Compared to the loss of hearing or sight, being unable to taste or smell normally may seem more an oddity than an illness. But those with such ailments would probably disagree.

142

There are several reasons why knowledge about how the "chemical senses" of taste and smell work lags behind what we know about the other senses. One reason is that a problem with taste or smell often is not perceived as a serious medical condition. "These disorders are not associated with significant morbidity and mortality and affect fewer than 5 percent of the population, so it is not a major public health concern," says Lucinda Miller, Pharm.D., in the division of family medicine at the Baylor College of Medicine in Houston. She adds that this attitude translates into skimpy research funding. In some situations, however, a poor or lacking sense of smell can be dangerous. Robert Henkin, M.D., Ph.D., of the Taste and Smell Clinic in Washington, D.C., recalls one patient who died in a house fire because he did not smell the smoke in time to escape.

Another hindrance to learning more about smell and taste is that the physical bases of these senses are difficult to study in a laboratory. Taste buds, for example, cannot easily be grown outside of the body as can visual tissue such as rod and cone cells. And, more often than not, laboratory animals cannot stand in for humans because their tastes differ. Consider sugars. We humans love sucrose (table sugar), but armadillos, hedgehogs, lions, and sea gulls do not respond to it. Opossums love lactose (milk sugar) but rats avoid it, and chickens hate the sugar xylose, while cattle love it and we are indifferent. These diverse tastes in the animal kingdom help ensure that there is enough food to go around.

Despite these hurdles, research into smell and taste is starting to open up. An exciting recent discovery, by Linda Buck, Ph.D., and Richard Axel, Ph.D., of Columbia University in New York, was that hundreds of genes are responsible for the sense of smell. This explains the capacity of the human nose to detect thousands of distinct odors.

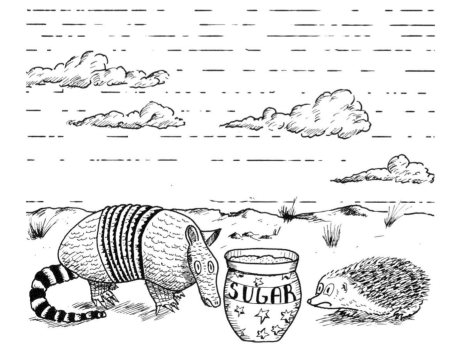

Many nonscientists have also helped explain our sense of smell. In September 1986, 1.5 million readers of *National Geographic* magazine scratched six scented patches in their issues, sniffed them, and sent the results identifying the aromas to biopsychologists Avery N. Gilbert, Ph.D., and Charles Wysocki, Ph.D., of the Monell Chemical Senses Center in Philadelphia. Although the investigators are still wading through the data, in preliminary results on a sample of 26,200 respondents published in the October 1987 issue of the magazine, the researchers said that two-thirds of the readers report temporarily losing their ability to smell at one time or another, and that 1 percent could not smell three or more of the sample scents.

Biology of the Senses

All senses work in basically the same way. Special nerve cells bearing sense receptors collect information from the environment. When these receptors are stimulated they send a message to the brain, where the cerebral cortex forms a perception, a person's particular view of the stimulus.

Most of what we call taste is really smell.

The ability to detect the strong scent of a fish market, the antiseptic odor of a hospital, the aroma of a ripe melon—and thousands of other smells—is possible thanks to a yellowish patch of tissue the size of a quarter high up in the nose. This fabric of sensation is actually a layer of 12 million specialized cells. The end of each cell sports 10 to 20 hairlike growths called cilia. Each cilium has a receptor that binds an odorant molecule—a bit of that fish or melon. The binding triggers a nerve impulse, and the message travels along the nerve cell, through a hole in the skull, to a part of the brain called the olfactory bulb. Although scientists do not know exactly how, the brain interprets the pattern receptors send it to register "hospital smell" or "cantaloupe."

The expert nose of the bloodhound is due to its 4 billion olfactory cells. Still, the human sense of smell is nothing to sneeze at—people can detect 1 molecule of green pepper smell in a gaseous sea of 3 trillion other molecules. Our 12 million smell cells and their many million more receptors allow us to discern some 10,000 scents. But, without air, there is nothing to smell, as astronauts can attest. In the vacuum of space, odorant molecules cannot reach their senses, and eating in space is a rather tasteless, not to say joyless, experience.

Most of what we call taste is really smell. We usually realize this when a cold hits our nasal passages. Even though the taste buds aren't blocked, the smell cells are, and this dulls much of food's flavor.

"Smell and taste are two distinct neurophysiological systems. The sense of taste is only sweet, sour, salty, and bitter. Other components of flavor are mediated by the olfactory system," says Beverly Cowart, Ph.D., director of the taste and smell clinic at Jefferson University Hospital in Philadelphia. A third sensory system delivers information to the brain about a food's texture, temperature, and chemical irritancy.

Ricki Lewis, a writer in Scotia, N.Y., has a Ph.D. in genetics and is the author of a college biology text.

144

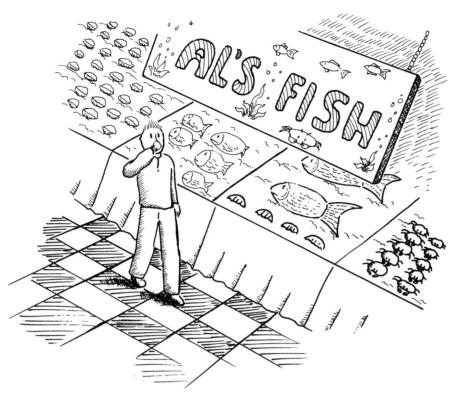

Taste comes from 10,000 taste buds, which are clusters of cells resembling the sections of an orange. Taste buds are found on the tongue, cheeks, throat, and the roof of the mouth. Each taste bud houses 60 to 100 receptor cells. These cells bind food molecules dissolved in saliva and alert the brain to interpret them. Cattle, with their 25,000 taste buds, are the bloodhound equivalent in the taste department.

The body regenerates taste buds about every three days. Although the tongue is often depicted as having regions in which taste buds specialize in a particular sensation—the tip tastes sweetness, the front saltiness, the sides sour, and the back bitter—researchers find that taste buds with all specificities are scattered everywhere. In fact, a single taste bud can have receptors for all four general types of tastes, says Henkin, who carried out much of the work describing the distribution of taste buds on the tongue.

Individual Differences

One person loves liver and onions; another gags at the thought. Of the 68 percent of women who can detect armpit odor (a chemical called androstenone), 72 percent report disliking it; of the 57 percent of men who can smell androstenone, only 50 percent dislike it. What accounts for these individual palates and noses? To some extent, what you taste or smell is in your genes. For example, the ability to smell a squashed skunk or freesia flowers is inherited.

Linda Bartoshuk, Ph.D., of the Yale University School of Medicine in New Haven, Conn., is fascinated by "why different people do not have the same experience when they eat." She and others have recently expanded upon a classical bit of genetic lore. It has been known for many years that 7 in 10 people inherit the ability to taste a bitter chemical called PTC (phenylthiocarbamide). PTC is a harmless chemical not found in food but impregnated into paper strips for use in laboratory teaching experiments. Bartoshuk finds that PTC "tasters" can detect many bitter substances that are tasteless to others.

"For example, tasters don't like the taste of saccharin, but nontasters don't mind it. Potassium chloride [a salt substitute] tastes nasty to tasters, like salt to others. Table sugar, too, is sweeter if you are a PTC taster," she says. Bartoshuk also finds that the protein in milk tastes different to tasters and nontasters, making cheese, for example, pleasantly tart to some, but bitter to others.

The ability to detect bitter tastes can show up very early in life, when smell and taste are particularly acute. "We believe the possibility should be checked that some babies who fail to gain weight may be responsive to this bitter taste in milk," Bartoshuk adds.

Treating Disorders

Because there are several steps to smelling and tasting, there are plenty of ways for things to go awry. The direct connection between the outside environment and the brain makes the sense of smell very vulnerable to damage. Smell and taste disorders can be triggered by colds and flu, allergies, nasal polyps (swollen mucus membrane inside the nose), a head injury, chemical exposure, a nutritional or metabolic problem, or a drug or disease. A cause cannot always be identified.

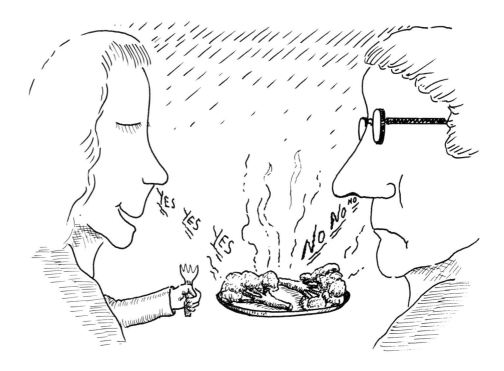

A Lifetime of Smell and Taste

We can smell and taste from birth. Regina M. Sullivan, Ph.D., and coworkers at the University of California at Irvine Medical Center in Irvine recently studied day-old infants to determine their ability to connect an odor with a pleasant experience.

Half the group of 66 newborns received citrus odors and simultaneous stroking several times for a day. The other 33 babies experienced the odor alone, stroking alone, or stroking followed by the odor. The next day, all the infants were exposed to the odor five times, for 30-second periods. The only babies who turned toward the odor were those who received the odor during stroking, thereby associating the citrus smell with touch.

Taste buds are most numerous in children under 6, which may explain why youngsters are such picky eaters. Recognizing that children's heightened sense of taste might account for compliance problems in giving antibiotic medication, Michael E. Ruff, M.D., and coworkers in the departments of pediatrics and pharmacy at Tripler Army Medical Center in Honolulu asked 30 adults to rank the pleasantness of the taste of the active ingredients in the 14 most often prescribed pediatric antibiotic suspensions. If parents, with their diminished sense of taste compared to their offspring, find a particular antibiotic distasteful, then perhaps drug manufacturers can be alerted to those products that need work in the palatability department—a major task when a medicine must contain a naturally bad-tasting substance. In this taste test, cephalosporins tasted best and penicillins the worst.

Taste and smell hold up remarkably well with age, probably because the body frequently replaces receptor-bearing cells, even in the elderly. Monell researchers concluded from the National Geographic Smell Survey that "detection ability remains near youthful levels well into the seventh decade," but they found that ability to detect the intensity of odors and to describe odors wanes with time. These deficits may reflect changes in thought processing, such as taste and smell recognition, rather than in the sense organs, suggests Richard Mattes, Ph.D., of Monell.

One disturbing finding is that older people are less likely to find the smell of chemicals called mercaptans offensive than are younger people. Mercaptans are added to odorless natural gas to serve as a warning if gas is escaping from an oven, for example.

Disease and drugs can affect smell and taste and may also account for the lessened acuity of these senses in older people, according to James Weiffenbach, Ph.D., sensory psychologist at the National Institute of Dental Research in Bethesda. "Among the participants in the Baltimore Longitudinal Study of Aging of the National Institute of Aging, we found that whether you are healthy or not is a more powerful determinant of taste complaints than whether you are younger or older. So maybe older people report more taste complaints because they are more likely to have medical problems," he says.

Weiffenbach also mentions a telling "overlooked point": that of senior citizens living in retirement centers where the food really isn't as tasty as home-cooked cuisine. "They know the food doesn't taste as good as it did ten years ago, because it really doesn't," he says.

Taste or smell, or both, can be absent, diminished, heightened, or distorted. Interestingly, Richard Mattes, Ph.D., and coworkers at Monell find that while those with taste or smell loss eat to compensate and gain weight, those with distorted smell or taste find eating so disturbing that they lose weight.

It is difficult to imagine how greatly enjoyment of life can be affected by a loss in the senses of smell and taste. Judith Birnberg, of Long Island, N.Y., wrote about her plight in the March 21, 1988, "My Turn" column in *Newsweek* magazine. Birnberg spent a year sneezing inexplicably and was suddenly left with the ability to sense only the texture and temperature of food. She was unable to smell or taste. For years, Birnberg lived on her memories of smelling piping hot coffee and peeled oranges. Her condition, attributed to "allergy and infection," mysteriously comes and goes. When taste and smell are intact, she rushes off to the nearest restaurant—but more often than not, her sensory acuity fades before the food arrives.

Birnberg had blood and urine tests galore, CT scans, and biopsies, had her sinuses drained, and took zinc supplements. Nothing worked. Finally, she found relief with prednisone. This strong steroid drug reduces swelling of the mucous membranes in the nose and may therefore improve the sense of smell, but its efficacy as a treatment for smell disorders has not been proven.

Feeling better, Birnberg went about smelling everything. "I inhaled

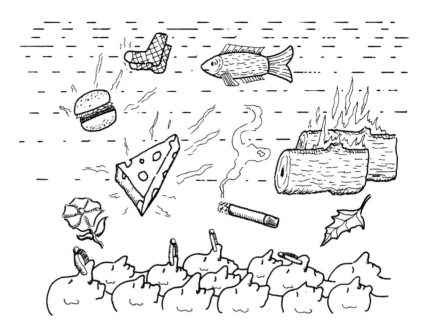

all odors, good and bad, as if drunk," she wrote. Prednisone, though, suppresses the immune system, so she is able to take the drug only intermittently.

Distorted Sensation

A group of 12 travelers touring Peru and Bolivia prepared for a day of hiking in the Andes mountains. A day before, three of them had begun taking acetazolamide (brand name, Diamox), a drug that prevents acute mountain sickness, which each had previously suffered. The headache, nausea, weakness, and shortness of breath of acute mountain sickness typically begins when one reaches 5,900 feet elevation and can progress to severe respiratory problems by 9,000 feet. These hikers planned an expedition to 12,000 feet. All went well, but the night after the climb, the group went out for beer. To three of the people, the brew tasted unbearably bitter, and a drink of cola to wash away the taste was equally offensive. At fault: acetazolamide.

The taste distortion caused by this particular drug makes biochemical sense. The drug inhibits an enzyme that normally dismantles bitter-tasting carbonic acid before it has a chance to register on the taste buds. "The drug stirs up anything with carbonation, enabling the person to taste the terribly bitter taste of carbonic acid," says Baylor College of Medicine's Miller. She has studied the drug's temporary effects on taste and believes the problem is more widespread than drug manufacturers realize. "Some people may not report it and may not make the connection to the drug. They blame it on altitude sickness," she adds.

Acetazolamide isn't the only drug to alter the chemical senses. "Drugs can alter taste and smell in many potential ways, affecting cell turnover, the neural conduction system, the status of receptors, and changes in nutritional status," says Monell's Mattes.

148

Drugs containing sulfur atoms are notorious for squelching taste. They include the anti-inflammatory drug penicillamine, the antihypertensive captopril (Capoten), and transdermal (patch) nitroglycerin to treat chest pain. The antibiotics tetracycline and metronidazole (Flagyl) cause a metallic taste.

Cancer chemotherapy and radiation treatment often alter taste and smell, but this is rarely reason to change therapy. "A taste and smell problem is probably not life-threatening, and treating something like cancer is the first priority," Mattes says.

Exposure to toxic chemicals can affect taste and smell, too. A 45-year-old woman from Altoona, Pa., suddenly found that once-pleasant smells had become offensive. Her doctor, Joseph Silverman, M.D., traced her problem to inhaling a paint stripper. Hydrocarbon solvents in the product—toluene, methanol, and methylene chloride—were the culprits responsible for her "cacosmia," the association of an odor of decay with normally inoffensive stimuli. She said she was helped by an antidepressant medication. However, since this type of drug is not approved for treating such disorders, this was an experimental use of the drug.

Taste distortions can be very upsetting. "It's easier for people to understand losing a sense than to suddenly have everything twisted. Since smell mediates a lot of food's flavor, when you don't smell at all, food tastes bland. You can perk it up by adding salt, sugar, lemon juice, or spices. But for dysosmics, food is actively unpleasant," says Cowart.

Sometimes a foul taste can persist with no food involved. This is a "taste phantom," a sensation that comes out of nowhere, says Bartoshuk. The condition is fairly common among women past menopause. At Yale, Bartoshuk helps pinpoint the source of phantom tastes. "Is it caused by a molecule in the mouth that shouldn't be there, or is brain stimulation abnormal? We can tell the difference by using anesthesia, which is a nerve inhibitor," she says.

If she anesthetizes the mouth and the bad taste goes away, then it's due to molecules there. If, following anesthesia, the patient gets worse, this points to the brain as the cause of the problem.

There are a number of special centers where people with absent or distorted senses of smell and taste can seek help. These include: Monell, facilities at Yale University, the State University of New York Health Science Center in Syracuse, the Hospital of the University of Pennsylvania in Philadelphia, Georgetown University in Washington, D.C., the University of Colorado in Denver, and the University of Connecticut Health Center at Farmington.

With researchers' increasing understanding of the complex interplays between the environment and our nervous systems that provide the nonessential but intensely enjoyable senses of smell and taste, it's likely that more and more sufferers of deficits in these systems will be identified and helped. Those of us whose senses are healthy can appreciate the complex neural connections that enable us to fully experience that April rain, July barbecue, and October's fragrant fallen leaves, and the myriad taste combinations that make dining such a pleasurable experience. □

Some people's sense of taste is so distorted that food becomes unpleasant.

What's Your Child's Play Style?

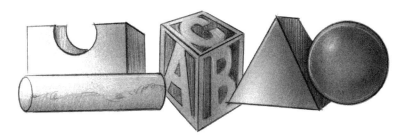

Karen Levine

ILLUSTRATION BY THOMAS TONKIN

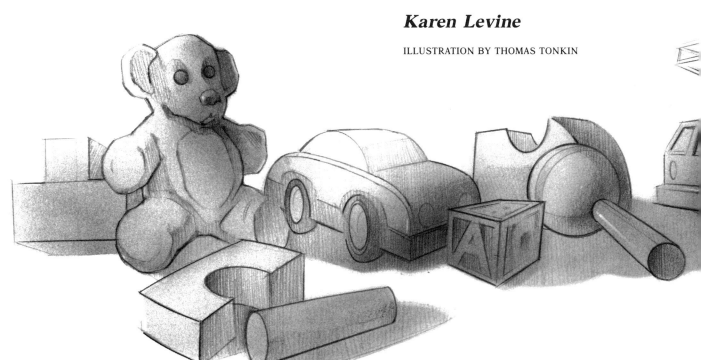

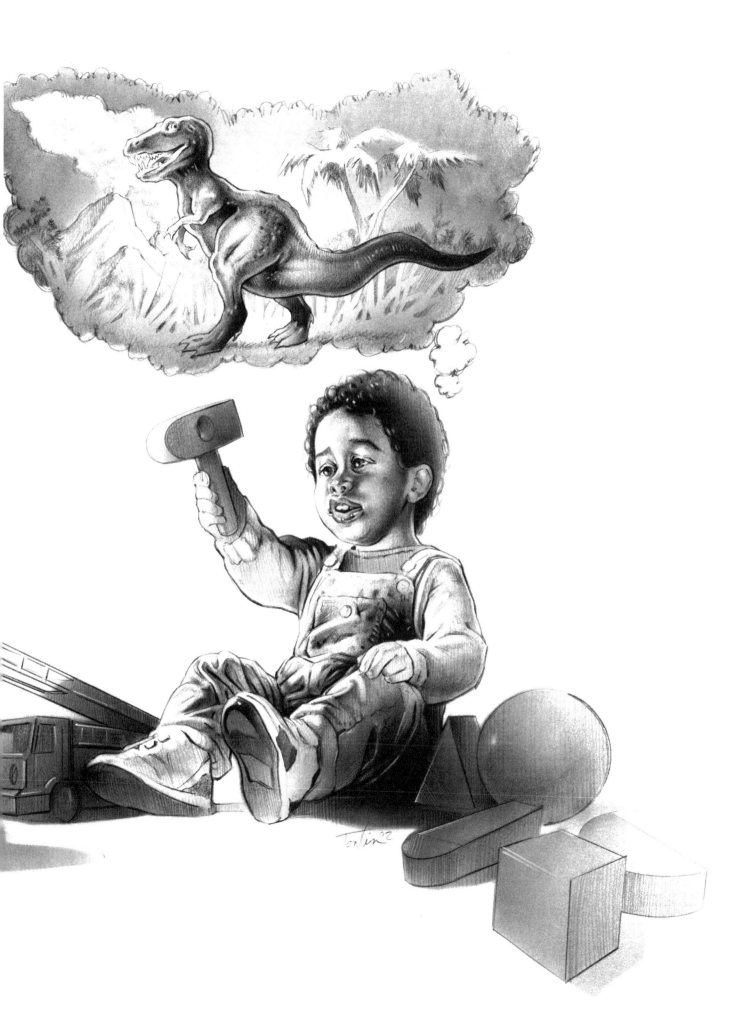

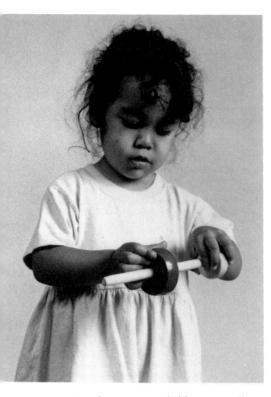

At play, some children are "patterners." They are interested in examining the physical properties of things, like the little girl above, and in using them in fairly realistic ways, like the busy child shown on the opposite page.

I remember once watching my older son, Noah, and his friend Gabri play together in a room strewn with action figures, small vehicles, and plastic blocks. There were two three-year-old boys and at least six different voices. Growling out orders or pleading for mercy, each figure had his own pitch. Noah ran over to a pile of the blocks and, with great care, began construction. "I'll make the fort," he called out to Gabri. "Yeah," said Gabri, approaching the blocks. He paused in front of them, picked up the two closest at hand, and looked at them for a minute before saying, "And this is the boat and this is the cannon." Gabri ran around the room, shooting the cannon and skillfully piloting the boat, while Noah sat amid his blocks, building the fort and narrating his progress.

As the afternoon progressed, Gabri found more cannons and boats, and Noah continued to build with his blocks and say such things as, "Okay, guys, this is where we put the prisoners." About 15 minutes before Gabri was to leave, Noah completed the fort. And for that last 15 minutes of their play, Noah's fort was a haven for all the good guys and their boats and cannons.

Patterners and Dramatists

Howard Gardner, Ph.D., a professor of education, and Dennis Wolff, a senior research associate, both at Harvard University in Cambridge, Mass., have studied children's play, particularly play styles. "Over the years," Gardner says, "we have identified two types of children: patterners and dramatists." Patterners, also called object-dependent children, have a tendency to focus on objects, typically playing with materials and toys in terms of investigating their physical properties rather than advancing social interaction.

Based on Gardner's description, Noah is clearly a patterner. If given a set of blocks at a very early age, he would be eager to examine them and would either sort or stack them. As he grew older, he would use his toys to support his play, but his use of them would always relate fairly concretely to their physical properties. A pencil, for example, might become a cannon for Noah, but it would never become a bowl of soup.

Gabri, on the other hand, is a dramatist. For him, the objects matter only in terms of how they can advance his fantasy. If he needs a cannon, he finds one in a nearby pile of plastic blocks. And if it is shaped nothing like a cannon . . . so what?

Both patterners and dramatists have the ability to transform one object into something else in a two-step process that experts refer to as distancing and object transformation. First the child creates the "distance" between reality and make-believe. Then he "transforms" what he has in order to make it what he wants. As most parents know, object transformation is at the heart of imaginary play. When my younger son, Nathaniel, was three, I found him sitting in my workshop holding an identical screw in each hand. "I'm a soldier," he said,

Karen Levine is a contributing editor of Parents *magazine.*

holding high the screw in his right hand. "And I'm a soldier too," he replied, holding up his left hand, "but I'm bigger than you are." With those words, he transformed two screws into imaginary combatants challenging each other to a fight.

According to Margery Franklin, Ph.D., professor of psychology at Sarah Lawrence College in Bronxville, N.Y., Nathaniel's words here were significant. Franklin has found that regardless of which play style children favor, they all go through specific verbal steps to immerse themselves in make-believe.

First they establish the play sphere by actually saying something like "Let's pretend." Next they verbally label the play objects and people by saying things like "This will be a soldier" or "I'll be the good guy." And finally they shape the progress of their play and maintain it by narrating and having a dialogue as they go along. Essentially, Franklin explains, the words take on the transforming power of a magic spell.

Although this verbal magic doesn't appear to differ among children with different play styles, there are some differences in how patterners and dramatists regard the objects they have transformed. "Physical realism is important to patterners," says Diane M. Horm-Wingerd, Ph.D., assistant professor of human development at the University of Rhode Island in Kingston. "Once they assign an identity to something, they're reluctant to switch it. If a patterner is playing carpenter, he'll find something long and slender to represent a nail. Later, if he plays pirate, he might find a use for the 'nail' from his carpenter days to fix

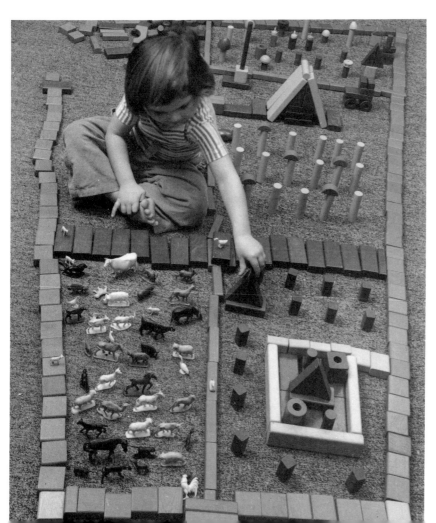

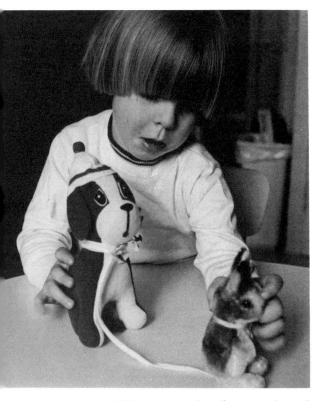

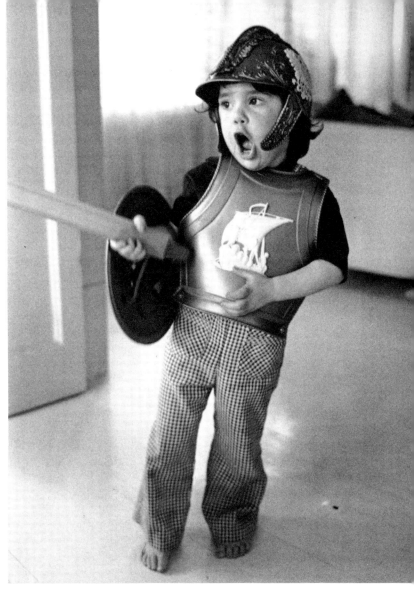

Some children act out their fantasies through little figures (above), and others like to dress up and become a make-believe character (right).

a broken plank on his ship, but he'd never turn that nail into a sword or something else more suitable to his new play theme.

"A dramatist," she continues, "can make the most outlandish substitutions. Anything can be anything. And when the direction of the play changes, so do the prop definitions."

Marilyn Segal, Ph.D., professor of developmental psychology at Nova University in Fort Lauderdale, Fla., has further differentiated play styles of preschoolers by observing that some children prefer to play "in miniature," which involves holding little figures and acting through them, while others show a preference for playing "in maxi," which involves dressing up and actually becoming the make-believe character.

One mother recalls that her oldest daughter's room was always full of dolls and stuffed animals that she would set up in different scenarios. "She'd always be narrating something or talking for all of her dolls and animals," the mother explains. "My younger daughter never had much of an interest in dolls, but I knew that if I was ever missing a pair of high heels or a belt or a hat, I'd find it somewhere in her room. If she played Mommy, she became the mommy. And once

154

when she was playing Baby, she went through half a box of her little brother's diapers before she managed to get one on herself."

All the World's a Stage

Play is more complex, however, than such broad categories imply. Researchers have found that other distinctive play styles coexist with a child's preference for mini-play or maxi-play. "We saw several types of play," Segal says. There were the actors, who generally picked a theme and stuck with it for a long time; the scriptwriters, whose play involved setting up a very detailed script that they enacted; the song-writers, who usually hummed or invented little ditties while they went about their play; and the set designers, who spent the greater part of their play preparing for play, sometimes never even getting around to playing!

Jake, the six-year-old son of Susan Engel, Ph.D., a visiting assistant professor of psychology at Williams College, in Williamstown, Mass., is a scriptwriter. "We were playing a game that involved Jake's being Spiderman," Engel recalls. "He was Spiderman, and I was the bad guy, but before we got to play, Jake had to lay it all out for me. He told me exactly what was going to happen and what each of us would say. He said, 'I'll say this, and you'll do that, then I'll say this, and then you'll shoot me. But I won't be dead, because I'm Spiderman, so I'll jump up, and then you'll fall down, and that will be the last time, and then it will be over.' We'd begin to play," Engel says, "but if I said something that wasn't in his script, he'd stop the action and say, 'No. You didn't do that right.' And we'd do it again until I got it right and until, according to Jake's script, it was over."

"Oh, I'm going to the doctor, and now I'm walking down the street because I'm gonna have a shot," sang three-year-old Mike, a song-writer, as he marched a little figure along the fringe of his living-room carpet. Indeed, even when Mike doesn't have lyrics for his activity, his father says that he always sings "da-da-da-da" when he plays with little figures.

Once, my son Noah and his friend Sasha—both set designers—spent an entire sleep-over dividing up an army of small "armed" animals. The negotiations were subtle and incredibly complex. By the time they fell asleep, they had spent more than three very happy hours in negotiations, and as far as I could tell, they weren't yet done. The next day held all sorts of promise. "Don't touch those piles," Sasha said as I turned off the light. "We're playing with them."

Parents often notice, whenever two or more children get together, that there are very clear leaders and followers. Research seems to indicate that there's an art to each of these roles. "Neither category is better or worse," explains Greta Fein, Ph.D., professor of early childhood education and psychology at the University of Maryland at College Park. "In fact, when you put an organizer, who can come up with a theme, together with a recipient, who can take the theme and run with it, you have the potential for very rich, nicely developed play."

Peggy Sradnick, director of Basic Trust Infant and Toddler Center in New York City, often sees this magical meshing among the three-year-

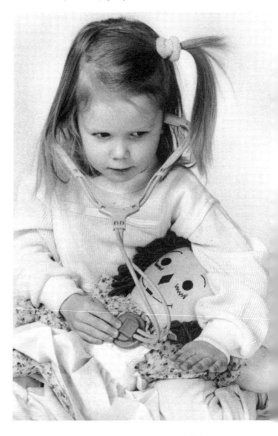

Imagining oneself as a doctor is a common form of play.

155

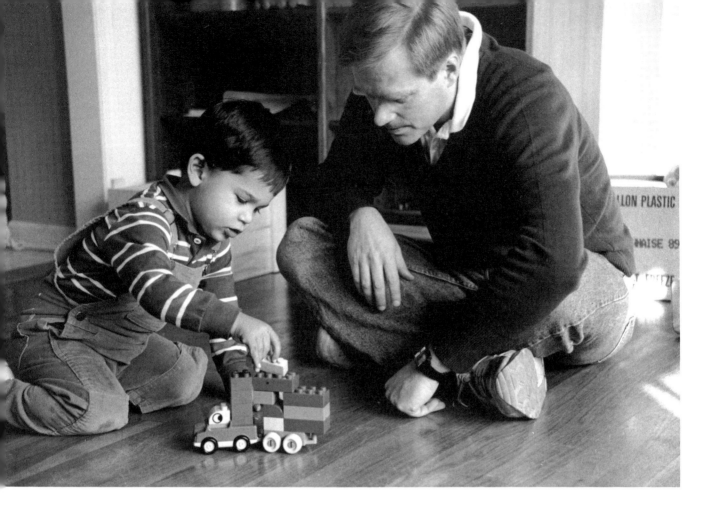

olds at her center. "I remember a period of several months when a three-year-old named Elana was totally absorbed with being a doctor. All of the other three-year-olds were patients, and their interest would ebb and flow, but Elana's interest was strong enough throughout the entire period to ensure a thriving practice.

"At one point," Sradnick continues, "Elana's practice became very full. In fact, it became more than she could handle. Kids were lined up waiting to see her. She handled it all very professionally for a long time, but finally she began to cave in under the pressure." Sradnick was watching one day when Elana stepped out of her office and, near tears, said, "There are *other* doctors. You have to see *another* doctor. It's too many patients for just me."

Elana's "practice" is a perfect illustration of the importance of initiators and receivers. Indeed, her "practice" would not have gone anywhere without her "patients," and her patients would have languished without their "doctor." Interestingly, at Basic Trust the roles became so real that even when Elana suggested that the patients in her waiting room see another doctor, no one answered the call. For that group of children at that time, there was only one doctor.

Parents' Influence

How much impact do parents have on their children's play styles? Margery Franklin draws an analogy between children and creative artists. "They forge their own style and their own way of doing things,"

156

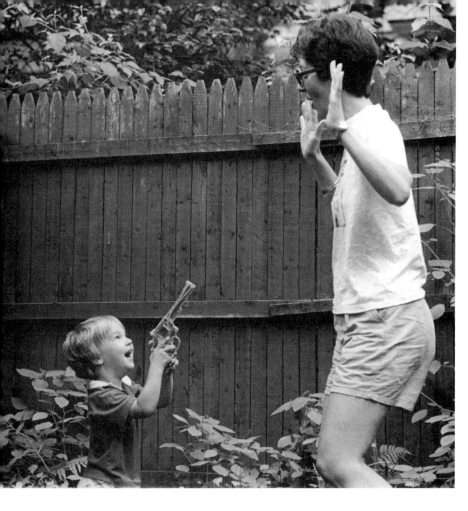

Adults have a tendency to communicate play styles to children. For example, those who enjoyed playing with blocks and Lego-type construction toys (opposite page) encourage that kind of play in their children. Parents who eagerly participate in fantasy activity (left) encourage the actor in the child.

she says, "but in the process, they take into account their environment and their experiences. The parts come from different places but are put together in the child's own way, shaped by who the child is."

Marilyn Segal, like Greta Fein, suggests that there is a more direct connection between parents and the play styles that their children adopt. "Some of it really has to do with the role of the adult," she says in discussing whether a child becomes an actor or some variation of a producer-director. "We found that adults had play styles also and that they communicated their play styles, either consciously or unconsciously, to their children."

Segal notes that a parent who makes a fuss the first time her child offers her an imaginary cookie—eating it up and asking for another—is encouraging the actor in the child. She calls such adults Appreciative Audiences, or AAs. Segal also suggests that parents who have a greater tolerance for mess—who aren't disturbed by having every belt and tie and shoe taken from its proper place, or by having chairs pushed together and draped with sheets—are more likely to have actor children.

Adults who are interested in the value of play as a form of emotional expression, and who use pretending as a way to help children work out conflicts or to mold ideas, are Therapeutic Adults—or TAs—according to Segal. TAs, she says, are more likely to have children who are producer-directors. Indeed, Segal found that the adults who enjoyed drawing, playing with blocks, setting up a dollhouse, or playing with miniature animals tended to encourage that kind of play in their children, both by buying the toys *they* liked and by showing their enthusi-

157

asm for those toys. "Even when parents don't think they're influencing their child, they are," Segal explains, "by the expression on their face when a child opens up a box of toys."

The Sibling Factor

The matter of how a child's play style is formed becomes even more complicated when we consider the impact of siblings. Fein believes that older siblings can play an influential role in shaping their younger siblings' play styles. "Big brothers and sisters may introduce their younger siblings to dramatic play," she notes; "and while I don't have any documentation, and I'm sure there are no hard-and-fast rules, I suspect that firstborn children are more likely to be organizers, and second-borns are more likely to be recipients."

One father told me that after visiting a safari park, his four-year-old son became very interested in animals. "We got him all sorts of plastic animals and books about them and even a safari hat," the father said, "and he used all of these props on imaginary jungle excursions. But it didn't take long to see that his very favorite prop was his little

---

Why Some Kids Can Play Alone

When Greta Fein, Ph.D., professor of early childhood education and psychology at the University of Maryland at College Park, talks about play styles, she distinguishes between children who tend to play alone and those who tend to play in cooperating groups.

I remember listening to Noah play in his room by himself when he was four. He was carrying on a dialogue in lots of different voices, and as the play progressed, the dialogue became more and more animated. At one point I made my way to his door and stood watching him. Finally he sensed my presence, looked up, and said, "Go away. *We* want privacy." I learned from Noah that just because I couldn't see his companions didn't make them any less real to him.

Recently, one friend complained that her daughter couldn't play on her own for more than a minute. "I like to play with Sally," my friend said, "but I'd also like to be able to sit and read a book while she plays in the next room."

I'd always assumed that the reason my children were so capable of playing on their own was that my husband and I spent so much time playing with them when they were very young. Interestingly, Sally's mother had come to the same conclusion to explain why her daughter could *not* play on her own.

Although Fein believes that the parent-infant interaction does, to a great extent, determine the child's play style—including the ability to play alone—she notes that the dynamic of the interaction is complicated and that the important issues are far subtler than "time spent."

"Some parents," she suggests, "are very anxious about their infant's development and express this anxiety by constantly entering into the child's activity.

"The rule that I suggest parents try to follow," Fein says, "is twofold. First: If a baby is doing well alone, then leave him alone. If the baby seems restless and bored, then intervene only to the extent that you get your baby hooked, and then back away and let him take over."

The second part of Fein's rule is to make sure that you engage your baby on a level at which he can participate. "If an infant is playing with a cup—waving it in the air, banging it on the floor, mouthing it—and a parent comes along, takes the cup, and begins to drop things into it," Fein explains, "the baby stops his own activity to watch and be entertained. Although this new game of dropping things into a cup is very entertaining to the infant, it's way beyond his developmental capabilities and ultimately distracts him from entertaining himself. After a while, the baby will come to rely on the parents for information and entertainment rather than rely on his own exploration of objects."

Fein makes the point that if the baby loses interest in waving and banging his cup, a parent can intervene with a rattle. "The rattle is different from the cup," she explains. "It makes a different sound and feels different in the baby's mouth. And if the parent waves it for a moment and hands it to him, the baby is capable of using it. The baby will be able to duplicate the parent's activity and get pleasure from his own actions rather than from observing his parent."

Margery Franklin, Ph.D., professor of psychology at Sarah Lawrence College in Bronxville, N.Y., is less willing to make a direct connection between the ability of children to play on their own and any one component of the parent-infant interaction. "It's clear that some kids can sustain very elaborate fantasy on their own, while other kids really see pretend play as being viable only as a shared activity. "In order to do the creative work of making believe," she explains, "children need to be able to live in their own heads. They are, after all, giving life to all of these characters. In order to develop that sort of richness, children need time and space, they need to be able to relax, and they need a sense of privacy. I would speculate," Franklin continues, "that children who aren't given enough time alone—who are constantly stimulated with entertainment of one sort or another—are less likely to be able to sustain make-believe play on their own."

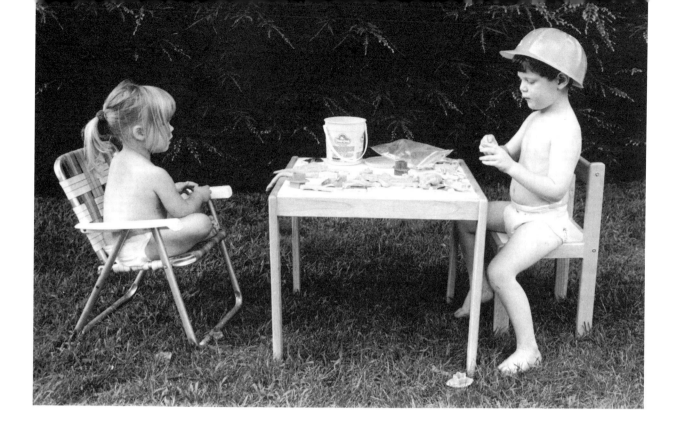

sister. Sometimes she was a lion, sometimes a zebra. In every case, she'd crawl along on the safari with him and stay with it a long, long time. She's not even two yet, but when her brother sets her up in a game, she has endless patience and enthusiasm for it."

It may appear that the only thing this boy is shaping is clay, but researchers say that older siblings often do a lot to shape younger children's play styles.

Play Styles and Intelligence

The question of just what these play styles mean for our children and for their future is a compelling one. Once we understand the implications of different play styles, we're in a better position to figure out what we, as parents, can do to help our children develop according to their unique potential.

Most researchers stress that no one play style is better or worse than another. When Diane M. Horm-Wingerd looked at the IQs of patterners and dramatists, she found no significant differences. Howard Gardner says that play styles reflect different types of intelligence— spatial, linguistic, logical, interpersonal, and intrapersonal. "What's important," Gardner stresses, "is for parents not to try to impose a style on a child because they like it. Rather, parents need to expose kids to as many different styles as possible—particularly during those first few years. The child will know, better than you, which one he likes."

Just a week ago, I handed each of my boys a bag of candies and sat down to talk with them as they tore the bags open. Noah poured the candies out on the table and began to sort them by color, then to arrange them in an elaborate pattern on the table. As he ate each candy, he redesigned the pattern to accommodate the new ratio of tans to reds to oranges to browns. Nathaniel also spilled the candies out, but that's where the similarity ended. He picked up a red piece and said, somewhat menacingly, "Okay, Mr. Red. You're gonna get eated." □

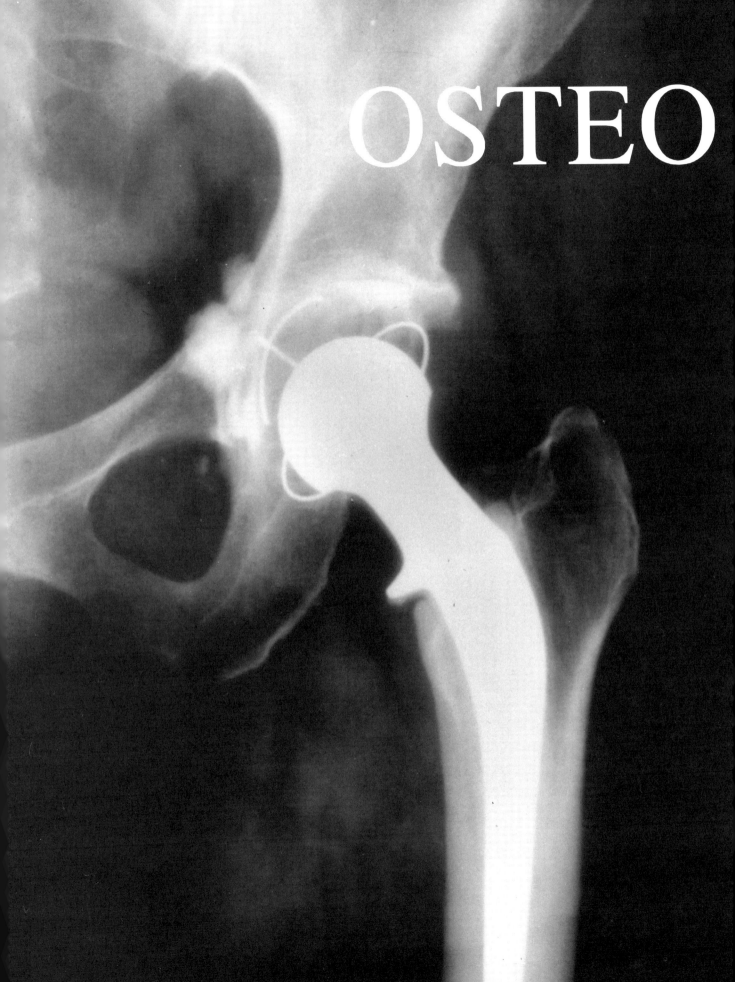
OSTEO

ARTHRITIS

"The thigh bone's connected to the—knee bone. The knee bone's connected to the—ankle bone..."

This religious folk song is hardly a lesson in anatomy, but it does make a key point. You depend on more than 300 joints, which connect your bones, for movement and mobility. Still, for many people, easy movement is no snap of the fingers. If you have severe arthritis, you know that holding a fork or opening the door of your car sometimes demands supreme resolve—or may be impossible.

Arthritis is one of the most common medical problems in the United States. It strikes one person in seven. There are more than 100 forms of arthritis, with varying causes, symptoms, and treatments. This article will focus on osteoarthritis (OS-tee-oh-ar-THRY-tis). It's the most common type of arthritis, destroying "shock absorber" cartilage that keeps bones from rubbing together.

Osteoarthritis affects nearly everyone past age 60. It may be so mild that you are unaware of it until it shows up on an X ray—or so severe that you'll need an artificial joint. People with osteoarthritis, and their doctors, once thought it was an unavoidable part of aging, with little help available. Today, effective treatment options replace resignation. Weight control, careful exercise, joint protection, medicine, and surgery can help. Facing this challenge, you can say, "I have arthritis, but it doesn't have me."

Signs and Symptoms

Nearly 16 million Americans have osteoarthritis. Musculoskeletal problems, including osteoarthritis, cost $35 billion a year—1 percent of America's gross national product—in lost wages and production.

Osteoarthritis can be deceptive. It doesn't cause a general feeling of sickness. There's no fever or weight loss and sometimes no visible change in your joints. Advertisements talk about minor aches and pains. But osteoarthritis can be much worse. A study in Framingham, Mass., showed that aside from stroke, osteoarthritis may cause as much disability as any cardiovascular disease. Following are the key signs and symptoms.

Stiffness. You're most likely to feel stiff for one or two minutes after you stand up. The stiffness usually subsides. If you have osteoarthritis, it's unusual for a joint to become completely stiff.

161

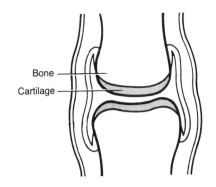

Normal Joint

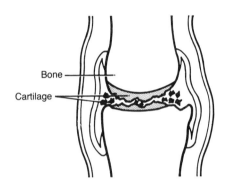

Joint With Osteoarthritis

Source: Arthritis Foundation

Pain. Many people describe osteoarthritis as a nagging pain. You may experience sharp pain when you move and a throbbing sensation at rest. Pain is worst if you've used a joint too much, or if you've been inactive. A few people have constant pain, even when resting. About 80 percent of people with osteoarthritis report pain that limits daily activity. You may find it increasingly difficult to swing a golf club or pick up your grandchild.

The origin of arthritis pain is not always apparent. "Referred pain" involves soreness at a distance from the affected joint. For example, you could have osteoarthritis in your hip and experience referred pain in your knee. Sometimes bones rub against each other. As the protective barrier of cartilage wears away, you may notice stiffness and a grating sensation, or pain, when bone ends rub together. But time may be your ally. Bones tend to "polish" each other in a process called eburnation. As the bone ends become smooth, movement may get easier.

The relationship between osteoarthritis and the weather is cloudy. Some people swear they can "predict" the weather. Although there is no documentation for this effect, rising humidity and falling barometric pressure may seem to worsen symptoms. A warm, dry climate may make you more comfortable, but it won't stop the disease process.

Inflammation. Redness and warmth are not common with osteoarthritis. When they occur, it's often because fragments of cartilage infiltrate the joint space. Fluid can build up.

Where Does It Strike?

What causes osteoarthritis? Nobody knows for sure. You're at a risk if you have injured or malformed joints. Your risk is greater if repeated

---

Don't Be Duped

Americans spend more than $1 billion a year on dubious cures for arthritis—about $25 for every $1 of valid research.

Copper bracelets are unproven cures but harmless. Colon cleansing and drugs with hidden ingredients can be dangerous. One person in ten who tries an unproven arthritis remedy reports harmful side effects.

Quacks rob you of money and the time and opportunity for effective care. Here are some popular, but false, nutrition claims:

- **Cod liver oil "lubricates" stiff joints.** It may sound logical, but your body treats cod liver oil like any other fat; there's no special help for joints. Large amounts of cod liver oil can lead to vitamin A and D toxicity.

- **Some foods cause "allergic arthritis."** There's no proof that food allergies cause arthritis. Also, you can't relieve arthritis by avoiding tomatoes or other foods.

- **Fish oils reduce inflammation.** Research on rheumatoid arthritis suggests omega-3 fatty acids in fish oils may give modest, temporary relief of inflammation.
  This finding is valid, but fish oil supplements are not advisable. You'd need about 15 capsules a day—and doctors don't know if that's safe. A lower dose won't help.

movement—or excess weight—puts strain on your joints. Osteoarthritis can strike joints from the base of your thumb to your big toe. But the disease is selective. Unless you've been injured or had unusual stress on a joint, it's uncommon for osteoarthritis to affect your wrists, elbows, shoulders, ankles, or jaw.

Osteoarthritis attacks three main locations. Most people have symptoms in just one place. But you could get the disease at two or even all three sites, at different times or together.

Fingers. Bony knobs called nodes or nodules enlarge your finger joints, creating a gnarled appearance. Injury to the finger can cause nodes, but they usually develop spontaneously. Heberden's nodes, the most common type, affect the end joints of your fingers. Nodes typically start in one finger but can involve all fingers to a greater or lesser extent. You may notice tenderness, numbness, stiffness, or aching. Opening a jar may be awkward or painful, but disability is rare. The condition runs in families and is more common in women. Heberden's nodes usually develop during several years, but women in their 40s sometimes develop the nodes in just a few weeks.

Spine. Osteophytes are bony outgrowths that often can be detected by X ray. These "spurs" develop near degenerated cartilage on your neck or lower back. They don't change your appearance.

Weight-bearing Joints. The most limiting form of osteoarthritis attacks your hips, knees, or feet, affecting both sides of your body. This problem develops during several years. It involves chronic or varying pain as you stand and walk. Fluid may collect in your knees. Your knees may swell and feel painful when you stand up. Osteoarthritis can injure either the inside or outer part of your knee joint cartilage. This can give you bowlegs or knock-knees and can impair walking. If your arthritis is severe, you may experience pain at night in bed.

Making the Diagnosis

Your family doctor usually can diagnose osteoarthritis from a physical exam. An exact diagnosis is important because you could have osteoarthritis along with rheumatoid arthritis, gout, or other problems. Your doctor may refer you to a rheumatologist, a physician who specializes in diseases of joints and muscles.

X rays usually are necessary to confirm the diagnosis. Because X rays pass through cartilage, an X ray of a normal joint shows bones separated by space. As osteoarthritis destroys cartilage, the space gets narrower. In advanced cases, an X ray shows bones touching one another. Many older adults first learn of osteoarthritis from routine X rays. But about two-thirds never develop symptoms. If you don't have symptoms, you don't need treatment.

Medications Control Discomfort

Here are the most common over-the-counter and prescription drugs for osteoarthritis:

Aspirin. Dosage makes a difference, so your physician needs to specify the amount that's right for you. Two tablets every four hours

Types of Joints

Your body has four types of joints:
- **Fixed.** These joints don't move. They absorb shock to help prevent bones from breaking. Fixed joints in your skull protect sensitive brain tissue underneath.
- **Hinge.** Like the hinge in a doorway, your knee joints let you move forward and backward.
- **Pivot.** These joints allow a rotating movement. Your elbow has both hinge and pivot joints.
- **Ball-and-Socket.** The large round end of a long bone fits into a hollow part of another bone. This makes swinging and rotating movements possible.

You get the most movement from ball-and-socket joints in your hips and shoulders.

163

may relieve pain. You might need up to a dozen tablets daily during several weeks for inflammation. But remember, aspirin can have serious side effects, such as gastrointestinal bleeding. Tell you doctor if you notice ringing in your ears or diminished hearing—the dosage may be too high. If aspirin causes heartburn or nausea, try fewer tablets more frequently. Taking aspirin with a meal or using an antacid may reduce stomach irritation. Ask your doctor about coated products. They protect your stomach but may limit how your body absorbs the aspirin.

Generic aspirin works well and is relatively inexpensive. Trademark brands have the same quality but are more costly. If aspirin smells like vinegar, throw it out. If childproof caps are hard to use, request a standard top.

Acetaminophen. This nonprescription product relieves pain as well as aspirin and is less likely to upset your stomach. But it doesn't help inflammation. Familiar brand names include Tylenol, Anacin-3, and Aspirin-Free Excedrin.

NSAIDs. The acronym (en-SAYDS) stands for nonsteroidal anti-inflammatory drugs. NSAIDs work as well as aspirin and may have fewer side effects. But they cost more, and you may need to take them several times daily, as you would aspirin.

There are more than a dozen types of prescription NSAIDs, with different chemical structures. Ibuprofen is a generic over-the-counter NSAID, also marketed as Advil, Nuprin, Medipren, and Motrin-IB. If you have stomach ulcers or other side effects from one type of NSAID, your doctor can suggest alternatives.

Corticosteroids. These prescription drugs are modified forms of hormones made in the adrenal gland. About 20 steroid drugs are now available; the most common is prednisone. Steroids can reduce pain

Tips for Coping

Severe osteoarthritis can strain the best of relationships. And it's usually a lifelong condition, so you need to learn to deal with it effectively. Some suggestions:

- **Accept your limitations.** Even with severe osteoarthritis, you still can enjoy a reasonably normal lifestyle. Recognize when you need to say, "No, I can't do that." And be firm. Expect some ups and downs in this balancing act.

  Don't let osteoarthritis take over your life. You still can participate in a regular exercise program. Swimming may be a good choice.

- **Be frank about your feelings.** It's OK to feel tired and even short-tempered because of osteoarthritis. But don't take out your frustration on other people. And let them know when arthritis is a problem. Otherwise, it's easy for people to assume you're upset with them. This tip is especially important if you have contact with children.

- **Build a network.** Don't hesitate to turn to others when you need help. A psychiatrist can help you cope with stress and depression. A social worker can suggest some appropriate support services, resources if you're concerned about job discrimination, and ways in which loved ones can adapt to your condition. An exercise group, your spouse, or a friend can help you take your mind off your problems.

164

and inflammation. Doctors do not prescribe oral steroids for osteoarthritis, but may occasionally inject a cortisone drug into an acutely inflamed weight-bearing joint—for example, your hip, knee, or ankle. Because frequent use of this drug may accelerate joint disease, your doctor will limit the number of injections to two or three annually.

Antidepressant Drugs. These prescription drugs may help treat the depression and insomnia that often accompany chronic pain. Even if you don't have depression, these medications can help relieve pain and improve sleep. They're not addictive, so you can use them for a long period of time. Possible side effects include sedation, dry mouth, constipation, or difficulty with urination.

Protecting Your Joints

Just as a lever and pulley help lift a heavy object, correct "body mechanics" help you move with minimal strain. A physical or occupational therapist can advise you regarding techniques and equipment that protect your joints while decreasing stress and conserving energy. Here are points a therapist might discuss with you:

Grasping and Twisting. Avoid grasping actions that strain your finger joints. Instead of a clutch-style purse, select one with a shoulder strap. Use hot water to loosen a jar lid and pressure from your palm to open it; or use a jar opener. Don't twist or use your joints forcefully.

Weight Distribution. Spread the weight of an object over several joints. Use both hands, for example, to lift a heavy pan.

Relaxation. Take a break periodically to relax and stretch.

Posture. Be sure it's good. Poor posture causes uneven weight distribution and may strain ligaments and muscles. When standing, pull in your stomach. Hold your shoulders back. A bed board can help keep your back straight when you're lying down. When sitting, never slouch. Make sure work surfaces are at a comfortable height.

Be Savvy. Throughout the day, use your strongest muscles and favor large joints. Don't push open a heavy glass door. Lean into it. To pick up an object, bend your knees and stoop while keeping your back straight.

Leisure Lessons. Plan each stage of your favorite activities; modify as needed. When you garden, plant in raised beds or install a window greenhouse to limit bending. Drip-irrigation with a timer is easier than watering. Cook double or triple portions, then freeze; shop for timesavers like shredded cheese and sliced vegetables. If you travel by air, reserve bulkhead seat for extra leg room.

Good Nutrition Can Help

Although food is neither a cause nor a cure for osteoarthritis, what you eat is important. Watch your weight. Excess pounds add stress to weight-bearing joints, worsening pain, movement, and inflammation. If ibuprofen or other nonsteroidal anti-inflammatory drugs cause water retention, ask your doctor or a registered dietitian about limiting sodium (salt). Eating a variety of foods will give your body the right

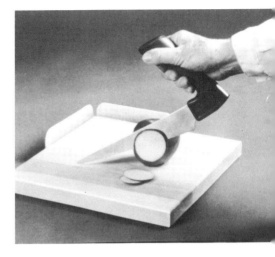

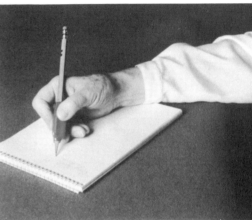

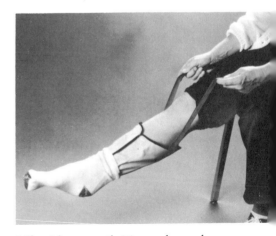

Life with osteoarthritis can be made easier with such inexpensive assist devices as a special knife and cutting board (top, spikes on the board hold objects in place), a pencil grip (center), and a "stocking aid" for putting on socks without bending (bottom).

165

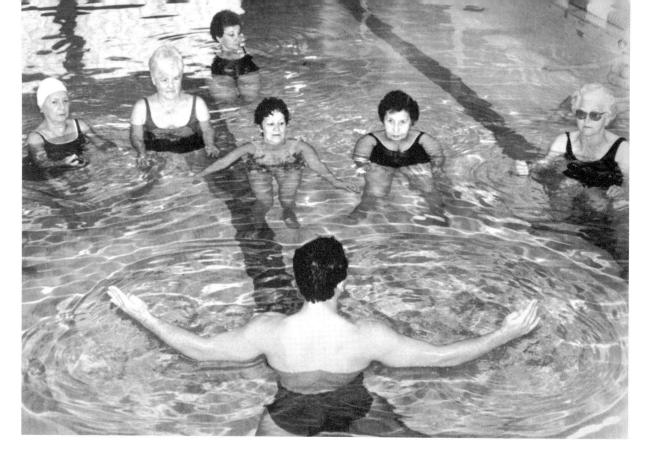

Arthritis patients take part in an exercise class sponsored by the Arthritis Foundation. Researchers say that low-impact exercises like swimming can help people whose joints are affected by osteoarthritis.

mix of nutrients for overall good health. A varied diet also can offset shortages that medications may cause. For example, regularly taking large doses of aspirin may increase your need for iron. You also may need more folic acid and vitamin C. Green leafy vegetables, asparagus, and whole-grain cereals are good sources of folic acid. Citrus fruits, tomatoes, cabbage, potatoes, berries, melon, and dark green vegetables contain vitamin C. Lean red meats, legumes, whole-grain breads, and cereals supply iron.

Sometimes getting enough of these nutrients, especially iron, is difficult. Ask your doctor or a registered dietician about a supplement with 50 to 100 percent of the Recommended Dietary Allowances for a variety of vitamins and minerals.

Exercise for Fitness and Fun

Rest is essential to control active inflammation. But don't let arthritis make you permanently inactive. Inactivity can make your joints stiffen. Your muscles become smaller and weaker. Weak muscles are less able to support joints. Your coordination and posture can suffer as well. Poor conditioning can worsen problems from heart disease to osteoporosis.

If a joint is sore, holding it in a slightly bent position may reduce pain. But if you keep the joint that way, pain can eventually increase. The health of your cartilage depends on how much you use your joints. For example, bending your elbow to touch your shoulder squeezes fluid and waste products out of your cartilage. When you relax the joint by lowering your arm again, fluid seeps back in, bringing with it both oxygen and nutrients.

166

Physical exercise doesn't hurt healthy joints. Studies show that joggers and aerobic dancers aren't more likely to develop osteoarthritis. But if you have arthritis, weight-bearing or high-impact activities like jogging or basketball may aggravate the problem.

If you hurt for two hours after exercising or doing a task, you've gone too far. Rest until the pain subsides. Next time, break the activity into smaller segments and alter the intensity or type of movement.

Consult your doctor before starting an exercise program. If you've had joint pain, joint surgery, or X rays that show osteoarthritis, your doctor may advise smooth, low-impact exercises like swimming, walking, stationary bicycling, and cross-country skiing. If you have arthritis in your back, floor exercises may help.

Other Methods To Relieve Pain

Ask your doctor, or physical or occupational therapist about:

Removal of Fluid. By draining fluid that collects around a joint, doctors sometimes can relieve painful inflammation.

Heat. Heat can relax muscles around a painful joint. You can apply heat superficially with hot water, a paraffin bath, an electric pad, or a hot pack; be careful to avoid a burn. For deep penetration a physical therapist can use ultrasound or short-wave diathermy to treat bursitis or tendinitis. Heating with ultrasound or diathermy can raise a joint's internal temperature. This technique requires monitoring and may worsen some forms of arthritis.

Cold. Cold acts as a local anaesthetic. It also decreases muscle spasms. Cold packs may help when you ache from holding muscles in a certain position to avoid pain.

Electrical Stimulation. TENS is an acronym for transcutaneous (across the skin) electrical nerve stimulation. A therapist places electrodes on your skin near the painful area. The electrodes are linked to a battery-operated stimulator. TENS stops pain by blocking nerve signals from reaching your brain. TENS may also help release hormones (endorphins) that fight pain.

Splints. Splints support weak, painful joints during activity and provide proper positioning at night, which promotes restful sleep.

Relaxation. Hypnosis, biofeedback, and other relaxation techniques are useful disciplines that require correct training and use.

Surgery: New Joints for Old

If conservative treatments don't help, your doctor may advise joint replacement surgery. This increasingly common procedure is called arthroplasty. During the last 30 years more than 80 percent of procedures have involved the hip and knee. Small-joint operations help the shoulder, elbow, wrist, and hand. Surgeons also repair tendons and ligaments for stability and mobility. Even with a successful operation, you won't be able to play vigorous sports. But you can expect less pain and swelling, as well as easier movement.

If pain keeps you awake at night or prevents you from doing important activities, your doctor may recommend an operation. Almost al-

Artificial joints, also known as prosthetic implants, can bring improvement when more conservative treatments fail. Among the available devices are implants for the hip (top), elbow (center), and knee (bottom).

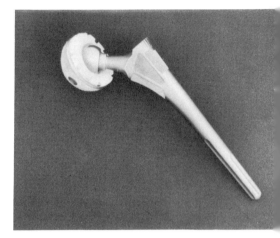

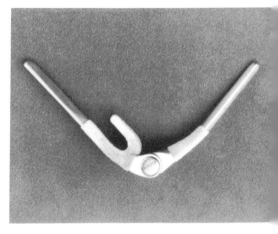

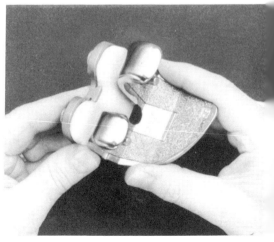

167

Other Common Forms of Arthritis

How They Can Affect You

Type	Joints Often Involved	Key Symptoms
Rheumatoid arthritis	Middle knuckles are most common site, usually on both hands. Also can affect your wrists and knees.	Prolonged morning stiffness. Inflamed, swollen joints. May rapidly erode or destroy joint or tissue in other organs.
Gout	Base of great toe; occasionally other joints. Usually affects only one joint.	Comes on rapidly. Red, hot, tender joint due to crystals in joints. (Often responds readily to medications.)
Infectious arthritis	Usually affects one joint. Tuberculosis affects the spine; gonorrhea attacks the knee. Staphylococcus may complicate joint surgery.	Warm, swollen joint. Symptoms usually acute. Can destroy joint. Fever common. (Causes include tuberculosis, sexually transmitted diseases, and Lyme disease.)
Lupus erythematosus	A systemic disease that commonly affects joints. Usually involves multiple joints, especially the hands, wrists, and knees.	Stiffness and discomfort usually worse than appearance of joints. Fever often occurs. Warm, swollen joints less common. (Can also involve kidneys, heart, lungs, and nervous system.)

ways, this is elective surgery. Your doctor will assess the degree of your pain and disability, the strength of your bones (osteoporosis prevents some older women from having surgery), the strength of ligaments supporting your joint, your weight, and your attitude. (Are you willing to participate in rehabilitation and accept the limits an artificial joint may pose?)

Prosthetic devices are made of various metals or polyethylene (a plastic-like material). At large medical centers, physicians sometimes use computers to custom design an implant and plan the operation. Large inventories of artificial joints enable surgeons to select the implant best suited to your needs. Traditionally, doctors have secured the prosthesis to existing bones with a special cement (polymethyl methacrylate). In recent years surgeons have been using implants with a porous surface. Existing bone grows into the prosthesis. This may help prevent loosening of the prosthetic components. Sometimes cement is still the best option.

Infection is rare but serious. With modern antibiotics, less than 1 percent of hip devices become infected. Blood clots can occur after surgery, and an implant may loosen with time.

What's Ahead?

Until recently many scientists viewed osteoarthritis as a simple "wear-and-tear" problem. New developments make the picture more complex—but also more encouraging:

Genetics. Scientists have identified a genetic defect that speeds cartilage decay. Researchers are studying how common this defect is, if it can be prevented, and if other gene problems also cause osteoarthritis. Physicians envision a test to tell who's at risk. Counseling about proper weight, exercise, and work might help minimize risk.

Cartilage Protection. Researchers hope to block the deterioration of cartilage. If you have a family history of osteoarthritis, future drugs may stop the disease before it starts.

Dissolvable Devices. Scientists also are working on drugs to stimulate the growth of cartilage. If these drugs are successful, doctors could insert a temporary joint replacement that dissolves as new cartilage forms.

What Can You Expect?

If your osteoarthritis is severe, don't ignore it. Get help. It won't go away—but you don't have to face this problem alone. Get involved in your treatment plan. You'll have less pain and more pleasure in daily activities. Remember this: If you have osteoarthritis, the outlook is good. It develops slowly. Crippling is rare. And the symptoms of the disease often subside. ☐

SOURCES OF FURTHER INFORMATION

Additional information on arthritis is readily available.

ARTHRITIS FOUNDATION. Offers information and programs to enhance quality of life for people with arthritis. Contact your local chapter or the national office: P.O. Box 19000, Atlanta, GA 30326. Telephone: 1-800-283-7800

PACE. This acronym stands for People with Arthritis Can Exercise. The Arthritis Foundation offers PACE programs at local chapters of the Arthritis Foundation and on videotape. Ask your doctor if PACE, or programs involving water workouts, are right for you.

SUGGESTIONS FOR FURTHER READING

ARTHRITIS FOUNDATION. *Guide to Independent Living.* This 416-page directory lists products to make daily activities easier.

FRIES, JAMES F., M.D. *Arthritis: A Comprehensive Guide to Understanding Your Arthritis.* Reading, Mass., Addison-Wesley, 1990. A practical look at the different types of arthritis and their treatments.

LORIG, KATE, R.N., DR.P.H., AND JAMES F. FRIES, M.D. *The Arthritis Helpbook: A Tested Self-Management Program for Coping With Your Arthritis.* Reading, Mass., Addison-Wesley, 1990. How to work with your healthcare team to manage arthritis.

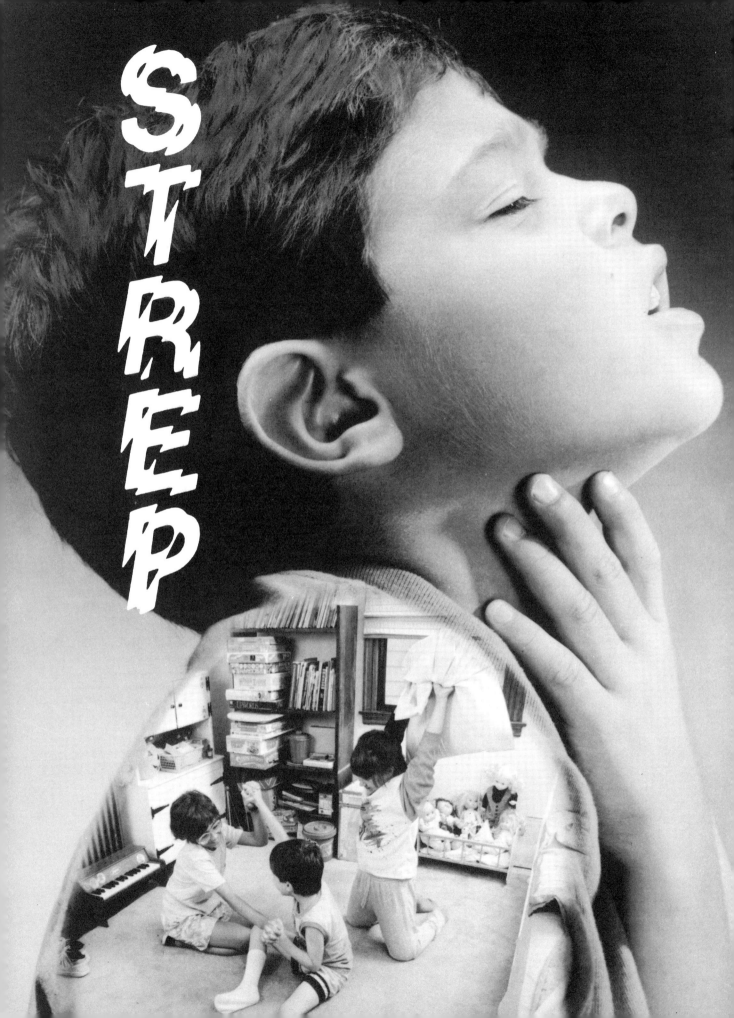

STREP

Margie Patlak

Few childhoods go by without the telltale fever and sore throat of a *Streptococcus*, or "strep," infection. Although these throat infections are common and easily treated, the recent rise of particularly deadly or troublesome strains of Group A *Streptococcus* has pushed the bacterium into the medical limelight—again.

In the past Group A strep has played a starring role in a number of deadly medical epidemics, particularly the scourges of rheumatic fever that swept across the United States in the first half of this century, killing or debilitating thousands of children each year. After World War II the number of cases of rheumatic fever dramatically declined until, during the 20 years between 1965 and 1985 alone, the yearly number of cases of rheumatic fever among school-age children dropped by more than 90 percent. The medical community had assumed that less crowded living conditions and the use of antibiotics were keeping the disease at bay. Some physicians went so far as to call rheumatic fever a "vanishing disease in suburbia."

That complacency was shaken in the mid-1980s when outbreaks of rheumatic fever were reported among children and young adults in various cities scattered throughout the country. Those reports were followed by other reports of a new and deadly form of strep infection that was afflicting adults. This disease, which is called toxic streptococcal syndrome, made the headlines when Jim Henson, creator of the Muppets, was reported to have died from it in 1990. There's also evidence to suggest that blood infections caused by Group A strep are on the rise.

"Group A *Streptococcus* seems to have taken a little twist again." says Dr. Rosemary Roberts, a medical officer with the U.S. Food and Drug Administration's division of anti-infective drug products. "We're seeing manifestations like rheumatic fever that we haven't seen for a while, as well as more invasive strains of Group A strep that are making people sicker much more quickly."

The jury isn't in yet on why Americans are experiencing such a boost in the severity of strep infections. Preliminary findings by researchers at the U.S. Centers for Disease Control in Atlanta suggest that a population increase among previously rare strep types may be behind both the recent rheumatic fever outbreaks and cases of the new toxic streptococcal syndrome. And heightened production of disease-causing toxins by more common strep types may also be responsible for the latest strep casualties.

There are more than 80 known types of Group A *Streptococcus*, which can cause more than a dozen different illnesses. Group A *Streptococcus*, in turn, is part of a broader category of strep organisms that cause an even larger number of diseases. Some of the more well-known Group A strep afflictions include upper respiratory diseases such as strep throat and scarlet fever, skin disorders such as impetigo, and inflammatory diseases such as rheumatic fever or kidney disease. In addition blood infections due to Group A strep are a serious and frequent complication of wounds or surgery.

Group A strep infections are treatable with antibiotics, the drug of choice being penicillin. Other antibiotics, such as erythromycin and various cephalosporins, are effective alternatives for patients allergic to penicillin. The FDA is responsible for ensuring both the safety and the effectiveness of all of these drugs.

Strep Throat

Strep throat (streptococcal pharyngitis) is probably the most well-known Group A strep infection. Although strep throat can occur at any age and at any time of the year, it mainly afflicts school-age children during the winter and spring. The many symptoms of strep throat include an extremely red and painful sore throat, ear pain, fever, enlarged and tender lymph nodes in the neck, white spots on the tonsils, or dark red spots on the soft palate. However, about 1 out of every 5 people with strep throat experience no symptoms.

Because nearly all the symptoms of strep throat can also occur with viral infections, laboratory tests are used to confirm a doctor's suspicion that a patient's sore throat is caused by Group A strep. The traditional laboratory test to identify strep is a throat culture. To isolate and identify Group A strep from a throat swab takes from one to three days using the culture method. In recent years a number of tests have become available that use antibodies to detect the presence of Group A strep directly on a throat swab, and these devices can provide test results in a matter of minutes. Many physicians feel that the rapid tests do not detect as many positive results as the culture method, so if the rapid test results are negative, a follow-up throat culture is recommended.

Strep throat is highly contagious among children because they are in close contact with one another. In addition, they have not yet developed resistance to any of the strains, as adults have.

The incubation period for strep throat is two to five days. During epidemics siblings of a strep throat patient have a 50-50 chance of also succumbing, whereas only 20 percent of the parents of such patients will develop strep throat. Children with strep throat should not return to school until their temperature returns to normal and they've had at least a day's worth of antibiotics.

Strep throat is easily treated with antibiotics. Treatment is usually not necessary for those individuals who harbor the strep throat microbe but show no signs of an active infection. These people are unlikely to spread infection to others, according to the American Academy of Pediatrics, or experience the complications of a strep infection, which include rheumatic fever and kidney disease.

Scarlet Fever

One of the more colorful variants of a strep infection is scarlet fever. The hallmarks of this disease include a bright red tongue, a brilliant scarlet rash (particularly on the trunk, arms, and thighs), a flushed face, sore throat, and fever. "Scarlet fever is simply strep throat with a rash," says Roberts. The red rash that typifies this disease is prompted by a toxin generated by the *Streptococcus* bacterium. The striking symptoms of scarlet fever make it easy to diagnose, but most physicians confirm their clinical diagnosis with laboratory tests.

Like strep throat, scarlet fever primarily afflicts school-age children during the winter and spring

months. Scarlet fever is easily treated with antibiotics, and, if left untended, the disease can foster the same complications prompted by strep throat.

Rheumatic Fever

Lurking behind several types of strep infections is the possibility of rheumatic fever. Although rheumatic fever is a relatively uncommon disease, its effects are serious enough to warrant concern. Signs of rheumatic fever include a red rash, pea-sized lumps under the skin, tender joints, fever, involuntary jerky movements, heart palpitations, chest pain, and, in severe cases, heart failure. Although most symptoms disappear within weeks to months, about half the time the disease leaves behind deformed heart valves that may limit patients' physical activities and foster premature death from heart failure.

The diagnosis of rheumatic fever is based on its symptoms in conjunction with a history of a recent strep infection, which can be confirmed by tests for strep antibodies in the blood. Rheumatic fever is thought to be triggered by an overly active immune system, which inadvertently destroys body tissues in its zeal to rid the body of a strep infection. Most symptoms of rheumatic fever crop up one to four weeks after a strep infection, although involuntary jerky movements may not surface for as long as six months after infection. About half of the recent cases of rheumatic fever, however, developed with mild to no previous signs of a strep throat infection, such as a sore throat with fever.

It's these signs of a strep infection that physicians rely on to prevent rheumatic fever. As many as 3 percent of untreated cases of strep throat can develop into rheumatic fever. But antibiotic treatment, even if it's not started until several days after the onset of symptoms, can squelch the possibility of rheumatic fever. Once rheumatic fever occurs, doctors can do little to prevent its damage. Anti-inflammatory drugs (such as aspirin or steroids) can ease many of the symptoms and possibly prevent some of rheumatic fever's more serious developments. Antibiotics are also used to treat any lingering strep infections. But even with such therapies, the disease often wreaks such damage on heart valves that they have to be surgically repaired or replaced with synthetic or animal implants.

Rheumatic fever usually recurs whenever its victims experience any new strep infections. To pre-

Margie Patlak is a freelance writer in Elkins Park, Pa.

vent such flare-ups, the American Heart Association recommends that anyone who has experienced rheumatic fever take prophylactic (preventive) doses of antibiotics. How long rheumatic fever patients require such a preventive drug regime depends on whether they experienced heart damage and whether they're likely to develop a future strep infection. Children who've had rheumatic fever, for example, generally take antibiotics on a daily basis until they reach adulthood, when the risk of a strep infection greatly diminishes.

Skin Infection

When Group A *Streptococci* literally get under the skin, they can foster a common skin disease known as impetigo. This contagious disease frequently afflicts mainly children during the summer, when insect bites, cuts, and scrapes are prevalent. These skin infringements serve as portals of entry for the *Streptococci.*

Impetigo starts out as a rash of pinhead-sized blisters or pimples that rapidly run together to form yellow, flaky crusts. The impetigo rash may itch or burn, but rarely causes pain. The disease is diagnosed with the aid of cultures of the fluid lodged beneath the crusts. If large numbers of strep bacteria crop up in these cultures, their guilt in causing the disease is firmly established. Impetigo can also be caused by other bacteria, including *Staphylococcus,* or by mixtures of staphylococcal and streptococcal bacteria.

Impetigo is combated with the use of topical or oral antibiotics, depending on its severity and frequency within a given population. Doctors advise impetigo patients to remove the skin crusts and wash their rash with soap on a regular basis. Occasionally, if not treated, streptococcal impetigo develops into a blood infection, and it can also foster kidney disease.

Kidney Disease

All kinds of strep infections can foster an inflammation of the kidneys (acute glomerulonephritis), although the disease most often follows impetigo. Less than 1 percent of all strep infections foster kidney disease, but because certain strains of strep are particularly prone to causing this complication, small epidemics of acute glomerulonephritis can crop up in private homes or in schools.

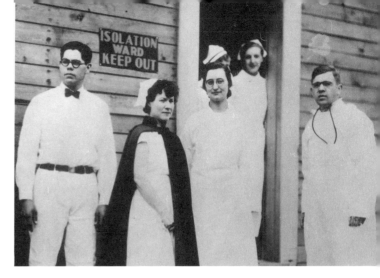

Before the advent of antibiotics, the spread of scarlet fever (a type of strep infection) was checked by isolating patients. Above, a scarlet fever isolation ward in Palmer, Alaska, in 1935. Below, health inspectors in New York harbor in 1921 remove suspected scarlet fever victims from a newly arrived ship so they can be quarantined.

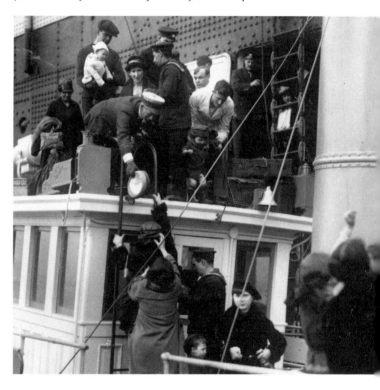

Symptoms of the disorder include a puffy face due to water retention, blood in the urine, pain in the loins, malaise, nausea, headache, and high blood pressure. These symptoms usually surface one to three weeks following a strep infection and subside within the same amount of time.

Diagnosis of acute poststreptococcal glomerulonephritis is based on symptoms, a history of a recent strep infection, and elevated levels of antibodies to strep in the blood. This form of kidney disease, like rheumatic fever, is thought to stem from an overactive immune response to strep.

Little can be done to prevent this heightened immune response once it's begun, although various drugs (such as diuretics) and dietary measures (such as restricted salt or protein intake) can ease many of its symptoms. Most patients recover without any permanent problems, although occasionally kidney damage inflicted by the disease may require dialysis or a kidney transplant.

Patients rarely experience a recurrence of acute glomerulonephritis following additional strep infections because of the immunity they develop to the specific type of strep bacterium that caused their disorder. (Only a handful of strep types can cause glomerulonephritis, and most cases of the disorder can be traced to a specific Group A streptococcal strain known as Type 12.)

Blood Infection

Although the number of bloodstream infections (septicemia) of Group A strep appears to be on the rise, they are still extremely rare. Only about 4 to 5 people out of 100,000 develop these infections each year, according to the Centers for Disease Control. But nearly one-third of all patients with *Streptococcus* blood infections will die from them.

Septicemia usually gets its start when streptococcal bacteria on the skin delve into an opening as large as a surgical or battle wound or as small as a minor cut or scrape. Normally, the body's immune system checks these bloodstream invaders before they wreak havoc in the body. In those individuals whose resistance is lowered, however, *Streptococcus* travels far and wide, causing such symptoms as fever, low blood pressure, chills, confusion, diarrhea, vomiting, or a red skin rash. Septicemia usually afflicts people over 60 who have an underlying disease such as diabetes or renal failure that compromises their immune defenses.

In addition to relying on clinical signs to diagnose septicemia, physicians use laboratory findings, including positive blood cultures, positive antibody tests, and extremely high numbers of white blood cells in the blood.

Toxic Streptococcal Syndrome

The new toxic streptococcal syndrome, first described in 1987 in the United States, is similar to septicemia. Patients with this disorder have many of the same symptoms as those of septicemia, but because of the disease's rapid progression, by the time they seek treatment they are often gravely ill. Toxic streptococcal syndrome patients frequently go into shock and experience multi-organ failure, as well as complications such as the pneumonia that reportedly killed Jim Henson.

Only 1 or 2 people out of 100,000 fall prey to toxic streptococcal syndrome each year. Unlike septicemics, most of these patients don't have any underlying diseases hampering their immune defenses. Of 21 cases studied extensively by researchers, most patients were in their 30s and the youngest was 25 years old. "The individuals who are getting strep septicemia and toxic strep syndrome," points out CDC epidemiologist Walter Straus, "are not the same ones who are getting strep throat."

Patients with toxic streptococcal syndrome are treated with antibiotics as well as with medical measures aimed at curbing its severe complications. The sooner patients are treated with antibiotics, the more likely they will recover from the syndrome, which kills about one-third of its victims.

Whether Group A *Streptococcus* infects the skin, blood, internal organs, or the throat, it is usually checked by prompt and appropriate antibiotic therapy. This is why, though recent outbreaks of serious strep infections are cause for some concern, they are not likely to prompt the extensive death or debilitation once tied to them. □

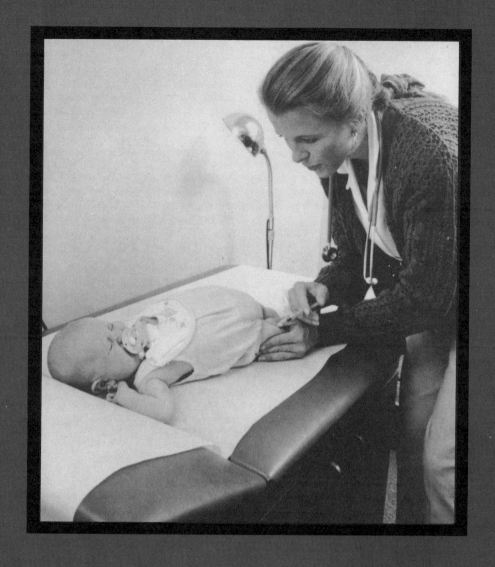

SPOTLIGHT
ON HEALTH

Contributors

Authors of articles in the Spotlight on Health section

Angier, Natalie. Science writer, New York *Times*. PROSTATE CANCER.

Bloomfield, Louise. Staff editor. OF CABBAGES AND KALE.

Brody, Jane E. Science writer; Personal Health columnist, New York *Times*. CONJUNCTIVITIS; COUNTERING SERIOUS SCARRING.

Cobb, Kevin. Free-lance writer specializing in health and travel. RSI: THE NEW COMPUTER-AGE HEALTH ASSAULT.

Dobkin, Bruce, M.D. Professor of Clinical Neurology, UCLA; Director of UCLA's Medical Rehabilitation Program. PLAYING FOR TIME: LOU GEHRIG'S DISEASE.

Fraser, Laura. Free-lance writer; regular contributor to *Health* magazine. GETTING THROUGH GRIEF.

Goldfinger, Stephen E., M.D. Chairman, *Harvard Health Letter*; Faculty Dean of the Department of Continuing Education, Harvard Medical School; Associate Clinical Director, Massachusetts Medical Health Center. CONSTIPATION.

Gustaitis, Joseph. Staff editor. MENACE OF THE MAT.

Halpert, Felicia E. Free-lance writer; co-author of *Mothering the New Mother*. THE DANGER OF MEDICATION MIXUPS.

Heller, Linda. Free-lance writer. YOGURT: BRING IT BACK ALIVE.

Lipman, Marvin M., M.D. Clinical Professor of Medicine, New York Medical College; Chief Medical Adviser, Consumers Union. SPEAK UP TO YOUR DOCTOR.

Munnings, Frances. Contributing Editor, *The Physician and Sportsmedicine*. EXERCISE: IS ANY TIME THE PRIME TIME?

Randall, Teri. Associate Editor, "Medical News," *Journal of the American Medical Association*. MUSIC THERAPY FOR THE ELDERLY.

Schultz, Dodi. Free-lance writer; Contributing Editor, *Parents* magazine. CONQUERING MENINGITIS.

Talan, Jamie. Staff writer, New York *Newsday*. PANIC DISORDER.

Wolpow, Edward R., M.D. Member of the Advisory Board, *Harvard Health Letter*; Assistant Professor of Neurology, Harvard Medical School. AFTER THE FALL: DEALING WITH HEAD INJURIES.

EXERCISE

Is Any Time the Prime Time?

Frances Munnings

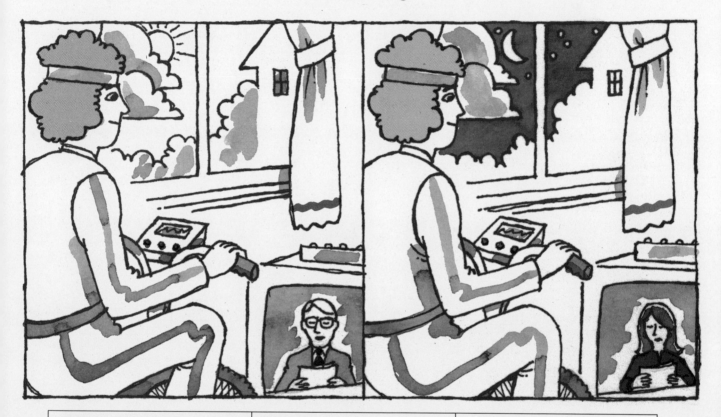

Finding time to exercise is often a struggle for many people. When trying to schedule exercise sessions, many wonder whether the time of day influences the benefits they derive from exercise. Some people want to know whether early exercisers get more from their exercise sessions than afternoon athletes or whether timing affects how safe their sessions are. A number of other questions arise: Are people more likely to be injured during different times of day? Are the risks of cardiovascular events greater in the morning? And does air pollution or weather alter exercise effectiveness? Answers aren't easy to come by, but research investigating these questions indicates that athletes need to think about their goals before deciding when to exercise.

The Rhythm of Exercise

A body in motion isn't independent of the rising and setting of the sun. "Almost anything you can name shows biological rhythmicity," says David W. Hill, assistant professor of kinesiology at the University of North Texas in Denton. "Hormones, body temperature, and sleep/wakefulness patterns all fluctuate predictably with time of day." The question is whether these biorhythms affect the body's response to exercise.

Hill has studied physiologic responses to exercise at different time of day. He found that

"Exercise: Is Any Time the Prime Time?" by F. Munnings. From *The Physician and Sportsmedicine*, May 1991. Reprinted with permission of McGraw-Hill, Inc.

177

strength peaked at about noon and that anaerobic and aerobic capacity were higher in the afternoon. In fact, the only response that was the same morning and afternoon was the ventilatory (anaerobic) threshold.

Unexpectedly, Hill found that although maximal oxygen consumption was 4.2 percent higher in the afternoon, the actual work achieved by the subjects was the same as in the morning. In other words, it took more oxygen to do a given amount of work during the afternoon. Hill thinks that part of the explanation may be that because body temperature is higher in the afternoon, some of the oxygen might have been used for actions unrelated to the measured work.

But athletes should not automatically switch to afternoon workouts. An exerciser has to think about goals when deciding what time of day to exercise, Hill says. "If competition is scheduled at a certain time of day, then train at that time," he says. "But if you don't know or care when you're going to compete, or if you're just trying to get in shape, exercise when you can get the best workout: in the afternoon. Because your strength and anaerobic and aerobic capacity are higher, you can get a more intense workout."

Weathering Effects

Athletes who are training for competition should weigh environmental conditions and physiologic responses carefully before deciding when to exercise, Hill says. It would seem that if a person were going to compete in, say, a hot and windy environment, then that is the best environment in which to train. But Hill says only some of the training should be done in those conditions. "If you train in better ambient conditions, you can achieve a higher intensity. You've only got so much cardiac output. You can put it into thermoregulation [temperature control] or you can put it into your running."

Another researcher who has examined physiologic mechanisms and time of day is Margaret A. Kolka of the Thermal Physiology and Medicine Division at the U.S. Army Research Institute of Environmental Medicine in Natick, Mass. She has looked at thermoregulatory functions—primarily heat dissipation.

Kolka says that body temperature, which is usually about 97°F in the morning, normally increases about 2°F during the day. Strenuous exercise can raise body temperature about 2°F, which would result in temperatures of 99°F in the morning and 101°F in the afternoon. Normally, the body can handle the increase in temperature, she says. "The body is very well adapted; it can dump the heat."

The rub comes when it's hot and humid. For example, Kolka says, "If your core temperature in the morning is 98°F and your skin temperature is 92°F and it's 75°F outside, the temperature gradient is 92°F to 75°F; so you'll dump heat well." But if in the afternoon your skin temperature is 93°F and the ambient temperature is 90°F, you have a gradient of only 3°F. Humidity further complicates the situation. If there are more water molecules in the air, sweat doesn't evaporate as easily from the skin surface, adding to the stress of exercise, she says.

Kolka says that if it's hot in the afternoon, exercisers have to take into account the consequences: a shorter and lesser effective workout because of the thermal stress.

Exercising for a Sound Sleep

Depending on when people exercise, fitness activities can affect sleep both negatively and positively, says Mark J. Chambers. "You need to exercise at a high energy expenditure rate and maintain it for quite a while to have a positive effect on sleep," he says. But, he cautions, the stimulant properties of the exercise will affect your ability to fall asleep if

you do it soon before you go to bed. And exercise won't help you sleep if done too far in advance of bedtime.

Chambers, who is a clinical psychologist at the Stanford Sleep Disorders Clinic in California, says that late afternoon is probably the best time to exercise if a good night's sleep is the goal. He explains that when people fall asleep, they are in the downward phase of the body temperature cycle. If a person exercises in the late afternoon or early evening, when body temperature peaks, the increase in temperature incurred by exercise causes a rebound drop that may facilitate sleep.

Get a Breath of Fresh Air

The quality of air, which varies throughout the day, also may affect exercisers. Air pollution is a special concern to people who exercise regularly, and the major culprit is the car, says Peter B. Raven, professor of physiology at the Texas College of Osteopathic Medicine in Fort Worth. "Some exposure comes from stationary pollutant sources, such as power stations and lumber mills," he says. "But cars pour out unexpended gasolines and hydrocarbons. In addition, the nitric oxides and carbon monoxide react with sunlight to produce ozone."

Raven says that urbanites should exercise when traffic patterns are light: early in the morning, if possible. If they exercise later in the day, say from 4:30 to 6:30 P.M., it's best to avoid major thoroughfares. Jogging in a naturally green environment would reduce exposure, Raven adds.

Exercisers have two reasons to avoid pollution, Raven says. First, exercise performance could be impaired. Ozone and other pollutants affect lung function, causing pain under the breastbone and more shallow and rapid breathing. Carbon monoxide, the most prevalent pollutant, binds with hemoglobin in the red blood cells, thereby reducing the amount of oxygen the hemoglobin can carry. Both of these factors inhibit oxygen delivery.

Second, exercising in polluted areas has important health effects too, Raven adds. "A person with coronary artery disease (CAD) would suffer from the reduced capacity of blood to carry oxygen because the heart would have to work harder at a given work load." In an atmosphere that had a high level of carbon monoxide, a person who had CAD would be prone to chest pain or a reduction in the pump function of the heart, he says.

A combination of sulfur dioxide and high humidity makes exercise particularly difficult for asthmatics. The mechanism is the same as for healthy exercisers: a narrowing of the tubes in the lungs—a condition known as bronchoconstriction—and pain.

A Time for Injury?

Because people tend to feel stiff in the morning, they may believe that exercise is safer later in the day, but Carol A. Macera says timing doesn't make much difference in injury rates. In a recent study, she found that the injury rate was not statistically significant between morning exercisers and those who exercised at other times of day—including in the dark. "Weekly mileage was probably the most important determinant of injury," says Macera, an epidemiologist in the School of Public Health at the University of South Carolina in Columbia.

Other researchers have addressed whether exercisers are at greater risk for heart attacks in the morning. Among a number of studies showing that cardiovascular events are more likely to occur in the morning is one that reported that there is marked increase in myocardial infarctions, a type of heart damage caused by a blocked artery, from 6 A.M. to noon. But experts say fear of morning exercise is unjustified.

"The chance of myocardial infarction during exercise is extremely low, so low that the ben-

efits of exercise outweigh the risks," says Paul D. Thompson, associate professor of medicine at Brown University Program in Medicine in Providence, R. I. "Even among patients with heart disease, the risk of myocardial infarction during exercise is low."

Thompson, who also is director of preventive cardiology at the Miriam Hospital in Providence, says that in his studies there was one death from cardiac arrest per year for every 15,000 healthy joggers. Another study showed a transient risk during vigorous exercise but an overall decreased risk of primary cardiac arrest in habitual vigorous exercisers.

Possible mechanisms for the reported increase in cardiovascular events during the morning, says Barry Franklin, are the pronounced increases in coronary vessel constriction, blood clotting tendencies, the percentage of blood red cells in the blood, blood viscosity, and certain blood chemicals, known as plasma catecholamines, that can stimulate physiologic activity. But Franklin, who is director of the Cardiac Rehabilitation and Exercise Laboratories at William Beaumont Hospital in Birmingham, Mich., also thinks that healthy people need not worry about morning exercise.

"I think that other factors are more important," Franklin says. "We need to be concerned about warm-up, cool-down, and staying within the training heart rate."

Exercisers should also be aware of three critical signs and symptoms of problems, says Franklin. "If a person experiences chest pain or pressure, light-headedness, or a markedly abnormal heart rhythm, it's best to stop exercising and investigate the cause of the symptoms."

Any Time Is Right

For Thompson and Franklin, exercise itself is more important than exercise at the "perfect time."

"For many people it's more convenient to exercise in the morning," says Thompson, "so if

people believe that morning exercise is dangerous, they may not exercise at all."

Hill seconds that notion. "Physiology aside," he says, "if the only time you're going to stick with it is at 6 in the morning, that's when you should exercise."

"Sticking with it" is yet another aspect of exercise that has been studied. Pamela S. Reed and colleagues looked at adherence in 263 patients in a cardiac rehabilitation program at William Beaumont Hospital in Birmingham, Mich. They found that the adherence ratio was significantly better for morning exercisers than for afternoon exercisers.

"The people in the afternoon classes skipped their exercise on busy days," says Reed, who is now a clinical nurse specialist at St. Joseph Mercy Hospital in Pontiac, Mich. "And sometimes they were too tired in the afternoon."

Reed believes that another factor, not actually measured, contributed to the better compliance among the morning exercisers. "These patients had been together longer," she says. "They were a closer-knit group."

Although the time of day is not as important as the exercise itself, a few guidelines prevail:
• Try to schedule exercise when it isn't hot and humid.
• Exercise during the afternoon for improved performance levels. (But be aware that heat and high humidity, which often are greater in the afternoon, may reduce the efficiency of exercise sessions.)
• Stay away from heavy traffic when exercising.
• Don't exercise vigorously just before bedtime if the goal is a good night's sleep.
• Look at factors other than time of day that might affect exercise. For example, exercise with a friend if the companionship makes it easier to stick with the program.
• Incorporate a warm-up and cool-down in exercise programs.
• Do not let the fear of a heart attack prevent engaging in a regular exercise program. □

CONQUERING MENINGITIS

Dodi Schultz

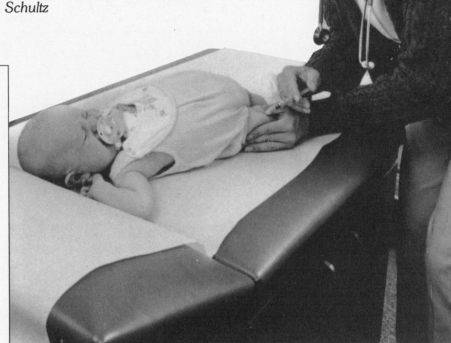

Bacterial meningitis is not solely a childhood disease, but a disproportionate number of its victims are infants and children. The symptoms and the speed of their onset can strike terror in the heart of a parent.

It may happen something like this: A child may have been suffering from a cold or a sore throat or, perhaps, nothing at all. Suddenly, the youngster is irritable, running a high fever, complaining of headache, and vomiting. Infants develop an eerie, high-pitched cry. Muscles in the neck and elsewhere may stiffen. The child may become delirious, slip into a coma, or have convulsions.

An alarmed parent's first impulse under these circumstances is to seek emergency medical care. It is precisely the right response. Without treatment the disease may be lethal, and the danger increases with youth; a very young child could die within hours of the time the first signs of illness appear. Whenever meningitis is suspected—in a child or adult—the patient should be rushed to the nearest hospital.

Before the advent of antibiotics, the vast majority of bacterial meningitis cases, in those of all ages, proved fatal. Now, with prompt diagnosis and treatment, more than 90 percent survive; among those who receive timely medical care, the relatively few fatalities now occur mostly among two groups: the extremely young and the extremely old.

Multiple Causes

Meningitis is an inflammation of the meninges, the membranes surrounding the brain and spinal cord. Sometimes, perhaps even most of the time, the infectious agent is a virus. Those cases, however, are cause for far less concern than the ones resulting from bacterial infection.

"There are probably more cases of viral meningitis than bacterial, " says Dr. Susan Alpert, a pediatric infectious disease specialist in the division of anti-infective drug products at the Center for Drug Evaluation and Research of the U.S. Food and Drug Administration. "But it can be so mild that the patient doesn't even see a physician, and many cases are never diagnosed. Bacterial meningitis is such a serious infection that it invariably comes to medical attention."

That serious infection may be caused by any of a number of bacteria. Many people would assume, from its name, that the bacterium called *Neisseria menin-*

Before antibiotics, most people with bacterial meningitis died; now, with prompt treatment, more than 90 percent survive.

180

gitidis (also known as meningo-coccus) is the major cause of the disease. In fact, it ranks second to another organism. The leading cause of bacterial meningitis is actually a strain, type b, of the confusingly named *Hemophilus influenzae*, so called because, when it was first identified, it was erroneously believed to be the cause of influenza or "flu" (which is actually caused by a virus). These two bacteria, together with the pneumococcus *Streptococcus pneumoniae*, account for four out of every five cases of bacterial meningitis.

Diagnosis and Treatment

Hospital diagnosis of bacterial meningitis begins with a lumbar puncture ("spinal tap") to obtain a sample of the cerebrospinal fluid that bathes the brain and flows down through the spinal canal. Normally clear, the fluid is ana-lyzed for the presence of bacteria and other evidence of infection. Samples of blood, urine, and res-piratory secretions may also be taken. But since the disease can progress so quickly, treatment—with intravenous antibiotics—is started even before any test results are available.

Among those drugs currently widely used to treat bacterial meningitis are a class of antibiot-ics called cephalosporins, espe-cially cefotaxime (brand name, Claforan) and ceftriaxone (Rocephin), and various members of the penicillin family. At least a week of treatment, and sometimes more, is needed.

When *H. influenzae* type b (Hib) or meningococcal meningitis has been diagnosed, household members and other close contacts may be placed on a short course of prophylaxis (prevention) with the antibiotic rifampin (Rifadin, Rimactane).

The dread of bacterial meningi-tis, whatever the cause, is based not only on its reputation as a killer but on the possibility of neurological complications—lingering deficits that can be espe-

Possible complications of bacterial meningitis include persistent hearing loss, recurrent convulsions, and mental retardation.

cially devastating in infants and children, who are still growing and developing. Those complica-tions may include persistent hear-ing loss, mental retardation, and recurrent convulsions, and they occur in 20 to 30 percent of those who survive a bout of bacterial meningitis.

An additional type of therapy has been proposed for children with bacterial meningitis, based on the possibility of staving off one of these neurological afteref-fects. One group of researchers has suggested that adding dexa-methasone, a corticosteroid hor-mone, to the antibiotic treatment may help prevent subsequent deafness.

"There have been numerous discussions of this question," says Susan Alpert, "and there are peo-ple on both sides. The original reports came from just one medi-cal center. Right now, there are studies being conducted around the country."

Why not just add the drug, in case it might help? As Dr. Alpert points out, "No therapy is totally

BACTERIAL BAD GUYS

Although meningitis can be caused by viruses, in the critical, potentially fatal form of the disease, the villains are bacteria. The first three listed here account for about 80 percent of all cases.

• *Hemophilus influenzae* type b ("Hib") is the most common cause of bacterial meningitis in the United States. Other strains of the bacterium—types a, c, d, e, and f, as well as "untyped" varieties—cause less serious illness, including middle-ear infections in children. There are now vaccines to protect infants and pre-schoolers, Hib's most frequent victims (most older people have developed immu-nity). Hib can also strike elsewhere in the body, causing pneumonia and other conditions.

• *Neisseria meningitidis*, also known as meningococcus, may strike at any age and has been epidemic at times in some parts of the world and under closed-population circumstances, such as barracks. There is a vaccine, but it hasn't been shown to be effective in very young children or proved safe during pregnancy. It's believed to be effective for three years, but this hasn't been definitely established. The vaccine is not considered necessary for routine use in the United States, except for the military. Vaccination is, however, recommended for those who travel to sub-Saharan Africa during the December-through-June dry season, when meningococcal meningitis has been known to be epidemic there; the hazardous area is a band covering most of Ethiopia and stretching westward through Sudan, Chad, Niger, and Nigeria to Guinea on the continent's west coast.

• *Streptococcus pneumoniae*, also known as pneumococcus, has an attack rate lower than that of *H. influenzae* and *N. meningitidis*, but the disease is just as serious. This bacterium is the main cause of meningitis in adults, although it can and does attack children as well. The meningitis is sometimes secondary to an-other condition caused by the same organism, such as pneumonia or an ear or sinus infection.

Other *Streptococcus* species, *Escherichia coli*, and *Staphylococcus aureus* are among a variety of common, widespread bacteria that are unlikely to cause critical illness in most children and adults, since most have developed immunity to them. They can, however, cause life-threatening meningitis in infants during the first four to six weeks of life, because newborns may not have protective antibodies. Low-birth-weight babies are most susceptible, and the mortality rate is high. Those with immune systems weakened by such conditions as AIDS are also vulnerable to infection by some of these agents.

benign." Corticosteroids can also have adverse side effects. And most of the children in the reported studies had Hib infection and were treated with one of two antibiotics; the outcome might be different with different bacteria and/or different antibiotics.

The Special Hib Threat

Over the past few years, there have been about 2,400 to 2,900 cases of meningococcal infection reported annually to the national Centers for Disease Control in Atlanta. Some 46 to 47 percent are in children and teens (who compose 27 percent of the population). And about a quarter of all the cases are in pre-school-age children (who represent about 6 percent of the population). The overall incidence is 1 to 1.5 cases per 100,000 population.

While there are no comparable figures for *Hemophilus influenzae* type b infection, CDC has studied comparative incidence in the spe-

---

The most common cause of bacterial meningitis in the United States is a bacterium known as Hib, which most often affects infants and preschoolers.

---

cific population subgroups of black non-Hispanics, white non-Hispanics, and Hispanics, reports medical epidemiologist Dr. Janet Mohle-Boetani of the CDC's Meningitis and Special Pathogens Branch. These figures consistently show that Hib cases outnumber meningococcal meningitis cases by about 3 to 1.

Among small children the comparative attack rate has been far higher. According to the CDC, before the introduction of the first vaccine, 1 in 200 children in the

United States developed an invasive Hib infection by the age of 5; 60 percent of those children had meningitis, and 3 to 6 percent died. (Aside from meningitis, the bacterium can also cause other serious illnesses, including pericarditis, or inflammation of the sac surrounding the heart, and pneumonia.)

The Hib Vaccines

Both physicians and parents have therefore welcomed the availability of effective vaccines to combat Hib. There have been a number of such vaccines; the earliest ones were different from those in current use.

The first Hib vaccine, known as Hemophilus b polysaccharide vaccine, was licensed by the FDA in April 1985 (polysaccharide refers to a viral component used in preparation of the vaccine). Within a year, a total of three manufacturers had been licensed to produce such vaccines, variously known as b-Capsa-1 (Praxis Biologics), Hib-imune (Lederle), or Hibvax (Connaught Laboratories).

Trials had demonstrated the polysaccharide vaccines' effectiveness in children at least 2 years old, but not under 18 months; their efficacy in infants between those ages was in question. The official recommendation of the CDC's Immunization Practices Advisory Committee was for routine vaccination at 24 months, with possible use in children as young as 18 months if they were considered to be at high risk of infection.

In December 1987 a new vaccine—known as a conjugate vaccine, a technical reference to a new method of formulation—was licensed by the FDA for children 18 months of age or older, in whom it was clearly more effective than the polysaccharide vaccines; one year later, a second conjugate vaccine was licensed for the same age group.

A third such vaccine was licensed in December 1989, with the statement that it could be administered to children as young

as 15 months. The following spring the advisory committee revised its recommendations, advising routine immunization of all children at the age of 15 months, using any of the three conjugate vaccines.

Late in 1990, after further clinical testing, the FDA announced

---

There are three vaccines available to combat Hib infections; two of them have been approved for babies who are as young as two months of age.

---

approval of two of the three vaccines for babies as young as 2 months of age. This was especially good news, since about two-thirds of all cases of Hib disease have struck children under the age of 15 months.

Vaccination against Hib infection is now considered part of the routine childhood immunization schedule, and is accomplished with the following conjugate vaccines:
• HbOC (HibTITER), made by Praxis Biologics, distributed by Lederle Laboratories
• PRP-OMP (PedvaxHIB), made by Merck Sharp & Dohme
• PRP-D (ProHIBit), made by Connaught Laboratories, only for children at least 15 months old.

Hib vaccine can be given during doctor visits at the same time as other routine protectives—DTP (diphtheria-tetanus-pertussis), OPV (oral polio vaccine), and MMR (measles-mumps-rubella) and all children under 5 years should receive one of the vaccines.

No serious adverse reactions to any of the three vaccines have been reported. Minor reactions, which occur in only 1 to 4 percent of children, may include a

HIB VACCINE RECOMMENDATIONS

Three vaccines are currently licensed by FDA to protect children against infections caused by the bacterium *Hemophilus influenzae* type b (Hib). Prominent among those infections is bacterial meningitis, of which *H. influenzae* is the major cause.

One vaccine, PRP-D, has been approved only for children at least 15 months old. For younger infants, either of the others may be used; since it's not known whether or not they are safely and effectively interchangeable, physicians recommend that when a child is receiving two or more shots before the age of 15 months, the same product be used.

This schedule is recommended by CDC's Immunization Practices Advisory Committee:

Age at First Dose	Vaccine	Vaccination Schedule
2-6 months	HbOC (HibTITER)	three doses two months apart, plus booster shot at 15 months*
2-6 months	PRP-OMP (PedvaxHIB)	two doses two months apart, plus booster shot at 12 months
7-11 months	HbOC or PRP-OMP	two doses two months apart, plus booster shot at 15 months*
12-14 months	HbOC or PRP-OMP	one dose, plus booster shot at 15 months or later (at least two months after first dose)*
15 months +	HbOC, PRP-OMP, or PRP-D (ProHIBit)	one dose only

*Any of the three vaccines may be used for the 15-months shot.

slight elevation of temperature and a bit of redness and/or swelling around the site where the vaccine was injected.

Most older children and adults do not need Hib immunization, and the advisory committee has not issued specific recommendations except for small children. The committee cites studies, however, suggesting good immunogenicity (development of antibodies) in high-risk people given Hib vaccines. They include those with sickle cell disease, leukemia, and human immunodeficiency virus (HIV) infection, as well as persons who have had their spleens surgically removed.

Unresolved Questions

The use of three Hib vaccines has caused some confusion (for most other routine childhood immunizations only a single vaccine is used). Only two of the three Hib vaccines are recommended for administration to small babies—and they are to be given on different schedules.

"There are differences in antibody response between the two vaccines approved for 2-month-olds—how soon antibodies appear, how high their levels go, how long they last," explains Dr. Bascom F. Anthony, director of the division of bacterial products of the FDA's Center for Biologics Evaluation and Research. "But they are both highly effective, and both have been judged worthy of licensure. If something good comes along, and it's both safe and effective, it's likely to be approved."

The vaccines are given on different schedules, Anthony says, because approval is based on the way studies supporting a maker's claims were conducted: "The efficacy data supported the two schedules. But this," he notes, "had no influence on the timing of the booster dose; many children in the studies simply weren't old enough for a booster dose when the study ended. The booster recommendation is based on antibody levels. The evidence shows that when the PRP-OMP vaccine is given at 2 months and 4 months, antibodies may be dangerously low by 12 months, and so a booster is recommended at that age."

This issue and others were addressed at a recent U.S. National Institutes of Health workshop on Hib vaccination. A major question is whether or not the two vaccines approved for infants under 15 months are safely interchangeable—that is, if one brand is given at 2 months, can the same baby be given the other at 4 months? (Since the answer isn't known, it's now recommended that the same brand be used.) The workshop participants agreed that further research is needed, and studies to clarify the interchangeability and scheduling issues are being designed.

Meanwhile, all children should be receiving Hib vaccine. It is hoped that Hib meningitis will soon take its place in the medical history books, along with polio and diphtheria, as a disease unfondly remembered and, thankfully, rarely seen. □

> **Vaccination against Hib infections is now considered a routine childhood immunization; all children under five should receive one of the vaccines.**

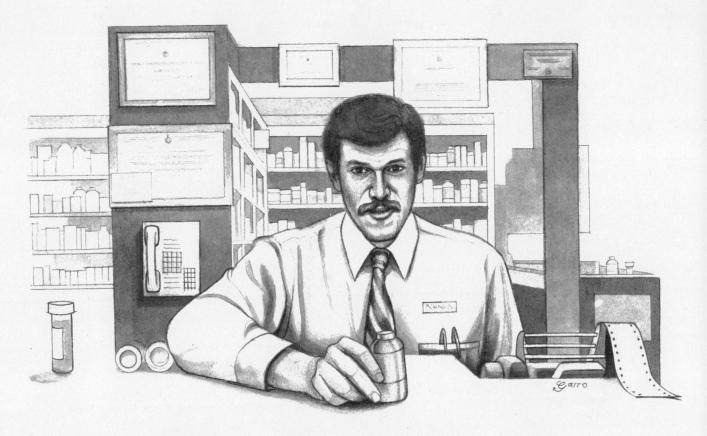

The Danger of Medication Mixups

Felicia E. Halpert

When our three-month-old daughter, Thalia, got sick for the first time several months ago, my husband and I dutifully gave her the antibiotic that our pediatrician had prescribed. He had diagnosed an ear infection and then had scribbled something on a prescription form. We drove directly to our local pharmacy, arriving just before closing time. A bottle of medicine was handed to us by the pharmacist, and that night we began administering it to Thalia.

Nearly a week later I raced back with Thalia to the doctor's office. The "antibiotic" had turned out to be a narcotic, an antidiarrheic drug for adults. "Is the child still breathing?" was the first response to my call to the local poison-control center. If we hadn't been dispensing a low dosage, my husband and I might unwittingly have fatally poisoned our daughter. A doctor's sloppy handwriting, a pharmacist's bad guess, and our own ignorance very nearly resulted in a nightmarish conclusion.

Mistakes Despite Precautions

Millions of prescriptions are written each year. A system of checks exists among doctors, nurses, and pharmacists, but it is not universally followed; nor is it foolproof. No one is perfect, and medical professionals are no exception to that rule. In a recent study reported in the *Journal of the American Medical Association,* physicians in a large teaching hospital were found to make, on average, two and a half errors every day in prescribing medication. Half of these errors were health-threatening to patients. The pro-

> **Millions of prescriptions are written every year, and although a system of checks does exist, mistakes still occur.**

fessional pharmaceutical journal *Drug Topics* reports that 13 percent of adult consumers say that they or a family member has at some time been adversely affected by receiving the wrong prescription medication, dosage information, or instructions.

Parents need to recognize the important role they play in preventing medication mishaps. We are the final checkpoint in the healthcare system, and we must be vigilant about monitoring what our children are taking and why. The error in Thalia's case could have been avoided—or rectified much earlier—if we had gotten better information from the doctor and pharmacist. We didn't because the hour was late, both men were hasty, and we wanted our daughter's misery to be relieved as quickly as possible.

"People are often passive about how they interact with medical professionals," says Richard Weisman, Pharm.D., director of New York City's Poison Control Center. "They should be encouraged to ask lots of questions." But often, parents are intimidated by health specialists who project an aura that blurs the line between knowledge and infallibility.

We were lucky: the dosage prescribed to Thalia resulted only in more frequent and longer naps,

not the overwhelming drowsiness and breathing stoppage that could have occurred. What lingered longer for us was the fear and guilt we felt about potentially harming our child.

Question Authority

Asking questions of a medical professional may make you feel awkward or as though you are wasting the doctor's or pharmacist's valuable time. But it is the only way that you can be certain your child is receiving the proper treatment. Get concrete answers to these questions:

1. What is the name of the medication? This is a basic, essential query that we neglected to ask the pediatrician. Certainly doctors should be responsible enough to provide this information, but if for any reason you're unsure or unclear about what's being prescribed, *ask.*

Since this was Thalia's first illness, we had no idea which types of children's antibiotics existed. And because we didn't know the name of the antibiotic that was prescribed, we could only assume that the bottle the pharmacist handed us contained the proper medicine. Head off potential tragedy before trouble begins— know exactly what you need. Keep in mind that drug names are often disturbingly similar and potentially confusing to a pharmacist who is having trouble reading the doctor's handwriting. The pharmacist is required to double-check with a physician if he has any questions regarding a prescription. It's critical that you receive the proper medication, not only because the wrong one can be harmful, but also because an illness can get worse if it's not being properly treated.

2. How does it work? Three-year-olds can drive their parents up the wall with the ceaseless question "Why?" Yet adults need to remember the value of critical questioning. It is important to understand why a particular medication is the right one for your

child. Make sure that the doctor's and pharmacist's explanations match. Learning how certain medicines work on the body helps you become more knowledgeable about your child's health and can help you interpret symptoms if something goes wrong.

Don't make assumptions about how the medicine should be administered. With medications, it is certainly true that everything has its proper place. One all too common mistake parents make, for example, is to treat an ear infection by putting a liquid antibiotic into their child's ear rather than her mouth.

3. In which form (pills, liquid, capsules) and strength will the medicine be dispensed? If the doctor tells you that he is prescribing a liquid medication and the pharmacist hands you a bottle of pills, you know there's a problem. The more specific the doctor can be about what the medicine looks like, the better. For example, the antidiarrheic medication we were given and the antibiotic that was prescribed both come in liquid form: one is a

> **Receiving the proper medication is critical; not only can the wrong one be harmful, an illness can get worse if it's not being properly treated.**

thin, clear liquid; the other is thick and pink. Had we known exactly what to look for, the error would have been easy for us to spot.

Many medications also come in different potencies, and you should read this information on your prescription form prior to handing it over to the pharmacist. Make sure that the strength noted on the form matches the one on the bottle you receive. Check refills to see whether they jibe with previous orders.

4. How often should the medicine be taken, and how large should the dosage be? Never guess about the amount or frequency of medication for your child. Medicinal benefits can turn tragic if you start playing around with dosages. Undermedicating may retard recovery; overmedicating can encourage or exacerbate side effects. Both the physician and the pharmacist should tell you how much of the medicine to dispense. The pharmacy's label on the bottle should also provide usage information. Question any inconsistencies in instructions. What saved Thalia was that we were giving her exactly the amount prescribed for the antibiotic, a dosage too low for the antidiarrheic to have really major repercussions.

When our suspicions began to grow, we checked the pharmacy's label, which contained the small-print statement, "Special Note: Use is contraindicated in children less than two years of age." A chart of recommended dosages for older children was listed.

5. When (such as at mealtime or before bedtime) should the medication be taken? Different medicines affect the body differently, and it is important to be aware of the optimal times for your child to take them. If you have the choice, it makes more sense, for example, for a medication that causes drowsiness to be given to your child at night rather than before she heads off to school.

6. How long should the medicine take to work? Know the time frame for seeing an improvement in your child's condition. If, after the appropriate amount of time, there has been little or no change, call your doctor. We had doubts about Thalia's medicine, but it was only after nearly a week had passed without seeing improvement in her condition that I asked a nurse friend about this particular "antibiotic." That's when I found out what we had actually been dispensing.

7. What possible side effects are there? You need to know what impact a medicine can have on your child. Awareness of potential side effects is the only way to monitor her safety. Some reactions aren't serious enough to warrant dropping a particular medication; others might mean that an allergenic response has set in or that your child's body has developed an intolerance to what is being administered.

Medications are generally accompanied by packaging information that lists possible side effects. The package insert that came with the antidiarrheic drug we were given included the warning "May cause drowsiness." Thalia, in fact, did sleep more. But we didn't realize that sleepiness is not one of the side effects of the antibiotic my daughter should have been taking.

Many people take time selecting a good physician but rarely consider their pharmacist's qualifications. Michael R. Cohen, who is adjunct associate professor at the Temple University School of Pharmacy in Philadelphia and co-founder of the Institute for Safe Medication Practices, in Huntingdon Valley, Pa., notes that we're "taught to shop around on price" when choosing a pharmacist, or else we pick whoever is closest to home or office. "But," he emphasizes, "there's also your health to consider."

All pharmacies are supposed to maintain patient profiles, and some states have passed laws requiring them. Such profiles include a medical history, a record of allergies, and a list of prescriptions and refills previously dispensed to the client. The pharmacist is doing an improper job if she doesn't ask any questions the first time you get a prescription filled. Look for a pharmacy where the pharmacist (and not a clerk) hands you the medicine, tells you its name and which disorder it's for, and explains exactly how to use it.

Cohen notes that some pharmacies now require their pharmacists to work under a quota system, filling a certain number of prescriptions per hour. This is a guaranteed stress enhancer that could increase the likelihood of the pharmacist's making mistakes.

If you think your child may be taking the wrong medication, call your doctor, pharmacist, or local poison-control center. Each of them can answer your questions about a particular medicine and what kind of impact it might have on your child.

Medical errors are serious, and they should be treated that way. Health professionals are required to be licensed, and organizations exist in every state to conduct investigations into fraud and malpractice. Review committees determine whether wrongdoing has occurred and whether the physician or the pharmacist should be fined or suspended or possibly even lose his license.

Don't have any qualms about wrecking someone's career by reporting an error. Severe penalties are meted out only when the person has a history of misconduct. If you never report an incident, the risk increases for other parents and children who are now using or will be using that person's services. □

PLAYING FOR TIME
LOU GEHRIG'S DISEASE

Bruce Dobkin, M.D.

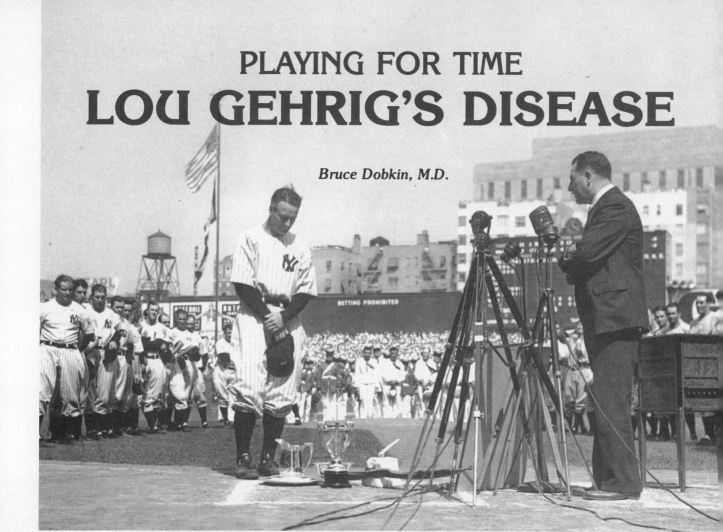

A ceremony honoring Lou Gehrig at Yankee Stadium in 1939, the year he retired because of ill health.

My seven-year-old twins made a tentative diagnosis. "Something's wrong with Sherry's daddy," one of them said. Their faces were earnest, their voices as wary as when they steel themselves to walk upstairs alone at night. "He sounds and walks funny," the other added. "Like a lobster."

They had seen him leaving a movie theater with his young daughter and son. When my children ran over to say hello to their schoolmates, my wife introduced herself. Bill, the father, did not seem self-conscious about his barely intelligible speech or his plodding gait, a stiff waddle that my wife associated with cerebral palsy or a stroke. When she mentioned Bill's name, I realized I knew this daddy. He had done his residency in medicine at the same hospital where I had trained in neurology. I had not seen him in 15 years.

My wife threw me a worried, interrogative look. I turned away from the kids, who were occupied

Amyotrophic lateral sclerosis, also called Lou Gehrig's disease after the ballplayer, is a nerve disease for which there is no cure.

with the cookie jar. "Your medical team hasn't given me enough data," I said, trying to end any speculation, but her worried look persisted. "It sounds serious," I said, under my breath. I was tempted to phone Bill, but I hesitated to intrude on his privacy. Instead, I put my wife on the case.

A few days later she bumped into Bill's wife, Caroline, at a school fund-raiser. At a quiet moment, she mentioned seeing him with the children. "It really tires him out, but he insists on being involved with the kids," Caroline said with a cracking voice. My wife asked if there was anything she could do. "I can't talk about it," Caroline sobbed. "It's been so hard." Almost

187

pleading, she asked, "Could Bill call your husband? He needs . . . we both need someone who has taken care of people with ALS." My wife, who had listened to my anguish as I watched my patients with this disease dwindle and die, immediately understood all too much about their future. Amyotrophic lateral sclerosis, also called Lou Gehrig's disease after the ballplayer who died from it, is a nerve disease with no cure. Many people are now familiar with it as the devastating disease that afflicts Stephen Hawking, the British physicist who wrote *A Brief History of Time*.

Downhill Turn

Several weeks later I received a call from Bill. I arranged to examine him on one of the days that my neurological rehabilitation clinic is held. It would give him and Caroline a chance to meet the nurse and therapists who would try to extend his ability to care for himself.

Bill greeted me like an old friend. He wore what could have been the same gray cardigan sweater I recalled from our hectic days as residents. It made him seem more mature then. He had been one of the steadiest, most compulsive young docs on the house staff. Now he seemed

The disease causes a degeneration of the nerve cells in the spinal cord and the brain that connect to the body's muscles via extensions called axons.

quite professorial; indeed, he had made a good name for himself as a researcher at a nearby university medical center.

Bill recounted his downhill turn with a doctor's clinical precision.

Almost a year ago, several co-workers in his laboratory kept asking whether he had a cold that he could not shake off. His speech had become nasal, like that of someone with a stuffy nose. He realized that he had been tiring easily, especially climbing stairs.

As the nerve cells they are connected to die, the muscles gradually waste away; nerve cells for the senses and for such functions as language are not affected.

Several months later he noticed telltale twitches over his shoulders and chest as he shaved in front of the bathroom mirror. These brief waves of flutters under the skin are fasciculations, unwilled contractions of tiny bundles of muscle fibers. While we all get an occasional repetitive twitch of a fatigued muscle, usually around the eye, Bill's were diffuse and unstopping, typical of what happens when muscles lose their nerve supply. A number of minor annoyances suddenly made sense to him: It now took a grunting effort to stand up from his couch. His voice had never cleared. His typing speed had slowed. His tennis racket kept slipping out of his hand when he hit the ball outside the sweet spot. Several times he had lost his grip on his children as he lifted them overhead.

Bill became convinced that he was suffering from ALS, a degeneration of the motor neurons, the nerve cells within the spinal cord and brain that send their elongated extensions, called axons, out to the muscles of the body. As these motor neurons die, the muscles they connect with gradually waste away as well. Neurons for the senses, such as vision and

touch, are not affected by this disease, nor are those involved in cognitive functions such as language and intellect. So the victim remains a lucid witness as the painless disease nibbles away at his body until paralysis and infection steal his breath and his life. Within the past eight months Bill had seen two neurologists, both of whom had confirmed his self-diagnosis.

In the meantime, though, his level of activity had continued to plummet.

"He's had to move into a downstairs bedroom because he can't handle the stairs," Caroline told me. "Two weeks ago, he fell in the bathroom after we had gone to bed. He was stuck between the toilet and tub until we found him in the morning. His forehead was bloody." She couldn't hold back her tears.

"I stopped the bleeding," he added, as if to reassure her that it was a minor mishap and every-

A virus may be to blame for the disease, or a mistaken reaction of the immune system, or even environmental toxins.

thing was under control. "The door was stuck closed, and when I pulled, it gave way and I fell."

I listened with increasing sadness. "Let me examine you," I said.

Bill pushed off the armchair with his hands, swayed a moment until his balance was assured, and walked to the exam table with a stiff-legged gait, landing more on the ball than the heel of each foot with every step. As I gently flexed and extended the joints at his hips and knees, I appreciated the muscle stiffness, called spasticity, that accounted for his pecu-

> **One in every 10,000 adults dies from Lou Gehrig's disease, and although there are exceptions, most patients die within five years.**

liar gait. His voice was soft, nasal, a bit breathless. The soft palate and tongue, both of which play a role in sounding words clearly, were weak. When I tested the strength in his shoulder muscles, Caroline's eyes again filled with tears. It was all too obvious that when I pushed down on his outstretched arms, the resistance he offered was far less than it should have been.

What Is Known

Bill had reviewed the medical literature on ALS, and he brought along reprints of some of the articles. Most were about efforts to find the causes of the disease. Five percent of cases are thought to be hereditary (but this was unlikely in Bill's case; no one in his family had ever been known to have ALS). Some studies have suggested that the neuronal damage can be caused by a virus or even inflicted by a misdirected immune system. Other epidemiological studies have found possible associations with environmental toxins, such as lead or mercury. On the Pacific island of Guam large outbreaks of a type of ALS have occurred among people who ground the seed of a local palm, *Cycas circinalis*, for food. No matter where they live, though, one in every 10,000 adults dies from ALS. And although there are exceptions like Stephen Hawking, most patients die within five years.

Rarely, someone who meets every criterion for ALS stops deteriorating after a year or two, as if the disease has been stalled. And

in fact, I'd had such a case, but Bill found no comfort in extraordinary cases and had no faith in experimental attempts to treat ALS. What he and Caroline wanted was my ear, my concern, and any practical help to prolong his independence in the hope that, maybe, some more promising treatment might yet turn up.

Coping

I talked with the therapists, and we set a plan to improve the intelligibility of his speech and work on his strength and balance. Before the couple left, I asked them to look into his disability and health insurance policies, to determine whether they paid for nursing care in the home. I did not wish to inject defeatism, but I had to begin to help them prepare.

Bill came alone two weeks later. I broached the decisions that would eventually have to be made. If he could no longer swallow without gagging, would he accept a feeding tube placed into his stomach? If tests showed that he was heading for respiratory failure, would he accept a tracheostomy, a tube in his windpipe connected to a mechanical ventilator? I looked for a sign—a shrug, something in his voice—that might tell me how far I should go to preserve his life when time caught up with us.

He paused. "If I was older, I wouldn't want to live on a respirator. But I really want to see the new millennium, see my kids finish high school in the class of 2000. Right now, I've got to believe that maybe I'll survive and know how they turn out." In Bill's sober face I envisioned other people with ALS. One man I'd known had somehow hung on for ten years, the last five hooked to a respirator. Remarkably, even when he appeared to be little more than a skeleton in a wheelchair, able only to blink his eyes, he seemed to cherish his participation in his family's life.

I also recalled an attorney I'd treated the year before. He had

given me a copy of his living will, adamantly stating that he would not allow a doctor to place him on a respirator. He worsened over the next six months, requiring the equivalent of a portable iron lung to sit in a wheelchair or sleep. Yet when his breathing deteriorated even further, faced with the imminence of death, he surprised me by letting the pulmonary specialist hospitalize him and connect him to a respirator.

The next day, when I came to see him, he wrote on a pad with his atrophied hand: "This was a mistake. I want to be off this machine." He repeated his wish to die to his wife and sons, who pressed us to abide by his choice. Quietly the pulmonary doctor and I disconnected our patient from the ventilator. When his breath-

> **In rare cases a patient stops deteriorating after a year or two, as if the disease had somehow been stalled in its tracks.**

ing deteriorated, we gave him a sedative. He died in several hours, as he had chosen.

Many difficult decisions loom ahead for Bill and Caroline. For the moment he pursues his research, and she fills her days with volunteer projects. Their minds are kept busy by the duties and gratifications of living. In the past three months of therapy Bill has reached something of a plateau. As a friend and a fellow father I try to share in the optimism he finds in not seeing himself go downhill too fast.

And when the frightening moment finally arrives—when the threat of death by suffocation can no longer be held back—I know Bill's family and doctors will be there to support his choice. That is what we are here for. ☐

Speak Up to Your Doctor

Marvin M. Lipman, M.D.

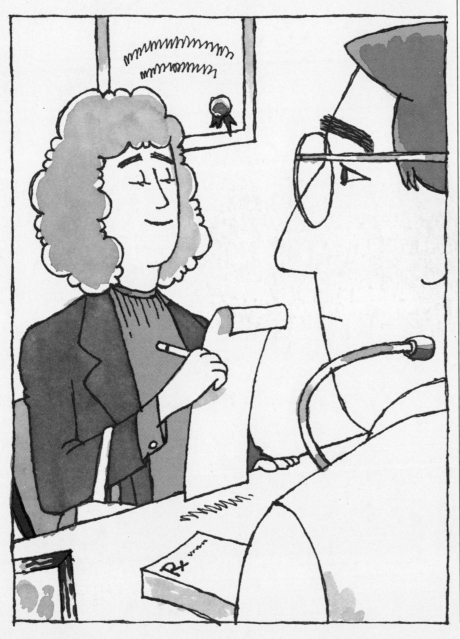

Are you satisfied with your doctor? If so, you're like most people. One survey found that even though people complain about the healthcare system in general, most are satisfied with their own physician. But the fact that you trust or feel comfortable with your doctor doesn't necessarily mean you're getting the best possible care.

A long-time patient of mine, a 48-year-old accountant, always insists that I take charge. I have to draw his symptoms out of him. Whenever I offer a choice of treatments, he smiles and says, "You're the doctor, you tell me." He generally seems quite satisfied with my care and has referred many patients to me over the years. On one recent visit, however, he seemed uncomfortable.

A month earlier, I had prescribed a diuretic to lower his elevated blood pressure. But the pressure stayed high. I asked him about his use of the medication. After several evasive answers, he blurted out that he'd stopped taking it because it made him tired. When I asked why he hadn't called me, he said he'd been reluctant to complain about a drug I'd recommended. He thought it might hurt my feelings.

While it's important to be satisfied with your doctor, satisfaction does not guarantee good health. In fact, one study found that satisfied patients were actually less healthy than dissatisfied ones. And in my experience, satisfied patients are no more likely to comply—for example, to take their medications or stick with their special diet—than dissatisfied patients.

A Compliant Patient

But it's also not enough just to comply with your doctor's orders. Consider this case: A 53-year-old teacher was started on hormone therapy by her gynecologist to help prevent osteoporosis and heart disease. Shortly thereafter, she became nervous, irritable, and

190

unable to sleep. The gynecologist, concerned that she might have an overactive thyroid, referred her to me.

Tests ruled out hyperthyroidism. Reassured that she had no serious disorder, the woman confided the source of her anxiety. A close friend had died recently of breast cancer. When the woman's gynecologist mentioned that hormone therapy might pose a small risk of the disease, she became frightened. But the gynecologist had made the therapy seem so important that she just took the pills and kept her fears to herself.

The woman's unquestioning compliance had not only kept her from discussing her fears but also from asking questions. Such questions might have led her gynecologist to reconsider the hormone prescription. Or they might have led the woman to seek a second opinion.

I suggested we measure her bone density and blood-cholesterol levels. The results, combined with her medical history, showed no need for hormone

While it's important to be satisfied with your doctor, satisfaction alone does not guarantee the best care.

treatment. I urged her to increase her calcium intake and to keep exercising.

The Active Patient

In both of those cases, the problem was a reluctance to speak up. In an elaborate series of recent studies, patients were taught to play a more active role with their doctor. The studies were the first experimental test of the idea that such active participation might actually improve patients' health.

Researchers from Boston's New England Medical Center pooled data from four separate trials, in-

volving a total of more than 250 patients who had either ulcers, high blood pressure, diabetes, or breast cancer. All of the patients were assigned to an experimental group or a control group. The breast-cancer patients were assigned according to when they showed up at the hospital; the others were assigned randomly.

In the experimental group, specially trained research assistants coached patients just before two separate office visits. To get patients involved in their own care, the assistants showed them the medical record of their previous office visit, identified issues that patients may not have understood the last time, and urged them to ask the doctor to explain.

The assistants described various treatment options and encouraged patients to inquire about those options during the visit and to negotiate the decision. They also emphasized that patients were free to bring up anything related to their problem, including its impact on their everyday activities or on their emotional, sexual, or family life. To help patients overcome their reluctance to speak out, the assistants had them rehearse their questions and negotiation strategies aloud.

In the control group, the assistants gave patients only general information about their disease.

Not surprisingly, patients who were urged to be more assertive obtained more information from their doctors. More important, the coached patients had significantly better outcomes. They reported fewer limitations in what they could do and better overall health. They also did better on the two objective measures that were taken: The coached patients with hypertension had lower blood pressure than the controls; and those with diabetes had lower blood sugar.

Becoming an Active Patient

Active, outspoken patients, who ask for explanations, seek infor-

Patients taught how to be more assertive with their doctors responded better to treatment; they reported fewer limitations on what they could do and better health.

mation, and aren't reluctant to get second opinions are usually less afraid of their disease and more determined to fight it. And they do indeed seem to do better than their passive counterparts. Here are some ways to become a more active patient:

• Don't worry that asking questions or expressing your reservations about treatment will annoy or disappoint the physician. You've come to the office to care for your health, not to please your doctor. If the doctor refuses to address your questions or reservations, consider asking another physician.

• Prepare for your office visit by writing down the key features of your problem and the questions you want to ask. If you tend to feel shy or nervous with the doctor, rehearse the questions at home and then again in the waiting room.

• Ask about the reasons for tests and X rays and about their meaning and accuracy; about the risks and benefits of treatment; and about the side effects of medications and their possible interactions with other drugs or with food or drink. Be sure you understand everything the doctor says. If the terms are too technical, request a translation.

• Ask for written information about your disorder. Or read about it at the library. Knowing about your problem will help you assert yourself in the doctor's office. And the more you know, the more intelligently you're apt to follow—or question—your doctor's advice. ☐

CONSTIPATION

Stephen E. Goldfinger, M.D.

The most common gastro-intestinal complaint in the United States, constipation occasions 2.5 million visits to the doctor every year. And, according to one recent estimate, it induces a national expenditure of $400 million on laxatives annually. Yet despite the magnitude of the problem, it is not an easy one to define.

Among a group of people surveyed in the mid-1980s, straining to pass feces was the symptom most frequently linked to constipation (52 percent). Other symptoms were cited less commonly: hard stools (44 percent), inability to defecate when the desire is present (34 percent), infrequent bowel movements (32 percent), and abdominal discomfort associated with defecation (20 percent). Of course, as the percentages indicate, these complaints often occur together.

In thinking about constipation, physicians and researchers tend to focus on the frequency of defecation as the crux of the matter. There is probably more than one reason for linking the medical definition of constipation to frequency of bowel movement. If nothing else, it is the easiest aspect of constipation to quantify (although not as easy as one might think). Also, when frequency diminishes there may be a serious medical problem warranting further investigation.

Even so, the importance of regularity to health has been greatly overestimated in Western culture for at least 3,500 years. The Egyptians associated feces with decay, by which they were obsessed and horrified, and they therefore placed laxatives (including dried fruit, castor oil, and senna), suppositories, and enemas high on their list of therapeutic agents.

As recently as the 1930s, Sir William Arbuthnot Lane championed the notion that feces retained in the colon would release

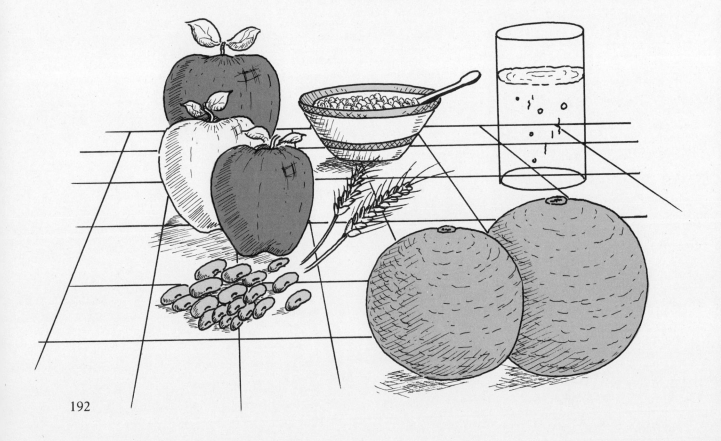

192

toxins into the system, leading to "autointoxication" and thus symptoms ranging from falling hair to premature senility. Lane was enormously influential in his time and no doubt persuaded the mothers or grandmothers of many of our readers that a bowel movement a day, more or less, is essential to good health.

The reality is different. Many adults defecate less than once a day and do fine. Around 1 of every 200 healthy adults has fewer than three bowel movements a week. It is also true, however, that such infrequent defecation is likely to be associated with a sense of bloating, distension, or other lower abdominal discomfort. Some people also link fatigue, achiness, and mental torpor to the sensation of retained feces. In general, defecation occurring anywhere from three times a week to three times a day is considered to be normal and not, in itself, anything to worry about.

The Kinds of Constipation

For practical purposes constipation can be divided into five main categories.

Normal Bowel Habits That Change Temporarily. Function may be disrupted during travel, in the aftermath of diarrhea from a viral infection, or by a change in activity level or diet. For some women constipation is a premenstrual symptom, and it is often a problem in pregnancy, perhaps because the colon reacts to the change in the level of sex hormones. There is, however, no direct evidence that this is the case.

Irritable Bowel Syndrome (Spastic Colon). Diarrhea and constipation often alternate in this condition; crampy pains, gassiness, and variation in the consistency of stool are other common features. Although it can produce lifelong symptoms, irritable bowel syndrome is not a dangerous condition. It is mainly associated with stress, but there is neither a

SOME CAUSES OF CONSTIPATION

Metabolic disturbances can lead to constipation. Among the most common are a high level of calcium or a low level of thyroid hormone. Diabetes or kidney failure can also cause constipation. Dehydration frequently contributes to constipation in elderly persons. In people of any age, sluggish bowel movements can be a sign of depression.

Severe discomfort at or near the anus can create enough spasm to hamper the evacuation of stool. Typically, the pain-spasm cycle is set off by a thrombosed hemorrhoid, a tender fissure (a raw slit in the skin), or a pocket of infection.

A cancer obstructing the lower bowel is the most worrisome possibility. Even if typical clues (blood in the feces, severe cramping, a tender, distended abdomen, and markedly narrowed stools) are absent, this diagnosis cannot be dismissed unless a proctoscopic examination or a barium enema has given assurance that there is no blockage.

Sometimes constipation results from medication. Calcium supplements are a common cause. Antacids with aluminum or calcium, antidepressants, diuretics, iron supplements, opiates, antipsychotic drugs in the phenothiazine group, and any of the many drugs with so-called anticholinergic effects can bring on constipation in colons that would otherwise function normally.

A very small minority of patients are constipated because nerves that would normally regulate bowel activity have been destroyed. Someone with a spinal-cord injury, for example, can neither sense a distended rectum nor initiate maneuvers to empty it. Other neurological causes include amyotrophic lateral sclerosis, multiple sclerosis, and Parkinson's disease. In a congenital condition known as Hirschsprung's disease, normal propulsion of feces is impossible because nerves within the bowel are missing.

known cause nor a detectable abnormality in the structure of the colon.

Laxative Habituation. People who have used laxatives for a long time come to rely on them for both psychological and physiological reasons. Some laxatives apparently can damage nerve cells in the wall of the colon. When this happens, the force of contraction is diminished and constipation is inevitable.

Symptom or Side Effect. Sometimes newly developed constipation can be a symptom of underlying disease or a side effect of a drug. If the basic problem can be

> **It is the most common digestive system problem in the United States and leads to 2½ million visits to the doctor every year.**

relieved, then the constipation goes away.

Chronic, Severe Constipation. Some people experience constipation as an isolated difficulty that persists for years or decades. It may fail to respond despite reasonable efforts to change diet and adjust toilet habits.

Chronic Constipation

The label "chronic constipation" is applied to several different conditions, which have only recently been distinguished from one another. A relatively simple procedure has helped to sort out the possibilities: the patient or research subject swallows about 20 small markers that show up on an X ray. At intervals during the following week, an image of the abdomen is made, and then the number and location of the markers are noted. Areas of slowing can be detected in this way. Studies using markers to determine transit time through the intestine have identified four types of abnormality and one paradox.

• The markers may move slowly

through the entire colon. When a bowel movement finally does occur, the feces are bulky and soft. This type of sluggishness, known as colonic inertia, is due to feeble contraction of smooth muscle in the wall of the colon. Possible causes for colonic inertia include diseases that injure nerves or suppress their activity; certain drugs; and prolonged overuse of stimulant laxatives, which destroys nerves in the colon wall. The condition can also occur for no known reason; perhaps there is a subtle disturbance in regulation by the nerves that control the bowel or an imbalance of hormones and other chemicals that help coordinate the colon's movements.

• The markers may move normally at first, then slow down considerably in the descending colon. The basic disorder appears to be

More fiber, plenty of water, and moderate exercise are the best answers to many cases of constipation.

similar to colonic inertia but is confined to the final portions of the intestine. This is known as hindgut dysfunction.

• The markers can move normally through the entire intestine, only to become delayed in the rectum. If the defecation reflex is inadequate, quite a large volume of feces may be required before an urge is felt. Normally, the optimal amount of stool to trigger the

defecation reflex is about 200 grams; the low-fiber diets typical of Western societies more typically produce stools averaging around 130 grams. Thus, lack of stool mass, either alone or in addition to inadequate rectal response, may contribute to accumulation of stool in the rectum.

Habitual disregard of the defecatory urge can lead to diminished rectal sensation and inadequate emptying. Over time, the rectum becomes so habituated to being stretched by feces that it fails to respond. Feces back up somewhat into the colon, which registers discomfort yet cannot empty itself.

• The markers may accumulate in the rectum not because the rectum itself is incapable of responding appropriately but because the outlet to the anus is obstructed. There appear to be two principle causes of pelvic outlet obstruction. In some cases the muscles surrounding the anus are incapable of relaxing to permit passage of feces. In others the problem appears to be an overly sharp angle between the colon and the rectum acting to retain feces, even though rectal contractions are about normal.

The Paradox

Studies of transit time through the colon have also produced one rather surprising finding. For several years Arnold Wald of the University of Pittsburgh School of Medicine has been investigating people who complain of chronic severe constipation that has no apparent cause outside the colon itself. These patients report having fewer than two bowel movements a week for a period of at least six months and as long as 25-50 years.

In two of Dr. Wald's studies, markers moved normally through—and disappeared from—the colons approximately one-third of such patients. As Dr. Wald commented when reporting this discovery in 1986, "These patients may have consciously or

SOME BASIC FACTS

Most of the work of digesting and absorbing food is completed in the small intestine. A slurry of fluid and indigestible particles passes from the small to the large intestine at their junction in the lower right corner of the abdomen. The material is then moved along the ascending segment of the colon by a series of slow, churning motions. In this phase, fluid and minerals are normally reabsorbed, so that only a small amount of each is lost in the feces. In diarrhea this recycling process is disrupted, and replacement of fluid and salts becomes very important.

Although our own digestive process ceases at the end of the small intestine, food continues to be processed in the colon by the bacteria normally present there. Compounds such as cellulose, indigestible to humans, are easily used by these bacteria as an energy source. In the process, the bacteria release various substances. Hydrogen gas and sulfur-containing compound may contribute to flatulence. Less conspicuously, small fatty acids released by bacterial digestion can be absorbed by the host and used as a very minor source of energy.

In the transverse segment of the colon, feces become formed. Bacteria constitute about a third of the fecal solids, undigested material another third. The remainder comprises sloughed material from the intestine and other components. Increasingly compact, feces are now propelled down the descending segment toward the rectum by periodic, firm contractions. When the mass reaches the rectum, the last segment of the colon, it is retained until a sufficient volume has accumulated to trigger the defecation reflex. In the interim, two factors prevent soiling. A ring of muscles at the anus—the internal sphincter—is kept tightly closed by its natural tendency to contract. In addition, there is an angle between the anus and rectum, maintained by tension in a muscle, the puborectalis, which pulls forward on the junction of the two. This arrangement serves as a partial valve to retain the feces.

When sufficient feces have accumulated, a new set of reflexes is triggered, relaxing the internal sphincter and signaling the urge to defecate. It is possible to override the urge by consciously constricting the external sphincter, a group of muscles under voluntary control that surround the anus. The internal sphincter ordinarily will not relax again for several hours, however. If the process of active resistance is repeated once or twice, stool may become increasingly dry and hard, and constipation is almost inevitable.

unconsciously misrepresented their bowel habits; documenting normal colonic transit enabled their physicians to reeducate them concerning normal bowel function and to curtail further diagnostic studies." In subsequent research, reported in 1989, Dr. Wald and his colleagues found that constipated patients with normal evacuation time "manifest a very high frequency of psychological distress"—with evidence of anxiety, depression, or somatization (the tendency to identify emotional discomfort as a bodily complaint).

Remedies

How to treat constipation depends very much on its type, severity, and duration. Even persistent constipation often responds to relatively simple measures. Under most circumstances the use of laxatives should be regarded as the last resort.

People with essentially normal bowel function who are going through a period of transitory discomfort can probably help themselves most effectively by increasing their dietary fiber intake, drinking plenty of water, and making sure they get moderate amounts of exercise.

There is substantial evidence that dietary fiber increases the bulk of the stool, softens it, and speeds transit time in an otherwise-normal bowel. On the other hand, there is really not much evidence that fiber has a similar effect in chronic constipation. There are two kinds of dietary fiber, both of which may prove to be helpful.

So-called *insoluble* fiber, such as wheat bran, has long been thought to work by adding bulk to the stool (because it is not easily digested by either people or bacteria) and by holding water. This explanation has, however, been challenged by Janet Tomlin and Nicholas W. Read at the Royal Hallamshire Hospital in Sheffield, England. In a study of 12 normal subjects, they provided supplements of either coarse bran or

---

ORAL LAXATIVES

All laxatives increase the bulk and water content of stool as well as soften it, although they probably achieve these effects in different ways. The following categorization is traditional but may need to be revised as these agents come to be better understood.

Bulk-forming agents are thought to be safe to take indefinitely on a daily basis.
• bran (in food and supplements)
• psyllium (many brand names)
• methyl cellulose (Citrucel, Cologel)

Stool softeners should be used sparingly and for short periods. As the name implies, they do merge with feces and soften their consistency, but they can have other effects on the body.
• mineral oil—use discouraged because it reduces absorption of fat-soluble vitamins and can produce lung damage if accidentally inhaled
• docusate (Colace, Dialose, Surfak, others)—may increase toxicity of other drugs taken at the same time; potential for liver damage has been cited

Osmotic agents are salts or carbohydrates that promote secretion of water into the colon. They are reasonably safe, even with prolonged use, but probably promote dependency.
• lactulose (Cephulac, Chonulac, Duphalac)
• sorbitol—much less expensive than lactulose and equally effective
• milk of magnesia, citrate of magnesia, Epsom salts

Chemical stimulants can lead to dependency and may damage the bowel with daily use for months or years.
• bisacodyl (Dulcolax)
• casanthrol (included in Dialose Plus, Peri-Colace)
• cascara (included in Nature's Remedy)
• castor oil (Neoloid, Purge)
• phenolphthalein (Correctol, Ex-Lax, Modane, others; included in Feen-A-Mint)
• senna (Fletcher's Castoria, Senokot, others)

---

plastic flakes milled to the same dimensions. The two substances had identical effects, including an increase of stool weight by more than double the amount of undigestible material (fiber or plastic)

---

consumed. Tomlin and Read concluded that mechanical stimulation of nerves in the bowel lining accounts for the effect of both plastic and bran. Indeed, coarse bran is a laxative, but fine bran is not. Their results are also consistent with those of two studies reporting that applesauce is no more laxative than apple juice, and peanut butter no better than peanut oil. In both studies, as K. W. Heaton of the Bristol Royal Infirmary has pointed out, the fiber "was all there in a chemical sense—but it was well nigh gone in a physical sense, like a violin that has been stamped on."

Soluble fiber, such as psyllium or the pectins in fruit, is known to swell with retained water, and this is thought to be the main reason for its stool-bulking and softening effect. But the story may be more complicated; some soluble fiber is digested by colon bacteria, which then help to increase fecal mass.

Although psyllium is sold in packages at drug stores, it is for all intents and purposes a dietary supplement. It can be taken for a lifetime without ill effects (except in rare instances of allergy, which can presumably develop from inhaling minute amounts of the powder).

Fluid intake reduces the need for the colon to dehydrate stools and is, in any case, harmless. So is exercise, which has a good reputation for regularity, although the evidence in support of it is slim. S. A. Bingham and J. H. Cummings, researchers at the Dunn Clinical Nutrition Centre at Cambridge University in England, carefully studied the bowel function of research subjects during a physical training program. They reported in 1989 that 14 healthy but sedentary men and women became physically more fit at the end of a seven- to nine-week training schedule, but no consistent change in bowel function could be detected.

Bowel retraining may provide relief for people who have gotten into the habit of ignoring the urge.

PRUNES AND CONSTIPATION

The common belief that prunes help maintain regularity has some, but limited, scientific support. Over half a century ago, Dr. George Emerson at the University of California in San Francisco investigated prune extract and discovered that a very dilute preparation stimulated contractions of rabbit intestines. This finding suggested that the active ingredient in prunes was a chemical, not just fiber. In the early 1960s researchers at Boston University School of Medicine confirmed the observation in patients whose intestinal drainage had been diverted to an ileostomy bag. Because of this arrangement, the daily output of fluid from the intestine could be measured after various foods were given. Of all of them, prune juice was by far the most potent in increasing the volume of fluid entering the collecting bag. A similar study conducted in 1987 has confirmed the effectiveness of prune juice in stimulating intestinal fluid output.

Many people rely on prunes to maintain regularity, believing that a "natural" remedy is better than a drugstore product. But it is not clear how different prunes are from over-the-counter laxatives. The active ingredient in prune juice is not known and is a matter of controversy. In 1951 three researchers at the Harrower Laboratory in St. Louis, Mo., reported an analysis of prunes. They found a compound resembling oxyphenisatin, a laxative drug. According to the California Prune Board, however, subsequent attempts to isolate such a compound from their product have failed. This work, said to have been done at the Sun Diamond Growers and at the University of California at Davis, appears not to have been published.

If a substance like oxyphenisatin is present, it could well be the critical ingredient in prunes and prune juice. This agent was used in laxatives in the United States for many years until it was discovered to cause liver damage and was taken off the market. A close chemical relative, phenolphthalein, is the stimulant cathartic in Ex-Lax, Correctol, and Modane, among other over-the-counter laxatives.

Existing evidence indicates that, at the very least, prune juice contains something that stimulates contraction of the intestinal wall and increases secretion of fluid. That substance has not yet been clearly identified.

The need for more research is apparent. It is unlikely that moderate consumption would cause any problems, but prune use, like everything else, should be prudent.

If a tight schedule has produced a tight sphincter, it may help to sit on a toilet, book in hand, for about 20 minutes each morning to encourage a return of reflexes that have disappeared. Straining, however, is not recommended, since it may lead to tightening of muscles that should be relaxed for comfortable defecation. When severe spasm of pelvic muscles prevents defecation, biofeedback training may be effective.

Stimulant laxatives contain chemicals that act directly or indirectly on the intestine to increase the secretion of water into the interior. Some of them also elicit more vigorous contractions from the colon. Using them daily over a period of months can lead to a flabby, inert colon that will always need a chemical fix.

Rectal suppositories are helpful in providing lubrication and in stimulating the defecation reflex. They are usually composed of glycerin, which is sometimes blended with sodium stearate, a fatty acid. Bisacodyl-containing suppositories have added potency because they act directly on the bowel to stimulate emptying.

Enemas usually become attractive only when oral laxatives cannot do the job. Introducing water into the colon helps to stimulate defecation. "Disposable" enemas deliver a solution of highly concentrated, nonabsorbable salts into the rectum and sigmoid colon. These salts attract an outpouring of fluid into the bowel and thus promote bowel contraction. Oil-containing enemas are sometimes recommended as softeners for feces that have become hardened within the rectum.

Can Surgery Help?

A few people with severe constipation remain plagued by bloating, pain, and failure to pass a stool for intervals of a month or longer. Patient and doctor alike may then consider the most drastic intervention: surgically removing the colon. Sacrificing the large bowel and connecting the small intestine directly to the rectum might be expected to solve the problem of constipation. Unfortunately, as a solution, surgery is far from perfect.

In 1988 a group of surgeons at St. Marks Hospital in London reported on the experience of 44 women who had their colons removed as a treatment for severe chronic constipation. Thirty-nine percent of them wound up with persistent diarrhea, and 11 percent continued to suffer from constipation. Persistent abdominal pain still plagued 70 percent of those who had complained of it before surgery. Additional surgery was necessary to diagnose or rectify lasting symptoms in 39 percent, and even then success was not guaranteed. Four of the women developed severe psychiatric disturbances after surgery. In light of these results, surgery should be regarded as a last resort, even for people with severe constipation that is not caused by a demonstrated anatomical abnormality. "Nevertheless," says Arnold Wald, a gastroenterologist at the University of Pittsburgh, "in appropriately selected patients who undergo careful evaluation, clinical results can be much better than these." □

> **The widely held belief that prunes and prune juice help maintain regularity has only limited scientific support.**

Getting Through Grief

Laura Fraser

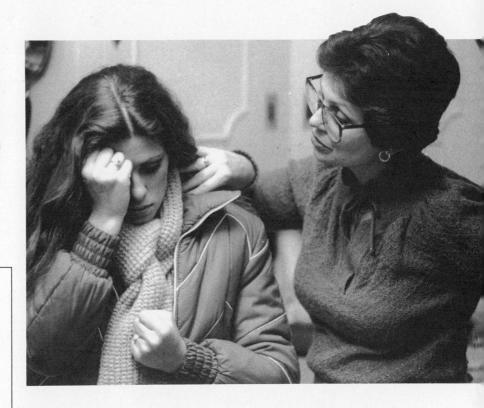

Hermione Davis, a retired Connecticut social worker with two grown children, knew for more than a year that her husband, not yet 50, was likely to die of a brain tumor. But that didn't make the reality of losing him any easier. "You can know intellectually that someone you love is going to die," she says, "but when it actually happens, it's still a shock."

Although grief is one of the most common of human emotions, most people who haven't gone through it themselves don't understand it very well.

"I don't think most people are aware of the extent of the trauma," says Anne Rosberger, executive director of the Bereavement and Loss Center of New York. "It's mental, it's emotional, it's physical, and it takes your whole being."

Psychotherapists say there is no way to prepare for the full impact of the death of a loved one, or for the ensuing tremors of anger, sadness, and longing that will be felt for years. But there is a growing body of advice on ways to work through grief once it hits.

The Stages of Grief

Grieving is now most often described as a succession of stages, first outlined by Elisabeth Kübler-Ross in her pioneering work *On Death and Dying*. But while the stages of grief may be somewhat predictable, our passage through them isn't. Most psychologists agree that grief proceeds at an individual pace.

The first stage is usually numbness and denial, when it seems as if the death just can't be real and the world feels distorted. "I felt like I was walking through pea soup," says Massachusetts psychologist Judith Souweine, whose mother died suddenly of a brain aneurysm at age 63. "I remember not wanting to get up in the morning, not wanting to remember that this had happened."

After the initial shock and denial, mourners may pass in and out of phases of anger, helplessness, depression, guilt, and fear. "I felt absolute rage," remembers Hermione Davis. "It wasn't fair. Why me? Why him?" Bouts of these emotions may last for a year or two—or even longer—before the person left behind finally comes to a stage of adjustment and acceptance.

"People are often afraid that they're losing control because these feelings are so strong and foreign to them," says John Stephenson, a family therapist in Portland, Me., and author of *Death, Grief, and Mourning*. Survivors may feel intense guilt for things they failed to do or say to the person who died, or somehow blame themselves for the death, endlessly running over the "what ifs." Hallucinations of the loved one, or even suicidal thoughts, are not uncommon. Those who have lost a mate often feel helpless, unable to take on the smallest tasks, or can feel that life isn't worth living.

Losing a Child

Perhaps the most difficult kind of death to overcome is the death of a child. "We expect our grandparents, and eventually our parents, to die, but we don't expect to outlive our children," says Therese Goodrich, executive director of The Compassionate Friends, a nationwide organization of support groups for bereaved parents and siblings. "The death of a child is out of synch, and it often takes up to five years for parents to start feeling normal again."

Children and Grief

Children who lose parents also require special understanding and help, say people who specialize in working with youngsters. Clear communication is the first step. If, for example, children hear that a parent has been "lost," they may wonder when the parent will be "found." Youngsters often believe, magically, that they've caused the death by something they've done or not done, and adults need to explain that they aren't at fault. Children usually heal well from grief, say psychologists, as long as parents and adults don't get in the way and tell them how they ought to do it.

Grief and Health

For young and old alike, grief can be physical as well as emotional. Peter Niland, an executive assistant for San Francisco's Shanti Project, which works with people with AIDS and their companions, remembers how sick he felt after his lover of 13 years died. "The depression affected me physically, through exhaustion, aches and pains, and an inability to sleep." Appetite loss, headaches, shakiness, indigestion, and heart palpitations are normal. Occasionally, more serious ailments crop up during bereavement. Studies of widows and widowers have found an increased death rate from cardiovascular disease; those who lose their spouses, it seems, are more likely literally to die of a "broken heart."

Most mourners adjust, but the adjustment may come slowly. "I finally came to some accommodation of my husband's death," says Hermione Davis. "I realized this is the way it is, and I'd better work on building a life for myself that doesn't include him. You accept that it's never going to be great, but you discover resources in yourself that you never knew were there." Davis took trips with friends to help her get a sense that her life was continuing afresh without her husband, and

she now helps others who've faced such loss by conducting bereavement support groups.

Working It Through

The best way to work through grief, say counselors who specialize in the process, is to sink into it, to grieve fully—allowing yourself and others, including children, time to cry, feel numb, reminisce with friends, be angry, or kick and scream if it helps. The problem is that such grieving isn't encouraged in American culture.

"Our culture deals with grief the same way we deal with food," says Robert Ostroff, an as-

---

SHARING THE BURDEN

Below are just a few of the organizations that either offer regional support groups or can steer you to help in your area. Also check with local hospitals and churches.

The Compassionate Friends. Support groups for bereaved parents and siblings; 708-990-0010.
Afterloss. Monthly newsletter focuses on grief recovery. P.O. Box 2545, Rancho Mirage, CA 92270; 800-423-8811.
Pregnancy and Infant Loss Center. Referrals for bereaved families experiencing miscarriage, stillbirth, and infant death. 1415 Wayzata Boulevard., Suite 105, Wayzata, MN 55391; 612-473-9372.
Parents of Murdered Children. Referrals to local chapters, plus a newsletter. 100 East Eighth St., Suite B41, Cincinnati, OH 45202; 513-721-LOVE.
Elisabeth Kübler-Ross Center. Workshops; regional bereavement groups. So. Route 616, Head Waters, VA 24442; 703-396-3441.
Theos. Groups (in both the United States and Canada) for those who have been widowed. 1301 Clark Building, 717 Liberty Avenue, Pittsburgh, PA 15222; 412-471-7779.
Center for Attitudinal Healing. Grief groups, including those for children with life-threatening illnesses and their families. Local offices in 50 cities. Head office, 19 Main Street, Tiburon, CA 94920; 415-435-5022.
National AIDS Hotline. Information and referrals to local counseling groups. 800-342-AIDS.

---

sistant professor of psychiatry at Yale University, who works with bereaved patients. "We think we ought to get a nutritious meal in 30 seconds. But the European notion of wearing black for 12 months speaks to the fact that grieving is a long process."

Rituals can help grievers cope, says Kübler-Ross. "It could be a totally nonreligious sharing of a group of human beings, perhaps with some flowers and music and some favorite songs. It is a closure to all the things that were never said and done."

John Stephenson often suggests that his bereaved patients write a good-bye letter to the loved one. "That helps them say perhaps what hadn't been said, and helps resolve unfinished business."

Judith Souweine says that the Jewish ritual of "sitting shivah"—when friends come visit and mourn with the bereaved for a week—comforted her after her mother's death. "What helped was having people who were willing to listen and talk."

For many people, however, there may be no neighbors who come by. "We don't have the kinds of family customs and culture that support the grieving process any more," says Ostroff. That's why it often helps mourners to find support groups of people who are undergoing the same kinds of painful feelings. Such groups have proliferated in recent years. "Grief groups are an unfortunate necessity for communities where there's nobody to talk to about the loss," says Ostroff. Local hospitals, psychologists, and even funeral homes can steer you to a grief group, including those that deal with specific kinds of loss—the death of a child, for instance. Some people, however, may prefer one-on-one counseling with a therapist.

But even with help, says Ostroff, know that when grief hits, you're in it for the long run. The ancient advice about grief still holds true, he says: "It takes time." And then some. ☐

YOGURT
Bring It Back Alive

Linda Heller

Back in 1906, when the Turkish massacres had just begun in Armenia, young Setrak Boyajian fled his country with only the clothes on his back, a letter with the New York address of a distant cousin, and a small jar of a tangy white substance said to bestow long life on anyone who ate it.

Today, at age 106, Boyajian talks eagerly about this salutary elixir. "Yogurt very nice thing for people," he says in a deep, gravelly voice. "Gives clear sleep, good health, everything else."

Boyajian reserves his praise for the tart delicacy he makes himself from his mother's original culture. As he moved from New York to Chicago to California, got married and raised three sons, became a carpet merchant and a dry cleaner before retiring at age 75, he continued to make yogurt from the same live culture, brimming with benevolent bacteria.

"First you boil milk in a big pot, then place pot in kitchen sink with some cold water to cool it down a little. Test the milk with the little finger. When it's the right temperature—not too hot or cold—add yogurt culture and stir a few times. Then pour it into a bottle, wrap the bottle in a blanket, and place it in oven with the heat off. In one or two hours you have yogurt."

Boyajian likes his yogurt straight up. He laughs at the thought of sweetening it with fruit, sugar, or honey. Instead, he spoons it right from the jar and downs about a pint every night before he goes to bed. He also adds it to water—for a traditional drink called *tahn*, which he sips throughout the day. "Better than coffee, soda, anything," he says.

Many Americans have come to agree with Boyajian on the virtues of yogurt. In fact, it's now the nation's favorite health food. We're eating six times as much as we did in 1970, almost ten cups a year for each citizen, according to New York market researchers Find/svp. At that rate, the com-

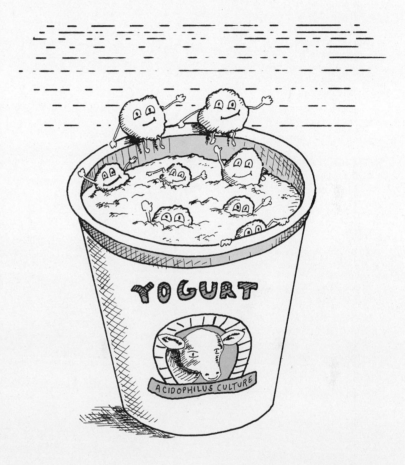

pany predicts, by the year 2000 each of us will be downing more than 20 cups a year.

Of course, no one promises that eating gobs of yogurt will give you Boyajian's extraordinary longevity. (He doesn't smoke or drink and makes a habit of exercising every day.) Basic yogurt is nothing more than milk to which a dose of harmless bacteria has been added. The bacteria pro-

duce an enzyme called lactase. This enzyme attacks the natural milk sugar lactose, giving off lactic acid. The acid then gently curdles the milk as it imparts a tart flavor. Though this workaday fermentation is anything but mystical, it does make yogurt special—and not just in the minds of ancient Armenians and come-lately food purists.

"Yogurt is nutritionally superior

199

to milk in several important ways," says Walter Mertz, the U.S. Department of Agriculture's chief researcher on food and health. First, each 8-ounce serving delivers 30 to 45 percent of the 1,000 milligrams of calcium we're advised to eat each day. (Cup for cup that's a third again as much as milk.)

Second, because yogurt is often thickened with extra milk solids, it has even more protein than does milk. And that protein is more digestible than milk's, because yogurt's bacteria break it down during fermentation.

The burgeoning bacteria also spin off vitamins B_6, B_{12}, niacin, and folic acid. "Years ago one of my graduate students measured the folic acid in milk, then turned that milk into yogurt," says Khem Shahani, a University of Nebraska food scientist. "He found the yogurt had a lot more folic acid." (Twice as much, in fact.) "I told him he was crazy, that he must have done the experiment wrong. But when we repeated it several times, we kept coming up with the same results."

Folic acid is essential for the production of red blood cells and is important in fetal growth. Though most of us get plenty of it—from leafy vegetables and from the yeast in bread—Shahani says that yogurt offers us nutritional insurance.

Further studies confirm that for many of us yogurt is indeed a better bet than milk. Consider a test run at the USDA in the mid-1970s. "We took a group of weanling rats, fed a fourth of them milk, a fourth buttermilk, and a fourth kefir [a custardy blend of milk, bacteria, and yeast]. The last fourth got yogurt," says food technologist Frank McDonough.

"Much to our amazement, the rats on the yogurt diet actually grew 20 to 30 percent faster than the others. We thought, 'Wow, we've discovered a growth factor in yogurt!' Well, we were excited about that for a year or two."

It turns out that baby rats, like two-thirds of the people in the world, are simply lactose intolerant: they lack the digestive enzyme lactase. When they swallow regular milk, the lactose goes through an unusual breakdown, causing intestinal distress and loss of appetite. Yogurt, however, has far less lactose, sometimes half as much. What's more, during digestion, yogurt's enzymes break down any lactose still remaining.

Cultured buttermilk and kefir aren't as good, according to McDonough. Not only do they start out with fewer bacteria, but their bugs don't churn out enzymes as quickly, if at all. The rats lapping up yogurt thrived because they were getting a more digestible food—not to mention more vitamins—than those eating the other dairy products. Plus, they felt better so they ate more.

To borrow from Boyajian, it all proves yogurt's a "very nice thing for people." So should the old Armenian's kudos be extended to *all* the ready-made versions now jumping off supermarket shelves?

Sadly, not all yogurts are created equal, and some are clearly inferior. Though the U.S. Food and Drug Administration requires yogurt makers to add at least one of two lactic acid-producing bacteria (*Lactobacillus bulgaricus* and *Streptococcus thermophilus*), it doesn't say anything about those cultures being alive or active in the containers you bring home. According to McDonough, a few makers heat their yogurt to hold down its tartness and extend its shelf life. This heat treatment

CULTURE BY THE CUP: MATTERS OF FAT, FRUIT, AND FREEZING

Despite its image as a light food, yogurt ranges from a stout 380 calories a serving to a slim 90—largely because some types are high in fat and others low. But yogurts are often loaded with sugar and preserved fruit, so low-fat and nonfat kinds can be even more caloric than their whole-milk counterparts. Here's the richness range for servings of one cup, the usual portion:

Plain. Second in popularity to strawberry flavor, plain yogurt is the most versatile. It's ideal with fresh fruit, can stand in for mayonnaise and sour cream in dressings, and goes well on potatoes and blintzes.

	Calories*	Fat**
Whole milk	170	39
Low-fat	150	20
Nonfat	105	less than 10

With fruit. The best seller comes with plain yogurt on the top and fruit preserves or puree on the bottom.

	Calories*	Fat**
Whole milk	220	29
Low-fat	235	11
Nonfat	200	less than 5

Pre-stirred. Also called European, French-, or Swiss-style, these yogurts come with their flavorings mixed in. They may be fairly high in fat while claiming to be "lite." Look for low- or nonfat kinds.

	Calories*	Fat**
Regular	up to 260	up to 31
Nonfat	125	less than 10
Breakfast style with nuts or grains and fruit	310	8

Frozen. A blend of milk, sweeteners, and stabilizers with a bit of "yogurt mix" (dry milk and inactive bacteria), frozen yogurt is basically economy-grade ice cream. Bacteria never actually ferment it, so it remains high in lactose—bad news for many people. The good news is that it generally has about *half* ice cream's fat.

	Calories*	Fat**
Regular	240	30
Low-fat	210	12
Nonfat	200	less than 5

*Per 8 ounces (1 cup), based on averages of products; based on information from the National Yogurt Association.
**Percent of calories

wipes out the bugs at the height of their powers, leaving much of the milk's lactose intact. (Labels must say if the yogurt's been heated.)

But even if you're not dodging lactose, it's worth scanning the fine print for yogurts with their cultures still kicking. Yogurt bacteria may actually protect you from illness—if they're *alive* when they reach your intestines. Heat treatment aside, many just can't get there. The two bacterial cultures in most supermarket yogurts aren't particularly hardy and generally won't survive the stomach's highly acidic gastric juices.

A third type of bacteria—*Lactobacillus acidophilus*—is a more robust bug. Khem Shahani and other food scientists have found that it endures passage through the stomach better than do the two more common cultures. And, he explains, it appears actually to take up residence on the walls of the intestines, where it can wage war against disease-causing bacteria. Acidophilus bacteria produce a slew of active compounds that provide a downright detrimental environment for salmonella, campylobacter, listeria, and other food-borne microbes. In 1972, Shahani isolated the first antibiotic in this culture, which he dubbed "acidophilin," hoping he'd bagged a new penicillin. "But once we took it out of the yogurt," he says, "it became very unstable. It needs an acidic environment and other qualities that only yogurt can provide."

Unfortunately, the culture shows up in only some American yogurts. (Check the label for *Lactobacillus acidophilus* or *L. acidophilus*.) "It's much more acidic and tangy than the other two bacterial cultures," Shahani says, "so most American manufacturers leave it out."

That's too bad. Many doctors recommend acidophilus yogurt for patients on antibiotics. Ordinarily, the vast populations of benign bacteria in our digestive tracts

Yogurt cultures hardy enough to survive the stomach's gastric juices may protect you from some intestinal illnesses.

keep the harmful invaders in check. But antibiotics can disrupt this balance—killing off the helpful bugs and allowing noxious, drug-resistant ones to prevail. The uncomfortable result is what doctors term "antibiotic-induced diarrhea." Acidophilus yogurt may help prevent it by recolonizing the gut with good bacteria. (When taking an antibiotic you should wait an hour or so before eating yogurt, or any dairy product, so its calcium doesn't interfere with the drug's action.)

Acidophilus yogurt may also help women suffering from chronic yeast infections, as Eileen Hilton, an infectious disease specialist at the Long Island Jewish Medical Center in New York City, showed in a recent study. For six months a group of 13 women ate one cup of the tart yogurt a day, then for six months went without. During the yogurt months, the women had a third fewer vaginal infections.

"The acidophilus bacteria is a natural enemy of yeast," says Hilton. "We think that it colonizes throughout the gastrointestinal tract, then migrates to the vagina, where it takes up residence and

Most yogurts sold in supermarkets don't contain cultures hardy enough to offer any specific health benefits, but they provide vitamins and minerals.

helps fight off yeast infections." Hilton isn't yet sure how all this works. Nevertheless, she tells patients who have chronic yeast infections to give the yogurt remedy a try.

Hilton's colleagues nationwide now dream of yogurt cultures engineered to meet specific health needs—while appealing to finicky American palates. Already, biochemist Barry Goldin and Sherwood L. Gorbach, a community health physician at Tufts University School of Medicine, have isolated a strain of bacteria that grows rapidly, withstands the flood of stomach acid, and takes up life in the intestines far better than do any commercial yogurt bacteria—including acidophilus. In several controlled studies the strain (*Lactobacillus* GG) helped end cases of antibiotic-related diarrhea in adults and severe diarrhea among infants.

The GG strain might someday offer consumers a hedge against cancer, according to Gorbach. In a recent study Gorbach and Goldin asked 21 healthy adults to drink two glasses of milk a day for a month, then switch to a GG-yogurt-and-whey drink. The doctors then measured the activity of certain bacterial enzymes linked to cancer of the colon. During the month on yogurt, the subjects' carcinogenic enzyme activity fell by half.

But you can't rush out and stock up on GG yogurt. So far, it's for sale only in Finland. As for the time-tested but possibly antiquated versions still widely available in American supermarkets, the yogurt visionaries pull their punches.

"I'm not sure if they offer any specific health effects," says Gorbach. "But from a nutritional point of view, they can provide you with plenty of vitamins and minerals, and they're certainly good for you, if they're low in fat."

"Besides," adds Goldin with a true yogurt-lover's bravado, "they taste good."

CONJUNCTIVITIS

Jane E. Brody

In the spring of 1991 my son complained that his eye was bothering him. The white of the eye was red and felt gritty and the eye kept tearing and releasing a pale yellow discharge. Two days later I awoke to the same symptoms. Within 12 hours my eye had swollen nearly shut and was constantly filling with the opaque discharge. The doctor's diagnosis was bacterial conjunctivitis, one of the many forms of what most people call "pink eye." Conjunctivitis is an inflammation of the conjunctiva, the transparent tissue that covers the white of the eye and lines the inside of the eyelids.

Ophthalmologists and pediatricians see many cases of pink eye in the spring, most of them the result of seasonal allergies. Although not contagious, allergic conjunctivitis can strike several members of a household if they have the same allergies. Allergic conjunctivitis is most common in

> **Conjunctivitis, or "pink eye," is an inflammation of the tissue that covers the white of the eye and the insides of the eyelids.**

spring and late summer into early fall, but it can occur at any time of year if the allergy is to pets or to cosmetics, perfume, molds, or dust.

For unknown reasons, viral conjunctivitis, which is highly contagious, was also exceedingly com-

mon that same spring. My 2-year-old niece and her baby brother got it, and then it hit their father and a babysitter. Outbreaks of viral conjunctivitis are common among young children in play groups, day care, and school. They also commonly strike campers and users of public swimming pools.

While most cases of conjunctivitis eventually clear up on their own, some can become very severe. Without aggressive treatment, some severe infections can permanently impair vision by damaging the cornea, the crystallike tissue that covers the colored portion of the eye.

Thus, it is important to know when you should seek medical attention for pink eye. Simply masking symptoms with over-the-counter eye drops that take away redness does nothing to control an infection.

Many Causes of Red Eye

Most of the time when eyes get red where they should be white the cause is not an infection. In addition to allergies, among the many noninfectious causes of redness are exposure to irritating chemicals, like those in soap or perfume or like chlorine in pools; fumes like cigarette smoke and smog; excessively dry air as on an airplane or when walking into the wind; sunburn, as might happen when sailing, skiing, or sunbathing without wearing protective lenses; overconsumption of alcohol; fatigue or sleeplessness; eyestrain from overuse of the eyes when lighting is poor; and a foreign object in the eye.

The best cure for such redness is to allow the tears to moisten and "disinfect" the eye with lyso-

zyme, the natural antiseptic they contain. People often awaken with bloodshot eyes that feel gritty because during sleep tearing stops. When eyes are healthy, the redness naturally clears on its own within half an hour.

More frightening in appearance but no more serious is the bright redness caused by a tiny hemor-

> **Most cases of "pink eye" clear up on their own, but sometimes aggressive treatment is needed to prevent severe infections.**

rhage just under the conjunctiva. While such hemorrhages can happen to anyone, they are more common in people who are overweight or have high blood pressure, diabetes, anemia, or atherosclerosis. They can also be caused by a blow to the eye, by heavy lifting, by straining during violent coughing, retching, or sneezing, or by straining when attempting to move the bowels.

The hemorrhages range in size from a pinhead to covering the entire white of the eye. They cause no pain or discomfort or blurring of vision. In fact, you cannot tell a hemorrhage is there unless someone tells you or you look in a mirror. Such hemorrhages result from a break in a tiny blood vessel on the surface of the eyeball, but since the blood lies under the conjunctiva it cannot be washed away. Instead, the body gradually reabsorbs it.

Infectious Conjunctivitis

Viruses, bacteria, fungi, and other organisms can infect the conjunctiva, resulting in an ailment that ranges in seriousness from completely self-healing to potentially

Allergies, viruses, and bacteria can cause conjunctivitis. Allergic reactions cause itching; viral and bacterial infections make the eye feel gritty.

blinding. Fortunately, most cases, even those that are highly contagious, do not threaten vision or cause anything more serious than temporary discomfort.

But only a doctor (not a pharmacist or optometrist) can determine for certain what is causing a particular case and how vigorously it should be treated. If you consult an ophthalmologist, the doctor should examine your eye through a slit lamp, which is like looking at the eye through a microscope, to see whether the cornea is infected.

Dr. Alan J. Friedman, an expert in eye infections at New York University Medical Center, explained that whereas allergic conjunctivitis causes itching, viral and bacterial infections do not. Rather, the eye feels gritty or scratchy. Bacterial infections typically cause a pus-like discharge. Most often these infections afflict small children, who tend to "stick their fingers in the wrong places and then put them in their eyes," Dr. Friedman said.

Bacterial conjunctivitis is very uncommon in adults, he added. It most often occurs as an offshoot of a viral illness. The bacteria invade while the eye's immune defenses are temporarily suppressed by the virus.

Stemming Contagion

To check the spread of infectious conjunctivitis, anyone with a red eye, especially if there is pus or a discharge, should not share towels or washcloths and should only use disposable tissues that are flushed down the toilet. If it is not possible to avoid touching the eyes or face, the hands should be thoroughly scrubbed immediately after. Parents who treat children's infected eyes should also wash thoroughly.

Since it is unlikely that young children will follow such precautions, it is best to keep those with eye infections away from other children and out of swimming pools until the infection clears completely.

Despite my concerted efforts to keep my infected eye from contaminating the other one, it, too, got infected a week later and the first eye became reinfected a few days after that.

After the fact, I realized that both my swim goggles and my makeup might be contaminated, so I disinfected the former and discarded the latter. Dr. Friedman said some viruses that infect the eye are so hardy that they can live on dry surfaces for weeks.

Where Conjunctivitis Strikes

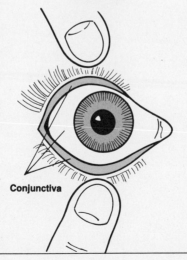

Conjunctiva

Bacteria too may live for days or weeks on inanimate objects, according to Dr. Friedman.

When to See a Doctor

See a doctor as soon as possible if a red, inflamed eye is also blurry or painful, sensitive to light, tearing, or producing a pus-like discharge.

When the causative organism is not determined by microscopic examination or a culture, doctors typically prescribe an antibiotic ointment or drops to cover the possibility of a bacterial infection or prevent a secondary infection. But there is no specific treatment for the common viral causes of

A prompt trip to the doctor is called for if a red, inflamed eye is also blurry or painful, is sensitive to light, is tearing, or is discharging pus.

conjunctivitis. Over-the-counter eye drops are not effective in treating infections and ophthalmologists say that these drops are of little use in countering allergic conjunctivitis.

Dr. Friedman is among a number of doctors who prescribe a topical steroid to relieve the discomfort caused by infectious conjunctivitis. He explained that while the steroid does nothing to cure the infection, by decreasing inflammation it makes the patient feel much better and it may lower the risk of a secondary bacterial infection, too.

Ordinary cases of infectious conjunctivitis may clear up in just four or five days even without any kind of treatment, or they may wax and wane for one to two weeks before the eyes heal themselves. ☐

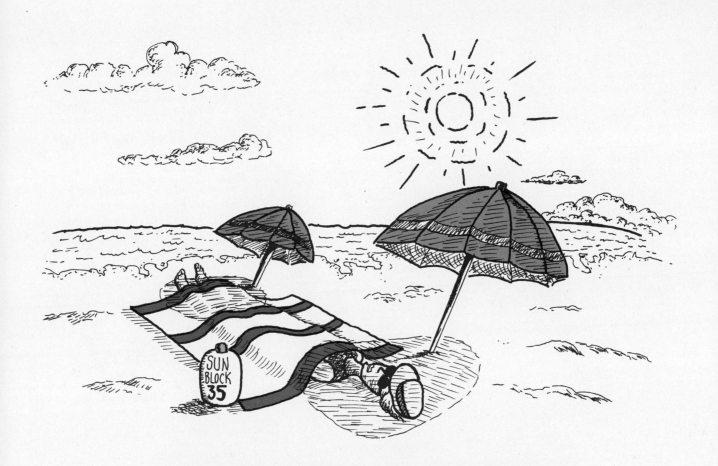

SKIN CARE

How to Handle Common Problems

As the body's largest organ, the skin is a massive playground for pimples, bumps, scales, swellings, and a host of other unwelcome visitors.

Most of these nuisances are harmless. Many eventually go away by themselves. But recurrent blemishes and other skin problems can be frustrating—particularly for mature men and women who thought that they had outgrown these little irritations years ago.

Skin Facts and Fiction

The causes of several common skin disorders aren't well defined—and some of the myths propagated to explain them hold little truth. For example, although regularly cleansing the skin is a good idea, dirty skin usually has little to do with the appearance of a blemish. The same is true for the use of cosmetics. Likewise, greasy foods and chocolate aren't the skin villains they've been made out to be. Long blamed for teenage acne and isolated pimples, they play a small role, if any. "Diet isn't a major factor,

204

and adjustments in the diet don't get rid of acne," says Houston dermatologist Dr. Madeleine Duvic, an associate professor of dermatology and internal medicine at the University of Texas Medical School at Houston. One

> **Greasy foods and chocolate, long blamed for teenage acne, actually play only a small role, if any, in causing that common skin problem.**

exception is iodides in shellfish, which may cause acne to flare.

Stress, on the other hand, has long been associated with certain skin problems—and recent research appears to support such a link. A University of Pennsylvania team studying inflammation at the cellular level has provided evidence that stress and anxiety can indeed trigger outbreaks of acne and eczema.

Other conditions that can trigger skin problems include puberty, pregnancy, and aging. And sun exposure can play a critical role.

Common Skin Problems

Although some skin problems can be stubborn, few are uncontrollable. Many can be managed at home. Others may be more effectively resolved by medical treatment.

Whiteheads. A small, white, pinhead-sized cyst called a milium may occasionally appear on the face. For a quick fix, a doctor can pierce and drain it. But a whitehead will disappear by itself, usually within a few weeks.

Acne. A greasy gang of blackheads, whiteheads, and pimples on the face or back brings more people to the dermatologist than any other skin disorder. Precious few teenagers escape the mortifi-

cation of acne. Although the condition usually lets up in the early 20s, it can last through the 20s and 30s or longer. And an occasional blemish can erupt at just about any age. Some women have perfect skin until their late 20s, when acne suddenly erupts.

Acne is caused by overactive sebaceous (oil) glands that become clogged. Bacteria that get trapped in the oil contribute to the formation of pimples. The oil glands' propensity to clog is controlled by hormones and is largely hereditary.

No treatment can cure acne. But some preparations can control it until it goes into remission. Dr. Duvic advises washing the face twice a day with a gentle soap and using oil-free cosmetics and hair products. For mild acne, a variety of acne creams and lotions are available on drugstore shelves.

If the condition doesn't respond to over-the-counter medications, a visit to the doctor may help, especially with severe cases, which can leave scars. Topical or oral antibiotics, such as tetracycline and erythromycin, can help eradicate the bacteria that colonize the oil duct and skin surface and promote formation of irritating fatty acids. If all else fails, more potent drugs may be prescribed—the

> **No treatment can cure acne, but creams and lotions from the drugstore can help control a mild case and antibiotics may help severe cases.**

topical wrinkle remover tretinoin (Retin-A) or an oral drug called isotretinoin (Accutane). Accutane is reserved for severe cases, as it can cause side effects in the user and severe birth defects if a woman who is using the drug becomes pregnant.

Dermatitis. Dermatitis (or eczema) is a term for pink, dry, scaly, and usually itchy skin.

Atopic dermatitis starts in infancy in families with a history of allergies or asthma. It appears on the face, in the bends of the elbows, and behind the knees. Atopic dermatitis often requires periodic treatment with antibiotics, as excessive dryness and splitting make the skin vulnerable to infection. Children usually outgrow atopic dermatitis.

Adult seborrheic dermatitis, which usually affects the scalp and face, is associated with stress and anxiety and may be caused by an allergy to yeast. This form of dermatitis usually itches.

> **Dermatitis is dry, scaly, and usually itchy skin. Among its causes are stress, allergies, chronic tension, and exposure to irritants.**

Over-the-counter hydrocortisone, a steroid cream, can control the condition on the face, although steroids shouldn't be used if acne is present. Strong steroids should never be used on the face. Mild seborrheic dermatitis of the scalp, which is commonly called dandruff, can be controlled with shampoos containing either tar or selenium sulfide.

Nummular ("coin-shaped") *dermatitis* appears on the limbs. It can be relieved with emollients, antihistamines, and prescription-strength topical steroids. Dr. Duvic says the round lesions may be caused by an allergy to nickel in jewelry or zippers. Nickel is also found in chocolate, buckwheat, baking powder, and orange pekoe tea. Chronic tension also has been identified as a cause.

"Housewife's dermatitis" occurs most often in people whose hands are frequently exposed to water

and irritants such as detergents and shampoos. Stress and a family history of atopic dermatitis may also play a role. The first step in controlling the condition is to avoid exposure to water and irritants by wearing gloves if necessary. Prescription-strength topical steroids may be effective. Allergy tests may determine whether the condition is actually *contact dermatitis*.

Contact dermatitis is dermatitis caused by exposure to an identifiable substance. A variety of substances commonly cause the condition—nickel alloys in jewelry, zippers, eyeglass frames, jean studs, and belt buckles; rubber in gloves, condoms, shoes, and elastic; perfumes and cosmetics; nail polish and creams containing lanolin; and plants such as poison ivy. Allergy tests may be necessary to confirm a diagnosis and to identify the allergen that's causing the reaction.

Over-the-counter steroids, cool compresses and, of course, removal of the offending allergen may help to relieve cases of contact dermatitis.

Swelling may accompany con-

tact dermatitis, and in some instance the face and eyelids also may swell. If swelling occurs, the doctor may prescribe an oral steroid, such as prednisone. In the case of extreme swelling or shortness of breath, however, call your doctor at once. It may be a sign of anaphylactic shock, a severe allergic reaction that can be life-threatening.

Skin Tags. Skin tags are small, brown or flesh-colored protrusions of skin that may appear around the neck, under the arms, along the beltline, or in other areas that rub. No one knows what causes them. Although some studies have shown an association between skin tags and colon polyps, which often precede the development of colon cancer, the tags appear to be benign. A doctor can easily clip them off if they're annoying.

Liver or Age Spots. Often developing on the hands and face, these flat or slightly raised areas of tan or brown color are caused entirely by sun exposure. Dr. Duvic says they can be frozen and treated with Retin-A. The best approach is to prevent further

The key to minimizing skin problems is a basic program of skin care that will keep the skin clean, moisturize it, and protect it from sun and wind.

discoloration by regularly applying sunscreen.

Seborrheic Keratoses. These rough, brown proliferations of skin are common and may be indistinguishable from liver spots. "Almost everyone over age 40 gets one," says Dr. Duvic. "It's a landmark of living." Seborrheic keratoses can appear most anywhere on the body. A doctor can scrape them off or freeze them if desired.

Preventive Maintenance

Though many skin problems are unavoidable, a good basic skin care program can help your skin look its best. Dr. Duvic recommends washing the face each morning and evening with water and a mild soap, such as Dove or Purpose. Dry skin should be patted dry—so that it remains damp—and then moisturized with a cream or lotion. Moisturizers act by sealing water in.

If you get a blemish, try to resist picking, squeezing, or scratching. Such assaults usually irritate the blemish and the surrounding skin.

Always protect your skin from sun and wind. Faithful application of a sunscreen with a sun protection factor (SPF) of 15 or greater can help prevent discolorations, blackheads, whiteheads, leathery skin, and wrinkles. Finally, make a habit of wearing gloves whenever you use household cleaning agents or other chemicals.

These few simple steps will go a long way toward keeping your skin clear and smooth. □

The best way to avoid skin problems on your hands is to wear gloves when using household cleansers and other chemicals.

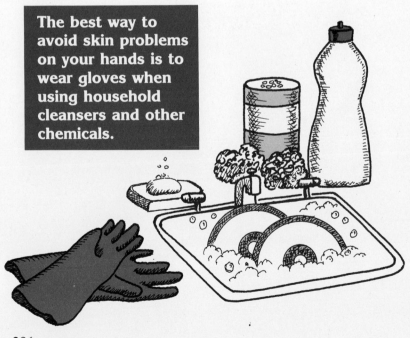

Chronic Muscle Pain Syndrome

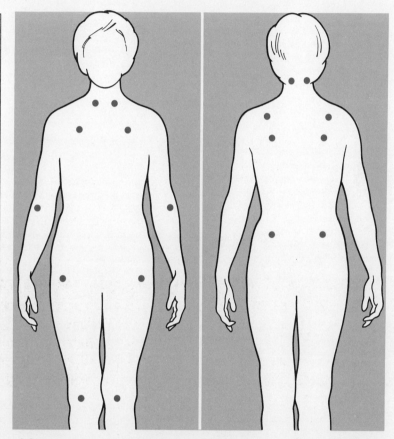

"I hurt all over." "My bones ache." "I'm tired all the time." Symptoms like these may characterize a chronic muscle pain syndrome called fibromyalgia or tension myalgia.

Although the condition has no cure, it isn't progressive, crippling, or life-threatening. You can reduce your symptoms or even make them disappear by correcting misuse of muscles, exercising, and controlling stress.

Muscles Ache When They Shouldn't

Fibromyalgia can occur within your muscles or where your muscles join their tendons, but not in joints. The results of laboratory tests, joint examination, and neurologic evaluation, including strength, sensation, and reflex testing, are normal.

The pain is chronic and widespread. Muscles ache when they shouldn't, remain tired and stiff after work or exercise, and continue to cause pain long after an injury has healed. You may "hurt all over" or just in a certain area, such as your head and neck, your arm and shoulder and the same side of your neck, or a leg and the same side of your lower back.

Doctors sometimes distinguish this pain syndrome from other causes of chronic pain by identifying tender points. A tender point is a spot in a muscle or area where a muscle joins its tendon. The spot is painful when pressed upon.

Although the pain of fibromyalgia may occur in different areas in different people with the condi-

If firm pressure applied to any of the tender points above (see dots) causes pain, you may have fibromyalgia.

tion, the location of these tender points is generally consistent from person to person.

In the absence of definite tender points, doctors may identify fibromyalgia or chronic muscle pain syndrome by the length of time of the discomfort (usually more than three months), the widespread area of discomfort, and the inability of a qualified physician, using appropriate tests, to identify any other cause.

Other Symptoms

You may also have one or more of the following problems as part of tension myalgia.

Tension and Stress. Poor posture, rapid repetitive motions, or

207

incorrectly using your muscles to lift, push, or pull can cause you to constantly hold your muscles tight when you should allow them to relax. This can predispose susceptible individuals to the aches, pains, and stiffness that are characteristic of this chronic muscle pain syndrome.

Many people with fibromyalgia constantly hunch their shoulders. They think they are completely relaxed but must be reminded to loosen their shoulders. Only then are they able to relax.

Emotional tension or stress can perpetuate fibromyalgia.

Difficulty Sleeping. More than 75 percent of people with various forms of chronic muscle pain have trouble falling asleep or awaken during the night with aching muscles.

Fatigue. Most people who suffer from this syndrome are physically out of condition. The cycle of pain, inactivity, and further deconditioning is aggravated each time you attempt some out-of-the-ordinary activity. Constantly tensing your muscles can make even everyday tasks painful or exhausting.

Temperature/Weather Sensitivities. Many people find that a hot shower or bath relieves aches and pains temporarily. Others say that cold drafts or changes in barometric pressure can make symptoms worse.

Treatment: Your Challenge

Numerous methods of treating chronic muscle pain exist, each with varying degrees of success.

Although fibromyalgia has no cure, it isn't progressive or crippling, and its symptoms can be controlled if you know what to do.

Myalgia Mimics

Several other conditions may mimic fibromyalgia.

For example, people who have rheumatoid arthritis often confuse their pain with fibromyalgia. Even though people with rheumatoid arthritis may also develop fibromyalgia, the two conditions are different.

Rheumatoid arthritis inflames joints. Fibromyalgia causes no damage to joints. There's no swelling and no deformation.

Epstein-Barr virus infection and the chronic yeast infection known as candidiasis are two controversial conditions that supposedly cause chronic muscle pain. Yet neither is proven to be linked to fibromyalgia.

The following approaches are based on the cumulative experience of physicians who have treated thousands of people with chronic muscle pain syndrome for more than 40 years in the Department of Physical Medicine and Rehabilitation at the Mayo Clinic:

1. Be active in your own care—If you're diagnosed with chronic muscle pain syndrome, take responsibility for participating in your own treatment. The time and effort you spend learning what chronic muscle pain is and what you can do to help relieve it are the most important steps in your care.

2. Learn correct posture and proper body mechanics—For long-term relief, you must learn how to correct improper use of your muscles. A qualified physical therapist can teach you proper body mechanics and stretching exercises to help relieve tensions that build in your muscles during everyday tasks.

Stretching allows your muscles

to relax periodically, breaking the cycle of muscle tension, aching, pain, and stiffness.

3. Condition your muscles with aerobic exercise—Research shows that conditioning muscles through moderate aerobic exercise improves signs and symptoms of fibromyalgia. Ask your doctor if exercise is appropriate for you. Then gradually develop your cardiovascular fitness with brisk walking or low-tension cycling. Aim for 30-minute sessions two or three times a week.

4. Relax—If stress is adding to your muscle pain, take advantage of stress management programs that may be available in your community.

Don't expect relief from medications. Learn to maintain correct posture and to use your muscles properly. Exercise and stress management may also help.

5. Don't expect a cure from medications; anti-inflammatory medicines and analgesics generally don't help relieve fibromyalgia symptoms.

If poor sleep is a major problem, your doctor may prescribe medications in the antidepressant category, such as amitriptyline, for their sleep-enhancing and pain-relieving properties. Depression is no more common in persons with chronic muscle pain syndrome than in other people.

People with fibromyalgia used to worry that their pain and fatigue were "all in the head." Now doctors recognize fibromyalgia as a common and real medical condition.

Through your commitment to exercise and lifestyle change, you can learn to understand and better control your pain. □

Music Therapy for the Elderly

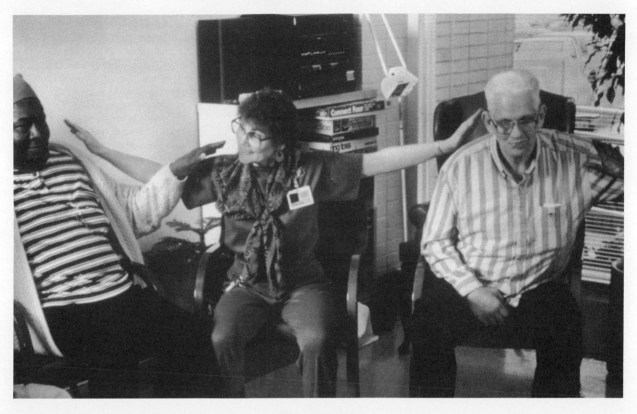

Teri Randall

Although illnesses vary, every patient at the geriatric day hospital at the University of Texas Medical Branch (UTMB), Galveston, receives one therapy in common.

This therapy is unusual in that it elicits immediate and positive effects in nearly all who receive it and has virtually no contraindications. Furthermore, it costs little more than a song because it is precisely that: a song.

"I'm in heaven when we're dancing cheek to cheek," Louis Armstrong and Ella Fitzgerald croon. As the tune emanates from the music therapist's portable tape player, 20 geriatric patients seated in two large circles reach out to pat their neighbors' shoul-

ders, look in each others' eyes, and smile.

Music for Mobility, Analgesia

In what is probably the highlight of their day at this specialized facility (one of only a handful of geriatric day hospitals in the United States) these patients are about to begin a half-hour music therapy session designed to increase their range of motion, renew motor skills, and ease pain. But they say that it doesn't feel like physical therapy when it's done to their favorite jazz, gospel, and country and western music.

As Armstrong sings *A Fine Romance*, patients tap their toes to the music, then launch into an alternating toe to heel step. They

clap their hands, then clap their neighbors' hands. The more agile execute little cancan kicks from their chairs. The less agile, and those in wheelchairs, pat their thighs in time to the music. Most of the patients have hypertension, or uncontrolled diabetes. Some have had strokes or amputations.

"Our goals are to reinforce the occupational therapy and physical therapy goals," says UTMB's Mary Rudenberg, RMT/BC (registered music therapist/board certified). But there are secondary goals that transcend the physical, and in terms of quality of life, are just as important.

"We get them to reminisce, and talk about when they went to dances, and when they heard these [musical] groups. It gets

209

them to socialize more with one another, to share, to draw on their long-term memories. It gives them a means of expressing themselves, of having a successful experience through music and movement," Rudenberg says.

Besides her daily group sessions at the geriatric day hospital, Rudenberg also works with individual patients with strokes, mental disorders, pain from hip fractures and arthritis, or chronic obstructive pulmonary disease. The latter sing and play the kazoo for respiratory therapy.

U.S. Senate Tunes In

Although music therapy as a modern profession began in the 1930s, and its use in the elderly population was widely discussed in the 1960s, it has gained renewed attention in recent years as an effective and inexpensive way to increase alertness and physical vigor while decreasing the isolation experienced by many geriatric patients.

In 1991 the therapeutic value of music was discussed for the first time before Congress. Physicians, music therapists, and patients testified in support of this approach before the Senate Special Committee on Aging.

Representatives from the National Association for Music Therapy urged Congress to allocate a "modest" amount of special projects money for the research and application of music therapy strategies for individuals suffering from Alzheimer's disease and various other forms of dementia, stroke, depression, grief, and other disabling conditions. They pointed out that the efficacy of music therapy has been demonstrated through extensive clinical practice, but demonstration projects, basic research, and clinical outcome research could extend and further validate music therapy applications.

They also asked Congress to include music therapy in the rehabilitative therapies section of the Health Care Financing Administration regulations, in the Medicare reimbursement guide, and in other federal legislation and regulations.

Senator Harry Reid (D, Nev) called music therapy "an innovative approach that won't widen the deficit, but can help millions of older people live happier, more fulfilling lives." After the hearing Reid asked the Committee on Aging to write an amendment to the Older Americans Act that would include music therapy in the list of services available to the elderly population in a variety of settings. By early 1992, such an amendment had been agreed to by both House and Senate.

UTMB is in the minority of teaching hospitals across the country that have music therapists on staff. Dr. Derek Prinsley, who was brought to UTMB in 1986 to further develop the geriatric program, is an internationally recognized expert on geriatric medicine and an outspoken proponent of music therapy in geriatric care.

In an editorial in which he describes the social, psychological, intellectual, and physical benefits of music therapy (*Australian Nurses Journal*, 1986; Vol. 15, pages 48-49), Prinsley notes that some patients—who are aphasic or dysarthric because of stroke damage to their left hemisphere—nonetheless can sing the words of a remembered song. The phenomenon occurs in patients who process music in the right hemisphere. (Musically naive individuals process and store music in the non-dominant hemisphere of the brain. But the musically educated do so in the dominant hemisphere, Prinsley wrote.)

Communication Through Music

Music therapists use a technique called melodic intonation to help aphasic or dysarthric stroke patients communicate their basic needs through singing. The technique was developed by speech pathologists and is now a mainstay of both speech therapy and music therapy.

The patient is taught to sing a short phrase, such as his or her name, "good morning," "I hurt," "water," or "help me."

The therapist assigns each phrase a different set of notes, Rudenberg says. Often the patient masters the notes first, then learns to say the words. Eventually, some patients can adopt a singsong way of speaking in which music serves as a supportive matrix for speech.

Prinsley suggests that music therapy for geriatric patients is particularly promising because these patients are of the generation that actively participated in music by attending concerts, dancing, singing in choirs, and playing musical instruments. He says this was much more the case than for the passive audiences of today who watch television or listen to the radio.

Among those who testified at the hearing was Dr. Oliver Sacks, neurologist and author of the books *The Man Who Mistook His Wife For A Hat* and *Awakenings*. Sacks has observed postencephalitic and parkinsonian patients demonstrate extraordinary responses to music. "One sees parkinsonian patients unable to walk, but able to dance perfectly well, or patients almost unable to talk, who are able to sing perfectly well," Sacks said.

Sacks described one parkinsonian patient, Rosalie, who tended to remain completely motionless for hours at a time, usually with one finger on her spectacles. But she can play the piano beautifully for hours.

"And, when she plays, her parkinsonism disappears. All is ease and fluency and freedom and normality," Sacks testified.

Chopin is Rosalie's favorite composer, and she knows all his works by heart. Sacks said, "One has only to say 'Opus 49' to her for her whole body, posture, and expression to change." Even her electroencephalogram, usually of almost comalike slowness, would become normal as she imagined, or played in her mind, Chopin's music.

Sacks said that the basal ganglia, sometimes called the "organs of succession," are damaged in parkinsonian patients. These patients therefore have great difficulty with sequences, or consecutive movement.

"But music can substitute for this basal gangliar function," he said. "It can become [while it lasts] a template for organizing a series of movements, for doing. Music is not a luxury but a necessity for such patients, and can [for a while] provide them with what their brains no longer provide."

Unlocking Memories

Sacks has also observed how music is a point of entry into the minds of Alzheimer's patients, a way to elicit memories and associations that have been long forgotten. "One sees that it is not an actual loss of memories here," Sacks said, "but a loss of access to these—and music, above all, can provide access once again, can constitute a key for opening the door to the past, a door not only to specific moods and memories, but to the entire thought structure and personality of the past."

To elicit these powerful responses, however, the music must have meaning and significance to the individual. Music therapists carefully select their music, usually through discussions with family members. (In fact, the only contraindication of music therapy, says Prinsley, is the possible emotional upsets of patients who have listened to music that elicits very unpleasant memories for them.)

Prinsley suggests that music therapists bear in mind the patient's ethnic background, and that an individual's " music memory" tends to be fixed during the ages of 15 to 25 years.

At UTMB, Rudenberg finds that her patients often respond strongly to folk songs and to spirituals. *Amazing Grace* is almost a universal favorite. ☐

A GERIATRIC DAY HOSPITAL

Geriatric patients who are discharged from inpatient care at the University of Texas Medical Branch, Galveston, may have the option of visiting a sort of therapeutic steppingstone between the hospital and independent community living. A geriatric day hospital, located on the university campus, allows patients to live at home while completing their rehabilitation at the facility 2 or 3 days a week.

The day hospital, thought to be the first of its kind in the United States, is distinctly different from day-care facilities, whose primary focus, essentially, is to keep content and safe those elderly persons who no longer can function independently.

"The main thrust of the day hospital is to try to get the patient back to some sort of independent living," says Dr. Jan MacGregor, instructor in internal medicine in the university's Division of Geriatric Medicine and the day hospital's primary physician.

Independence Has Many Meanings

The meaning of independence varies with each patient. For some, it may mean learning how to feed themselves. For others, it can mean diminishing their disability somewhat through therapy, or simplifying their environment and medical regimen so that they can continue to live at home.

The patient's care is coordinated by a team that, depending on the patient's needs, includes physicians, nurses, physical therapists, occupational therapists, speech pathologists, dietitians, social workers, and music therapists. Transportation to and from the day hospital is provided by the Galveston County Community Action Council or by family members.

Geriatric day hospitals are commonplace in Europe, particularly in England, and also in Australia. Previous attempts to begin such facilities in the United States have failed due to limited financial support.

The university opened its day hospital in November 1988 under the leadership of Dr. Derek Prinsley, a geriatrician who pioneered day hospitals in Great Britain and Australia. At the time it was the first facility of its kind in the United States. A few others have opened across the country since then.

Prinsley served as director of the UTMB Division of Geriatric Medicine in the Department of Internal Medicine from 1986 until August 1991, when he returned to the University of Melbourne, Australia, as professor emeritus.

The day hospital cares for 15 to 20 patients a day, most of whom have experienced strokes, complications of diabetes, amputations, or fractures. A few have neurological disorders.

Referring Physician Relationship

Patients are accepted only from physician referrals, both from the community and within the medical branch. Referrals from every medical department have increased over time, a sign to MacGregor that physicians are viewing the day hospital favorably.

Besides the physical benefits, MacGregor says that the emotional benefits may also contribute to the patients' well-being. The day hospital environment is friendly, supportive, and optimistic. She says she has been told by a patient that the staff and other patients are like family.

"At the same time," says MacGregor, "we inject a bit of realism, because they [patients] are around other people who have similar problems. They see that, yes, they are indeed disabled, but life goes on. They learn to measure their improvement on a new scale, not the scale they used before they were disabled." To assist in this process, a social worker regularly leads group discussions on adjusting to disease and disability.

The Division of Geriatric Medicine is conducting a study to determine the clinical and cost benefits of the day hospital. It is hypothesized, but not yet proven, that treatment there prevents or postpones nursing home placement or readmission to the hospital.

AFTER THE FALL

Dealing With Head Injuries

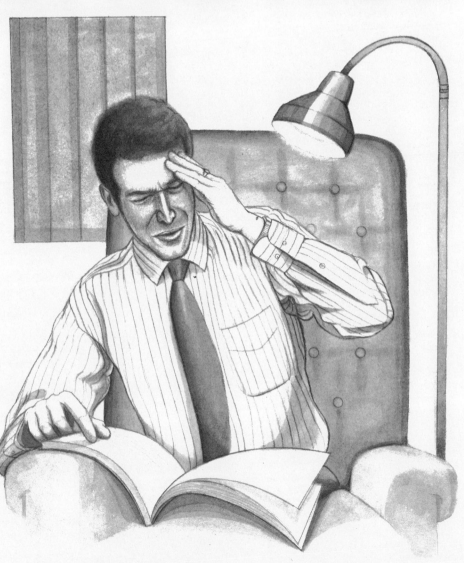

Edward R. Wolpow, M.D.

Modern life is hard on the head. One estimate is that there are 325,000 cases of mild head injury a year in the United States, costing over a billion dollars for hospitalized patients alone. Motor-vehicle accidents cause 42 percent of mild brain injuries. Falls account for another 23 percent, and assaults 14 percent. Falls are most important among the very young and the elderly; adolescents and young adults are more vulnerable to injury from other causes.

Many of these injuries are mild and seemingly of little consequence, but some cause persistent, subtle disruption of brain function. For anyone who must regularly handle demanding mental tasks—say a college student—a few months of thinking less well is bad enough. But worse, in a way, can be the reaction of the injured person's family, employer, and physician, who often fail to recognize that mild head injury may be followed by as much as a year of difficulty from the post-concussion syndrome.

Telling Blows

When someone loses consciousness for hours or days, has a skull fracture, or undergoes surgery to have a blood clot removed, nobody is much surprised when it takes a long time for that person to recover. Everyone's expectation is, appropriately, that such injuries take a long time to heal.

> Many head injuries are mild and of little consequence, but some cause a subtle disruption of brain function.

Much more common is the scenario in which a person gets whacked on the head and momentarily loses consciousness, or feels briefly stunned and disoriented but then comes to and appears to be essentially normal. If the episode is sufficiently frightening, the person is brought to a hospital or a physician; the appropriate examination reveals nothing clearly wrong. This patient has suffered a concussion—a blow to the head producing momentary loss of consciousness, or something close to it, without detectable anatomic damage to the brain.

Although researchers have investigated concussion, no one is entirely clear as to the nature of the injury. It appears there is some damage to the white matter of the brain, where long-distance traffic is carried through bundles of nerve fibers known as axons. Such damage can evidently occur whether or not consciousness is lost, and it leads to the postconcussion syndrome.

Not all blows to the head will do this. Boxers, for example, appear not to have postconcussion

syndrome every time they are knocked out (although the cumulative damage from boxing is well documented). To be injurious, a blow to the head must presumably strike at a particular angle and speed. The vulnerable portions of white matter appear to shear against each other in certain directions but not others. An analogy is a diamond that is cleaved along a specific plane when it is struck in a particular manner.

The Makings of a Syndrome

Postconcussion syndrome has several elements. Headache is a prominent complaint, even after tissue swelling and bruising from the direct blow have abated. Perhaps the most common is the muscle tension type, usually felt around the back of the head and neck. Contracted muscles are evident to an examiner. Medication can relieve this type of headache, which may last quite a long time. Sometimes a nerve under the scalp is directly damaged, and it will spontaneously cause pain (neuralgia) referred to the area it

> The injury done by a concussion is not entirely clear, but it appears there is some damage to the brain's white matter.

serves. Head injury can also precipitate a period of migraine attacks. It is not at all unusual for a bad siege of migraine, which may last for months, to be set off by even a trivial head injury.

Subtle intellectual deficits can develop. People most commonly have difficulty with memory, which becomes apparent as they try to learn new things. Tied to this change is a reduction in creativity—the ability to have new ideas—and in motivation to use the mind. This set of symptoms, often seen after head injury, may be mistaken for depression but is really a temporary reduction of intellect. Because the deficit tends to be slight, it is most noticeable in people to whom mental activity is important.

BESIDES THE BRAIN

The brain is not the only structure that can be damaged by a head injury. Broken teeth and noses are fairly obvious and relatively easy to treat. Some other potential problems are not so readily detected or fixed, however.

The Ear. The two delicate structures of the inner ear, the cochlea (for hearing) and the labyrinth (for balance), are protected by a bony enclosure but can still be injured. Even with modern imaging techniques, it is impossible to tell whether a few drops of blood have escaped into the chambers or a membrane has been torn. Preventing this type of trauma was the major reason for adding an ear flap to the batter's helmet in baseball.

Hearing loss or tinnitus (buzzing or ringing noises in the ear) can result from damage to the cochlea. And injury to the labyrinth sometimes causes dizziness and difficulty with balance—the most disabling symptoms for many head injury patients.

The Eye. If the eye is struck directly, the damage may be apparent to an ophthalmologist, who can see whether the retina is torn, the cornea scratched, or there is bleeding into the eye. But even if there is no obvious structural break or leak, patients sometimes complain of blurring or of vision that isn't quite right. This may result from the ocular counterpart of a concussion (presumably nerves in the retina are sufficiently injured to cause less-than-perfect vision, but no damage is apparent to the examiner).

The Sense of Smell. A blow to the front of the face can cut some or all of the fine nerve endings running from the nose to the brain. The loss or reduction in the sense of smell is often experienced as a dulling of flavors in food.

Fatigue—intellectual, physical, and emotional—is another important component of the postconcussion syndrome. The term "fatigue" is hard to pin down with a simple definition. In essence, people with fatigue may start a project feeling full of energy, but this sense quickly disappears. They can't stay with a task long enough to complete it. A typical example is picking up a book with the intention of reading a couple of chapters, but putting it down after getting through a page or two. Whatever the brain normally does to sustain commitment to a task fades out. It's also very

> **The effects may range from headaches and cognitive problems to a reduced tolerance for alcohol.**

common for patients to say that they get a headache after concentrating on the task for a short while and that this prevents them from continuing.

Underlying many of these cognitive difficulties is a loss of the ability to process more than one kind of information simultaneously. An example of the problem is given by Dorothy Gronwall, a researcher at the concussion clinic of the Auckland Hospital in New Zealand. As she points out, "the normal 3-year-old child can unwrap a toffee and can walk but cannot do both at the same time. In contrast, an adult can walk and hold a conversation while unwrapping the sweet." Gronwall points out that patients become slow to respond because they can only process "smaller than normal chunks of information," distractible because they cannot monitor irrelevant stimuli as efficiently as before, forgetful because they may ignore what they aren't focusing on, and inattentive because they

take in a limited amount of information.

An odd, but very typical, feature of the postconcussion syndrome is a reduced tolerance for alcohol. Someone who could drink two or three beers at a party now takes a few sips and feels drunk or drowsy. It's important that people be very careful about drinking after a head injury. The diminished capacity for alcohol will last as long as the other symptoms do.

People with postconcussion syndrome may also lose some insight. It is fairly common for them to believe that they can resume a normal work load soon after the injury and then to be surprised and disappointed when they can't.

Finally, and perhaps most strangely, personalities are likely to change. Typically, people become more assertive and less diplomatic than they have normally been. This may not be detectable

> **Patients need to know that they aren't crazy. Their symptoms are real. And they will get better.**

in someone who is usually brazen, and it might not show up in some cultural backgrounds. But in a setting where it is not tolerated, such assertiveness can have devastating effects.

Picking Up the Pieces

Recovery may come rather quickly after a long period of little progress. It typically takes longer in older people and in those who have had a previous head injury. One of the more specific signs may be the return to normal capacity for alcohol, which often accompanies the reappearance of normal intellectual function and energy. What may not be so easily reversible is a difference in personality. If you change for a while, and then come back to your "old self," the people around you are no longer the same. The world alters when it alteration finds, to misquote and contradict Shakespeare. You can't simply say a year later, "I didn't mean it at all." Bridges may have been burned.

There is no specific treatment for postconcussion syndrome. Reassurance and support are, however, critical. Patients need to know that they aren't crazy or malingering. Their symptoms are real. And they will get better. Sometimes the symptoms are nearly gone in a month, but it is not at all unusual for someone in an intellectually demanding role to lose a year from his or her life before returning to normal. Meantime, physicians, employers, coaches, teachers, and family should respect the fact that the working of the brain can be seriously affected by even a bloodless blow to the head. □

THE MIDDLE OF LIFE:
A Good Place to Be

Because life expectancy in the United States has increased so dramatically in this century, the definitions of middle age and old age are undergoing significant change. The postwar "baby boomers" are entering middle age; the population over 65 is expected to double by 2007. And thus, because so many of us expect to live a long life, the notion of 65 as the gateway to old age has begun to seem old-fashioned.

In 1890 life expectancy in the United States was only 42 for men and 45 for women, so that 65 indeed seemed—and was—a venerable age. Average life expectancy did not rise to 65 until 1940. Today people may regard themselves as still middle-aged in their fifties and sixties—the peak of accomplishment and satisfac-

> **Traveling, reading, and taking classes can help keep the mind in good shape. Regular physical exercise also aids mental functioning.**

tion for many. People in their seventies and older often retain their health, their energy, and their "psychic aliveness," as some psychiatrists call the zest for life. Dr. Arnold Modell, a psychoanalyst at Harvard Medical School, writes that "the middle years"— which begin at about 35 and may last the rest of our lives, until very old age sets in—are "life itself, or what living is all about." Of

course, for older people who are in poor health, lack access to adequate health care, or live in poverty, the picture may not be so rosy.

Nevertheless, recent research has done something to demolish the stereotypes of aging. None of the propositions listed below would have been taken seriously 30 years ago, yet all are now re-

garded as valid. (Note: The quote from Dr. Modell above, as well as citations below from Dr. Steven Roose, Dr. John Oldham, and Dr. Elizabeth Auchincloss are from *The Middle Years*, a collection of papers presented at a symposium organized by the Association for Psychoanalytic Medicine and published in 1989 by Yale University Press.)

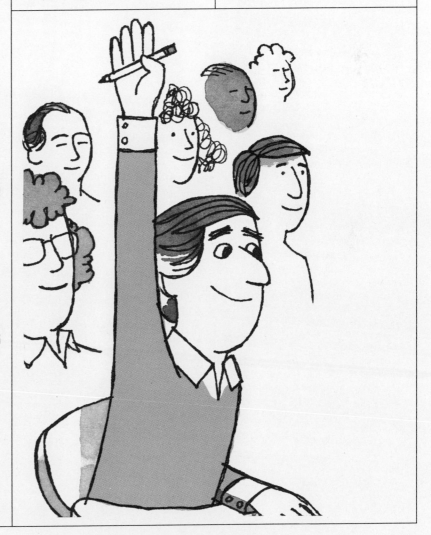

215

Some Mental Functions May Improve

Biologists used to believe that the end of early childhood marked the end of brain development and that the brain was complete and static until it began to decay. Now we know that the brain is dynamic and adaptable well into middle age and beyond, unless disease intervenes. Some brain changes occur during the middle years, specifically in the locus coeruleus, an area in the brain stem associated with anxiety and perhaps in some people with panic attack disorders and depressive diseases. According to Dr. Steven Roose of the New York State Psychiatric Institute, the deterioration of this area may account for the "mellowing" during middle age, the "decrease in intensity . . . a reduction in anger, anxiety, and impulsivity."

Anyone over 45 or so is also familiar with a slowdown of memory: names and facts may become harder to retrieve, although temporary memory lapses can be ameliorated with training. Yet studies of animals show that the brain remains open to development. Knowledge and good judgment are cumulative; they can and do increase with experience. Studies have found that many mental capacities are surprisingly stable across the years. One thing that makes a difference is keeping the mind in shape: working, reading, taking classes, talking to others, cultivating a hobby, playing games, traveling. Another thing that can help is regular physical exercise, which seems not only to help preserve neurological functioning into old age, but also potentially to enhance it in older people who had been sedentary.

Menopause Can Have a Positive Side

Menopause, marked by the cessation of menstruation, is a process, not an event. It may bring certain worries to the fore (fear of aging, for instance, or of being defeminized or desexualized). Yet most women find the passage relatively smooth. Some of the changes are for the better: no more menstrual cramps, no need for contraceptives, and no more worry about pregnancy. A woman's interest in sex may actually increase after menopause.

The great majority of women don't have medical problems caused by menopause. But for some women, estrogen loss may result in hot flashes or vaginal dryness—as well as a decline in bone density, putting them at risk for osteoporosis later in life. Most women will want to seek advice from a doctor about hormone replacement therapy, though not everybody needs it.

Sexuality Need Not Wane

An active sex life, contrary to myth, is by no means unusual in mid-life or even old age. Ongoing research indicates that 80 percent of men in their 60s continue to be interested in sex. At 78 or older, one out of every four men is sexually active. Women, too, retain their sexual abilities and interests into the 70s and beyond. Indeed, sex may be freer and more satisfying, since it is now separated from reproductive worries. Decreased sexual activity in older women usually arises from lack of a partner, rather than lack of interest.

It is true that sexual capacity in men (the ability to achieve and sustain an erection) can be altered by age. Women may experience a decline in vaginal lubrication after menopause. But these problems are not necessarily permanent and can be treated medically, if necessary—they need not limit sexuality. Coital performance is not the only expression of sexual love. Sexual love can endure, change, be renewed and developed throughout the life span. In middle age and later, people may renew a relationship with a lifelong partner or may change partners. They may change their sexual practices or feel able to express a lifelong but hidden preference. For instance, some heterosexuals may find companionship in a homosexual relationship.

And Going Strong

- **Verdi** composed his *Ave Maria* at age 85.
- **Martha Graham** performed on stage until she was 75 and choreographed her 180th work in 1990 at 95.
- At age 98 the noted pianist **Mieczyslaw Horszowski** played a full program and three encores to a sold-out house at Carnegie Hall in 1990.
- At age 80 *Marilla Salisbury* set a record for her age group in a five-kilometer walk. Her time was 40 minutes, and her pace just under five miles per hour.
- **Michelangelo** was carving the *Rondanini Pietà* six days before he died at age 89.
- **Marion Hart,** sportswoman and author, learned to fly at age 54 and made seven nonstop solo flights across the Atlantic, the last time in 1975 at age 83.
- **Anna Mary Robertson Moses** (Grandma Moses) had her first one-woman show when she was 80.
- **Titian** painted into his 90s.
- In 1981, at the age of 62, **Eugene Lang** launched his pioneering "I Have a Dream" program (now operating in 20 cities) to finance college educations for inner-city black and Hispanic children.
- Four new books on the recommended reading list in a recent issue of the *New York Times Book Review* were all by authors in their 80s or 90s: **Isaac Bashevis Singer** (Nobel Prize for literature in 1978), **Victor Weisskopf** (physicist), **V.S. Pritchett** (short-story writer), and **Isaiah Berlin** (historian).

The Benefits of Exercise Tend to Intensify

According to a recent editorial in the *Annals of Internal Medicine*, "functional aerobic age is probably lowered by the conditioning effect of repeated exercise." In other words, exercise makes you younger. Major studies have indicated that exercise prolongs life. In one study of 16,000 men, those who walked nine or more miles a week had a lower mortality rate than those who walked three miles or less. Those who engaged in light sports for two hours a week also increased their life expectancy.

More and more people in their fifties and sixties—and beyond—retain a zest for life as they explore new opportunities.

In another study, conducted at Washington University School of Medicine in St. Louis, heart function in men and women in their 60s improved by 25 percent to 30 percent after a year of endurance exercise. Men in their 70s showed increased muscle strength after just eight weeks of strength training. A recent report from the Medical College of Pennsylvania cited growing evidence that older people can start an exercise program at any age and have short-term physiological benefits as well as a reduced incidence of chronic diseases. Exercise can improve cardiovascular fitness, respiratory capacity, and strength. It can help lower blood pressure, raise HDL ("good") cholesterol levels, relieve emotional stress, and help with weight control. Weight-bearing exercise (such as running or walking) may delay or prevent the bone loss that comes with

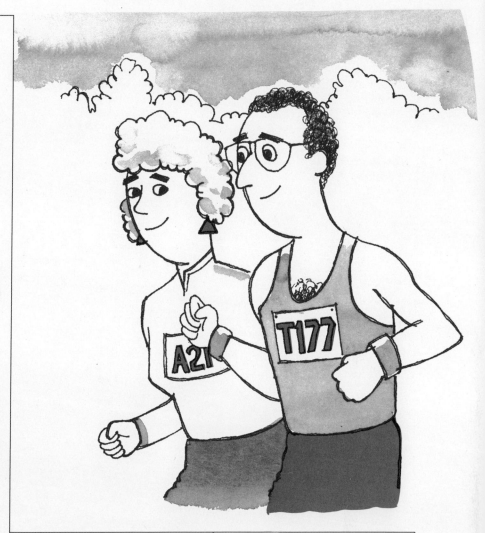

aging (osteoporosis). And people who exercise regularly almost always say it improves their sense of well-being.

If you are starting an exercise program in mid-life, you need to start slowly and increase the length and intensity of your workouts gradually. It's probably a good idea to check with a doctor before you significantly increase your exercise level.

Good Nutrition Has the Same Importance

It's just not true that older people need nutritional supplements, or lose their ability to digest high-fiber foods, or should stop eating

protein, or have to live on laxatives. Yet these and other myths persist.

In fact, older people need the same healthy diet as would any healthy adult—plenty of fruits, grains, and vegetables, which supply not only vitamins and minerals, but fiber as well (you need about 25 grams of fiber a day, a level that, when consumed with adequate fluid intake, will ward off constipation for most people and provide other long-term health benefits). Carbohydrates should supply most of your calories; protein should account for 12 percent to 15 percent of your caloric intake, and fat for no more than 30 percent. You don't need

217

supplements of zinc or vitamin C. It is true that caloric needs seem to diminish somewhat with the years, beginning as early as age 20 and decreasing by about 2 percent with each passing decade. But this change may be partly because people tend to become less active.

Retirement Can Have Positive Effects

It's a myth that retirement itself can take years off your life, although many of us worry about being bored or feeling useless when we're no longer part of the workaday world. Studies support

Older people need the same healthful diet as any healthy adult—plenty of fruits, grains, and vegetables, which supply vitamins, minerals, and fiber.

the idea that deterioration after retirement, when it occurs, is usually caused by some *prior* illness or disability. Many people actually thrive on a more leisurely way of life. Retirement, for many, presents an opportunity to reexamine their life goals and do new kinds of work.

The Empty Nest Is Often a Happy Nest

The departure of grown-up children from home—once thought to result in severe depression for mothers—may actually improve the lives of parents. One study of women with "empty nests" found that they often emphasize their opportunities to take on new roles, to function assertively and independently, and to enjoy their freedom once the daily responsibilities of parenthood are behind them. Though the study did not

look at the effect on fathers, they too might welcome what Dr. John Oldham, a psychoanalyst at Columbia University College of Physicians and Surgeons, calls a "much needed breather." The nest may quickly be filled up again by dependent parents, or sons or daughters returning with or without young children. Yet the respite can be welcome.

You Now Have Time to Be Altruistic

Although, according to the stereotype, older people are seen as needy rather than generous, a recent study suggests that concern for others increases with age. An estimated one-third of the elderly do volunteer work. In one study, reported in *Psychology and Aging*, almost 1,400 passersby were observed in a shopping mall as a pregnant woman solicited donations to fight birth defects: older people gave more often than the young, and those 65 and older gave more often than any other group. As you get older, too, you may have not only the time to be generous but also more available resources. There's some evidence that people who take an active role in their community tend to be healthier than those who live in

The departure of grown-up children may actually improve the lives of parents, giving them the chance to take on different roles.

social isolation. Thus altruism may benefit the giver as well as the receiver.

A recent survey found that many people go through a period of "major re-orientation in or by their 40s." More than half of those aged 56 to 65 said they completely agreed that "middle

age is a more caring and compassionate time."

You Finally Understand Your Parents

According to Dr. Oldham, emerging from adolescence into adulthood involves learning to interact with your parents from your own vantage point. Parents, as perceived by middle-aged offspring, are less "magically omnipotent." They become almost peers. As parents grow very old and die, however, children may idealize

In middle age, people see their parents as peers, not as "magically omnipotent," and forgive them for their shortcomings.

them once more. "Parents are gradually forgiven for their shortcomings, since one can no longer secretly hope for them to change or make amends for earlier mistakes," writes Dr. Oldham. As people grow older themselves, they tend to see their parents as having done their best and largely to forgive them their real limitations and mistakes.

Life May Stabilize in Pleasant Ways

According to Dr. Elizabeth Auchincloss of Cornell University Medical College "middle age is not only less eventful but also less stressful than youth. . . . As men and women are freed from the constraints of social roles that are currently typical of family life, men often shift toward a more nurturing, sensual, and affective orientation, while women, in contrast, begin to explore more 'socio-expressive roles'." In other words, you have a chance to think about and express new aspects of your ideal self. ☐

RSI
The New Computer-age Health Assault

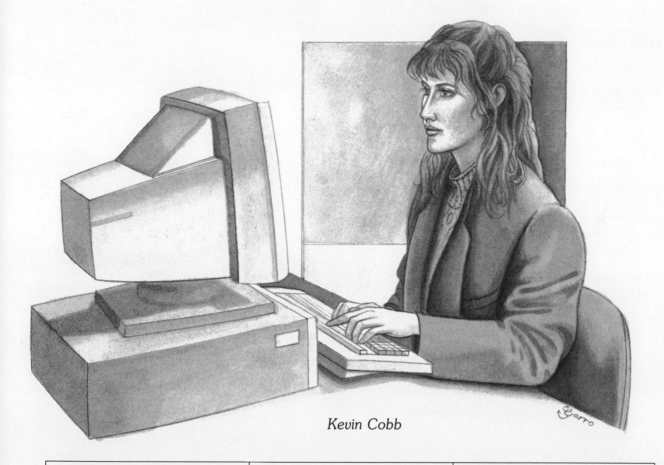

Kevin Cobb

October 12, 1988, is a date Deana Bunis will never forget. "That morning I woke up with incredible pain in my hands," says the 37-year-old business writer at *Newsday*, a daily newspaper on Long Island, N.Y. "They felt like they were on fire."

She immediately made an appointment with an orthopedic surgeon. Follow-up visits to an occupational-medicine specialist, two more orthopedic surgeons, and a rheumatologist finally helped nail down the diagnosis: repetitive strain injury, or RSI.

Two months later, with no relief in sight, Deana had to stop working. It was her job—typing her news stories at a computer terminal—that was causing the pain.

Deana is not alone—not by a long shot, it seems. Surprisingly, the new high-tech tools of her trade—the very computers that were to bring an era of unparalleled productivity—are also bringing a radical upsurge in ailments like hers.

Writers are by no means the only victims of RSI, whose pain strikes anywhere from the neck to the fingertips. Data-entry workers, computer programmers—anyone who spends long hours typing on a computer keyboard is at risk. So are other workers whose jobs require them to use their hands in repetitive motions for prolonged periods of time, including meat packers, auto and other factory workers, supermarket checkout clerks, even musicians. But it's the rapid proliferation of

219

computer-keyboard use that threatens to make RSI an industrial epidemic.

There are medical treatments that can ease the pain of RSI, and it's generally not a crippling disease. Many people do recover and return to their jobs, as Deana Bunis did, for example. But some find that while their condition may improve somewhat, it never goes away. The good news, though, is that RSI seems entirely preventable.

Getting a Handle on the Problem

" 'Repetitive strain injury' is the catchphrase used by many experts to describe disabling upper-limb pain caused by repetitive activities," explains Dr. James S. Thompson, formerly associate professor of orthopedic surgery, Johns

Many kinds of workers, from meat packers to musicians to the rapidly growing army of computer keyboarders, are vulnerable to RSI.

Hopkins University School of Medicine, and chief, hand/upper-limb reconstruction in the department of orthopedic surgery at Johns Hopkins Hospital, Baltimore. (Some experts, though, use the term Cumulative Trauma Disorder, or CTD.) The common factor in all RSI, he says, is overuse of muscle tendons, which causes inflammation followed by

pain and swelling, and which can impinge on nearby nerves. When RSI progresses to that extreme, a writer can become as disabled as a construction worker.

Why would computer keyboards cause RSI, when no such problem surfaced with decades of typewriter use? After all, keyboards seem much gentler by comparison—no paper to insert, no return lever to throw at the end of each line.

Ergonomists, scientists who study how people adapt to the workplace, believe that's precisely the problem. Instead of performing various tasks, someone working at a computer keyboard holds his hands, arms, back, and neck in the same static position, stressing the same muscles and tendons relentlessly for hours at a time, explains Steven Sauter, Ph.D., an ergonomist with the National Institute for Occupational Safety and Health (NIOSH) in Cincinnati. (It is possible that typists suffered these disorders, too, but they were not reported or recorded.)

The opportunity for injury increases if poor workstation design leads to awkward body positions that put extra strain on muscles and tendons, or pinch nerves. Add stress to the equation—with its muscle-tensing, shoulder-hunching effects—and there's even a greater chance of RSI, ergonomists say.

No one yet knows exactly how pervasive RSI really is. CTD occurring anywhere in the body now accounts for roughly 48 percent of all reported occupational injuries, according to the Bureau of Labor Statistics.

In a recent NIOSH study of 1,000 data-entry operators in New York State, 12 to 15 percent reported almost constant discomfort in their arms or shoulders. And in a recent NIOSH Health Hazard Evaluation at *Newsday*, 40 percent of the 834 workers surveyed reported symptoms consistent with RSI during the previous year. Reporters, who spent most of their day working at a keyboard, were

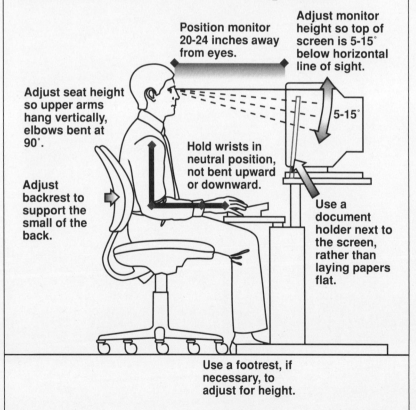

How to Sit at a Computer

Position monitor 20-24 inches away from eyes.

Adjust monitor height so top of screen is 5-15° below horizontal line of sight.

Adjust seat height so upper arms hang vertically, elbows bent at 90°.

Adjust backrest to support the small of the back.

Hold wrists in neutral position, not bent upward or downward.

5-15°

Use a document holder next to the screen, rather than laying papers flat.

Use a footrest, if necessary, to adjust for height.

more likely to report such symptoms than classified-sales representatives. The more time spent typing, and the faster the typing speed, the higher the prevalence of RSI.

These studies aren't absolute proof of a connection between keyboard use and RSI, says Dr. Sauter, but "it seems apparent there's a relationship there."

Recognizing RSI

There are many different forms of RSI. Carpal tunnel syndrome, whose pain is caused by pressure on the median nerve where it passes through the bony "carpal tunnel" in the wrist, has gotten the most press. Others include tennis elbow, tendinitis, and tenosynovitis (inflammation of a tendon and its sheath in the forearm or wrist).

No one yet knows for sure which types hit keyboard users most often. "There are no exact figures available for the United States," says Dr. Sidney Blair, professor of orthopedics at Loyola University Medical Center, in Maywood, Illinois. "But it appears that neck and shoulder pain are the most common. Hand and wrist problems account for 15 to 20 percent of all cases."

It needs to be said that many keyboard users never have a problem. And some get only mild symptoms that come and go. Others, though, have pain severe enough to warrant medical intervention. And in rare cases, RSI can lead to complete disability—where workers can't use their hands because of pain, nerve damage, or muscle loss.

The key for keyboarders, then, is to be aware of the signs of RSI and seek medical advice as soon as they notice the earliest symptoms, says Dr. Thomas Hales, occupational physician with NIOSH, in Denver. At that point, RSI can be nipped in the bud; the damage can be halted or even reversed, he says.

The symptoms to watch for are pain, numbness, or tingling in the

fingers, hands, forearms, shoulders, or neck, swelling of the hands, pain when moving your hands, or trouble using your fingers (clumsiness, dropping things).

Orthopedic surgeons and hand surgeons (a subspecialty) are experts in treating such musculoskeletal disorders. But many other groups—family physicians, rheumatologists, neurologists, for example—can treat these conditions, too. The key is to find a

It is important for keyboarders to be aware of the signs of RSI and seek medical advice as soon as they notice the symptoms.

doctor who's competent and experienced in dealing with computer-related RSI. One way is to check with your local medical society, says Dr. Blair.

Preventing the Pain

Doctors don't agree on which are the best medical treatments for RSI (see "Soothing Tender Tendons and More"). But all of the experts we spoke with agree that prevention makes sense. If overuse of muscles and tendons leads to RSI, then it stands to reason that easing the strain on those muscles and tendons can prevent or alleviate it.

That's exactly what NIOSH research has been finding. Recent studies show "indications of improvement in terms of reduced musculoskeletal discomfort in major companies that have made

SOOTHING TENDER TENDONS AND MORE

When it comes to treating repetitive strain injuries, doctors seem to agree on one thing: give it a rest. Either a reduced workload or some time off is usually recommended to give necks, shoulders, arms, or hands time to recuperate.

Beyond that, though, there doesn't seem to be a consensus on the best way to treat RSI. Some doctors prescribe nonsteroidal anti-inflammatory drugs to reduce pain and inflammation. Others prescribe muscle relaxants, splints, ice, aspirin, and physical therapy. Many doctors recommend the use of wrist splints to help relieve pressure on the median nerve. The splints keep the wrists in a neutral (not bent) position. Patients are usually advised to wear them only at night—locking the wrists during the day may cause you to compensate with abnormal elbow or shoulder motions, causing more problems.

Doctors may suggest applying heat or cold to relax muscles. "But be aware that heat may aggravate the condition in some patients," says Loyola University hand surgeon Dr. Sidney Blair. Occupational therapy or physical therapy with ultrasound, massage, or stretching exercises may also be prescribed. "Some doctors even believe in weight lifting exercises for the hands to rebuild muscles," says Dr. Blair, "but I think this is a bad idea. Repetitive motion is what's causing the problem in the first place."

Elevating the hands may help reduce swelling in some patients and thus relieve pressure on nerves, says Dr. Blair. He is also careful to treat any underlying medical problems that can contribute to swelling, such as thyroid disease. He recommends restricting salt intake for the same reason.

A few doctors believe that vitamin B_6 is helpful in relieving carpal tunnel syndrome, a type of RSI, "but there are no well-controlled studies that support this," says Dr. Blair. "Some people have been helped slightly by small doses—50 milligrams twice a day." Reports linking high doses of B_6 to nerve damage have made most physicians shy away from this option, however. Self-medicating is unwise. Talk with your doctor.

Patients who are disabled and are not helped by more conservative measures may find some relief with cortisone injections. Surgery to relieve the pressure on squeezed nerves is a last resort. It's best used only in cases of proven nerve entrapment and after getting a second opinion.

appropriate ergonomic interventions," says Dr. Sauter. Interventions range from reorganizing VDT workstations to correcting posture to making schedule changes. "We do advise applying these steps," says Dr. Sauter.

In recognition of this fact, the city of San Francisco recently enacted a law requiring proper adjustment of video-display terminal (VDT) workstations. If you are concerned about RSI or are already experiencing some discomfort, you may want to take some action to make your workstation and work habits kinder and gentler to your body. Here are some guidelines:

Set your sights on the screen. NIOSH recommends that you position the monitor 20 to 24 inches

> **The city of San Francisco recently enacted a law requiring proper adjustment of VDT workstations.**

away (about arm's length). Otherwise, the characters are too small to read comfortably, causing eyestrain; and you'll be likely to lean forward to see the letters more clearly, straining your neck and back.

Look for the best angle. The top of the screen should be a bit below your horizontal line of sight—between 5 and 15 degrees is comfortable for most people's necks. If you don't have an adjustable stand for your monitor, use whatever is at hand—a pile of books or 2 X 4s can do the trick in a pinch.

Get a document holder. If you must switch your gaze between a document and the screen, place the document in a special holder positioned right next to the screen.

See your way clear. If a vision problem causes you to strain your neck, consult your eye-care specialist about getting the proper glasses for the kind of VDT work you do.

Sit up straight. A stooped, hunched posture with your head extended forward can increase stress on the cervical (neck) spine and shoulders.

> **Think what you can do to make your workstation and work habits kinder to the body.**

Get a comfy chair. A well-designed, fully adjustable chair is a must for preventing poor posture, says Susan Isernhagen, a physical therapist and consultant in ergonomics from Duluth, Minnesota. The chair should have a backrest that maintains the normal arch of your back, she says. And the height of the chair and keyboard should be adjusted so your elbows are bent at about a 90-degree angle when typing.

Keep your wrists in line. Place the keyboard straight in front of you and keep your wrists in a neutral position—not bent upward or downward—while you type. A thin keyboard or wide, soft wrist rest can help minimize backward bending and reduce the strain on shoulders, neck, wrists, and arms. You can buy a wrist rest or custom-make one out of a firm piece of foam rubber.

Take a break. Get up and move around at least once every hour. Exercise breaks should gently work the kinks out of hands, arms, shoulders, and neck. This rests the muscles from the stressful static posture of hovering over the keyboard. It helps uncramp muscles, bringing better blood flow to nourish them and remove waste products.

Don't be so forceful. Striking the keys harder than necessary may lead to increased wear and tear, says Dr. Sauter. Depress the keys just hard enough to be sufficient.

Reschedule your work. Alternate highly repetitive tasks with other normal tasks. If you normally type for 20 minutes before proofreading, for example, try proofing every 10 minutes instead to give your arms and hands a break more often.

Build variety into your job. Try moving your phone or printer to a position you have to walk to, suggests Dr. Sauter. That way, sore hands and arms get a rest. This may seem inefficient, he says, but because it helps relieve fatigue, it may actually boost performance.

Don't let your VDT reflect poorly on you. Reflection or glare from your monitor can cause you to crane your neck to get a better view of the characters on the screen. Some VDT screens come with antireflection coatings. Attaching a mesh antiglare filter to the screen can also help fight glare. It's best if your monitor is placed perpendicular to windows. You can also use window blinds or curtains to help control glare. Finally, you can adjust the tilt of the screen slightly to aim reflections away from your eyes.

> **Exercise breaks and relaxation techniques can help uncramp muscles and ease tension.**

Learn to relax. You may not be able to prevent emotional stress at work. But taking a break to reduce muscle tension may help, says Dr. Sauter. One helpful technique is called progressive muscle relaxation. Sit or lie down comfortably. Tense and relax the muscle groups of the shoulders, neck, and back until you can identify when they are tense. Then let your back, neck, and shoulders go limp and concentrate on remaining relaxed for several minutes. It may take a few weeks or more for you to master this trick of relaxing. □

PROSTATE CANCER

Natalie Angier

When Frank Zappa's daughter, Moon Unit Zappa, told a concert audience in New York in November 1991 that her father was suffering from prostate cancer and could not attend the celebratory performance of his music, a disease that is often ignored or dismissed as an "old man's cancer" suddenly took center stage.

Mr. Zappa, an icon of progressive rock music since his days with the Mothers of Invention in the 1960s, has refused to discuss the details of his illness. His press agent said he was "fighting it well," was neither hospitalized nor bedridden, as had been rumored, and was working at home on his next musical project.

Mr. Zappa's case, together with the death in October of the producer Joseph Papp from prostate cancer, focused attention on a disease that unbeknownst to most people is one of the biggest causes of cancer death in the United States. Since 1973 the rate of prostate cancer has climbed by more than 50 percent, and it is now the commonest malignancy among American men and their second biggest cancer killer, after lung cancer.

In 1992, 122,000 men will develop the tumor and 32,000 will die of it, making prostate cancer the masculine equivalent of a far more publicized illness, breast cancer.

Detecting a Nascent Tumor

Although the disease tends to strike men over 65, the increase extends beyond what can be accounted for by the aging of the population. Mr. Zappa, for example, was only 50 at the time his illness became public knowledge.

As with most malignancies, the best way to treat prostate cancer is to catch it at its earliest possible stage. Many nascent tumors can be detected during a routine rectal exam; if a malignancy is removed when it is still confined to the prostate, the cure rate is essentially 100 percent.

Researchers are also making strides in the use of ultrasound as a noninvasive means of detecting prostate tumors, and they are fine-tuning blood tests that measure levels of a protein associated with the onset and evolution of the cancer.

Even for those suffering from advanced cancer, doctors now can tame the disease with a combination of potent hormones, putting a patient into remission for a decade or longer. The new drug therapy is a considerable improvement over the traditional and rather extreme treatment for advanced prostate cancer: orchiectomy, or removal of the testicles.

But doctors complain that male stubbornness prevents such advances from proving of much use. "The main obstacle to detecting prostate cancer early is that men are not as progressive as women are about getting routine checks," said Dr. William J. Catalona, chief of urologic surgery at Washington University Medical Center in St. Louis. "The fact is that 85 percent of men will not submit to a rectal exam unless they're having problems, usually related to urination." As a result, he said, "seven out of ten cases have already spread beyond the prostate gland by the time we detect them," at which point they are harder to treat.

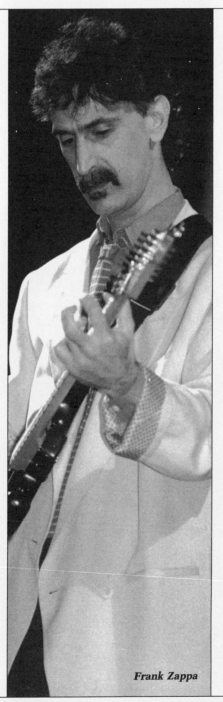

Frank Zappa

223

> **If detected early through rectal exam, prostate cancer is almost 100 percent curable. But most men shun routine rectal exams.**

Prostate cancer afflicts a walnut-size gland at the base of the bladder, which generates semen needed to transport and nourish sperm cells. Like breast cancer, which can be stimulated by estrogen, prostate cancer is often stimulated by sex hormones, androgens like testosterone. The two cancers are also thought to be at least partly the result of a diet rich in animal fats, although the link remains to be proved.

For reasons that remain mysterious, prostate cancer is two to three times as common in blacks as in whites, even when differences in socioeconomic status are taken into account. And the tumor generally is a slower-growing malignancy than is breast cancer, sometimes developing so gradually that it is never noticed while the person is alive.

But in other patients, particularly men younger than 60, the tumor can be swift and aggressive, which is one reason why the American Cancer Society now recommends annual rectal exams for any man aged 40 and up. In the exam a doctor inserts a gloved finger into the rectum to palpate the prostate gland in search of little nodules that may prove to be malignant.

Treatment

Beyond the unpleasantness of the rectal exam, many men stay away from the doctor's office because, until recently, surgery to remove the diseased gland usually destroyed an adjacent network of nerves that control erections, leaving a man impotent.

But in the last few years urology surgeons have perfected a delicate technique that excises the gland without disturbing neighboring nerve fibers. Assuming the tumor is still confined to the prostate, most men can soon resume a normal sex life.

"Today it's possible to treat localized cancer and preserve sexual function in 60 to 70 percent of patients," said Dr. Patrick C. Walsh, who is the urologist-in-chief at the Brady Urological Institute at Johns Hopkins Hospital in Baltimore.

For those in whom the cancer has spread to distant sites, like lymph nodes, surgery is no longer enough. To treat advanced disease, doctors cut off the body's production of androgens, depriving all stray tumor cells of the male hormones that fuel their growth.

Many physicians now use a combination of two drugs, one that prevents the brain from sending signals to the testicles to generate new androgens, and another that blocks the activity of any existing androgens that are still in circulation. Unfortunately, the drug treatment amounts to chemical castration, often extinguishing libido and potency.

Through anti-androgen treatment, a patient with advanced prostate cancer may live anywhere from 2 years to 15 years or more, long enough for many older men to die of something other than their cancer.

New Test

On a more experimental basis, some urologists are trying to ferret out new cases of prostate cancer with a test that measures a blood protein called prostate-associated antigen. The normal task of the protein is unknown, but researchers have found that levels of it often rise with the onset of prostate cancer and continue to soar as the tumor grows. But the experimental blood test still misses about 30 percent of tumors found through a rectal exam, and many researchers said the test needs considerable improvement before it will prove useful for large-scale screening.

"There's a lot of controversy about these markers right now," said Dr. Ruthann M. Giusti, a medical oncologist at the National Cancer Institute who treats many men with advanced prostate cancer. "Many of us feel that their specificity and sensitivity are just too low." For the time being, she said, men should learn to accept the sort of poking and prodding with which women are all too familiar. ☐

SIGNS AND SYMPTOMS

Most signs and symptoms of prostate cancer are nonspecific, that is, they are a warning that there is some kind of problem with the prostate, whether it's an infection, benign enlargement of the prostate gland, or cancer. One or two of the symptoms can mean problems completely unconnected with the prostate. Only an examination by a physician, accompanied sometimes by tests, can tell for sure. Also, early prostate cancer often shows no symptoms, so regular checkups for men 40 and up are essential. The nonspecific symptoms include:

- Weak or interrupted urine flow
- Inability to urinate or difficulty in starting urination
- Frequent urination, especially at night
- Blood in the urine
- Urine flow that is not easily stopped
- Painful or burning urination
- Persistent pain in the lower back, pelvis, or upper thighs

Source: American Cancer Society

PANIC DISORDER

Jamie Talan

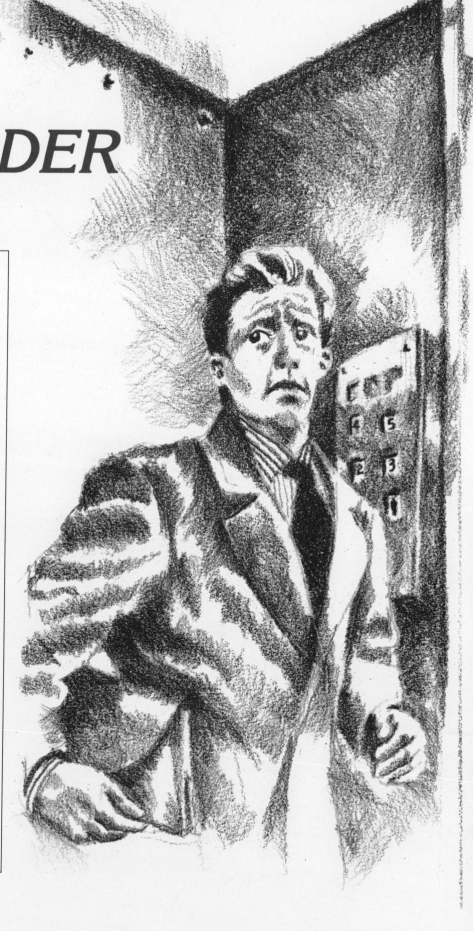

What if the doors don't open? Or the train gets derailed and crashes? What if I have a heart attack when the train is moving and nobody can save me? What if I don't make it out alive? Do I have enough insurance? How will my wife make it without me?

Life for Peter Pecere used to be a succession of such thoughts, accompanied by rapid heartbeat, nausea, shaking, numbness, hyperventilating, and sweating. He said he thought he was having a heart attack, but visits to emergency rooms and internists, neurologists and cardiologists, all left him with a clean bill of physical health. Then came the psychiatrists and psychologists, who had their own ideas. But analysis did nothing to prevent the panicked states from consuming his life. Prescribed drugs were also useless, offering nothing more than a two-week hospital stay to break his addiction.

Now, after two decades, Pecere said he is free of the thoughts and physical sensations that paralyzed him. He can ride elevators without fear that his heart will stop. He takes the train 16 stops from his home in Port Jefferson to New York, without worrying that he will die. He even took his first airplane flight, to Boston, with his therapist in tow, just in case.

"It wasn't that I was fearful of the train, or the elevator," Pecere said. "I was petrified of experiencing the racing thoughts and physical symptoms."

For Pecere and others who seek specialized treatment for their disorder, the what ifs are turning into so whats. Pecere is one of millions of Americans who suffer the debilitating effects of panic disorder, a psychiatric condition that can keep a person bound to the limits of their fears, the biggest of which is the panic attack itself. Studies suggested there is a biological explanation for such attacks, and researchers are finally taking seriously the warning signals experienced by up to 2 percent of the population with panic disorders.

The federal government is embarking on a national campaign to educate doctors and the general public about the symptoms of panic disease and how they can mimic many physical illnesses, including brain tumors and heart attacks. "Getting the medical community to accurately diagnose the illness and utilize the available treatments has been a tremendous problem," said Dr. Thomas Uhde, director of the Anxiety Research Program at the National Institute of Mental Health, the federal agency funding the educational effort. "We have the treatments, but they are not being delivered to patients."

In September 1991 a consensus panel charged by the federal government to make recommendations about the treatment of the illness found that physicians are unaware of the symptoms of panic disorders, often misdiagnosing and failing to treat patients.

According to Dr. Layton McCurdy, professor of psychiatry and dean of the Medical University of South Carolina in Charleston, only one in four people ever gets the proper treatment, and many end up so frustrated by the medical system that their condition drives them into hiding.

"I think there is significantly more money wasted on medical tests than it would cost to treat the condition," McCurdy said. Another problem, he added, is that many insurance companies

Millions of Americans suffering from panic disorder are bound to the limits of their many fears—the biggest of which is fear of the panic attack itself.

fail to reimburse for the treatment of such conditions. The panel also urged researchers to carry out more studies to figure out how common the disorder is and the best methods for diagnosing and treating it.

According to the *Diagnostic and Statistical Manual of Mental Disorders* (Third Edition, Revised), the diagnostic bible of the psychiatric profession, anyone who has four attacks in a given month has a panic disorder. The attacks, which occur twice as often in women as in men, come on sud-

SIGNS AND SYMPTOMS OF AN ATTACK

Spontaneous jolts of intense fear or discomfort accompanied by at least four of the following symptoms:

- Shortness of breath or smothering sensations
- Dizziness, unsteady feelings, or faintness
- Accelerated heart rate or palpitations
- Trembling or shaking
- Sweating
- Choking
- Nausea or abdominal pain
- Depersonalization—the feeling that you're removed from your own experience
- Numbness or tingling sensations
- Hot or cold flashes
- Fear of dying
- Fear of going crazy or losing control

Source: American Psychiatric Association

denly and are generally over within 10 minutes.

Causes

Researchers have few clues about the nature of the illness. Some believe that the attacks—a sudden feeling of doom accompanied by increased heart rate and blood pressure, profuse sweating, shortness of breath, and light headedness—may actually be a state similar to hyperventilation, taking in more oxygen than needed and blowing off too much carbon dioxide. This physical phenomenon, according to Dr. Jack Gorman, scientific director of the Phobia, Stress, and Anxiety Disorders Clinic at Long Island Jewish Medical Center (LIJ) in New York City, may induce the increased heart rate, altered blood pressure, and breathing difficulty seen during panic states.

Unlike generalized anxiety, these attacks occur spontaneously and not in response to undue psychological stress, researchers say. Indeed, studies are finding that these attacks are triggered by a chemical imbalance in the brain. Panic attacks can be both induced and prevented by administering chemicals that act on certain brain centers.

Studies are showing also that the condition may run in families. According to Myrna Weissman, an epidemiologist at the New York State Psychiatric Institute in Manhattan, panic disorder occurs at a rate of 15 percent in family members, compared with less than 2 percent of the general population. The institute is just beginning genetic studies of families with at least four relatives with the disorder to identify any markers linked to the illness.

Children and teenagers may also suffer from these panicky states. Also troubling is the recent finding that as many as one in five panic patients will attempt suicide, placing the condition on the same life-threatening scale as depression. Sufferers are also more likely to drink, a form of self-medication that may in itself exacerbate the disorder.

Treatment

According to Gorman, there are many therapies that work to diminish the fears of panicky patients, helping as many as 90 percent of patients.

The most common drug treatment is Xanax, a high-potency benzodiazepine. Certain antidepressant drugs such as imipramine also reduce symptoms. These drugs have side effects, including addiction, and doctors find that symptoms return soon after the medication is stopped. Surprisingly, some anti-anxiety drugs—Buspar and a drug called Ritserin that blocks the brain chemical serotonin—do not work in treating the disorder.

Roche Pharmaceuticals is now testing a new compound called bretazanil, a so-called partial benzodiazepine that acts within five minutes and could possibly be taken at the first sign of an attack, slipped under the tongue in much the same way an angina patient

> **Recent studies have shown that panic attacks can be both induced and prevented by giving chemicals that act on certain brain centers.**

uses nitroglycerin. The drug has just been tested in 160 patients in Basel, Switzerland, and researchers are still analyzing the results.

Few panic patients will be helped by medication alone, said Julian M. Herskowitz, director of TERRAP Anxiety and Phobia Care in Huntington, N.Y. There are a variety of cognitive and behavioral approaches that work, he said.

At LIJ, Gorman and his colleagues are involved with a large, multicentered treatment trial

studying the effectiveness of a combination of drugs and a form of behavioral therapy. The therapy was developed by researchers at the State University of New York at Albany and is based on the belief that panic sufferers are just more sensitive to their own

> **The average victim of panic disorder consults ten physicians before receiving a correct diagnosis of the condition.**

sensations. Head pounding may be interpreted as a brain tumor, a racing heart as a threatening cardiac arrest. Patients are taught to reproduce the sensations common during an attack, and in time they learn not to attach doom to these feelings. The program takes 12 weeks and says it has a cure rate of 90 percent.

Traditional psychotherapy, according to the federal consensus panel, is probably ineffective in treating the disorder.

One of the goals of the federal campaign will be to help doctors better diagnose the disorder and deliver appropriate treatments. According to Dr. Wayne Katon, a researcher at the University of Washington Medical School in Seattle, there is an overutilization of the healthcare system by people trying to figure out what is wrong with them.

The average person sees ten physicians before a correct diagnosis is made. And about one-third of patients who visit a cardiologist with atypical chest pain actually suffer from unrecognized panic. In one study Katon examined 74 patients referred for angiography and found that 43 percent of the patients with normal arteries had a panic disorder, compared with 5 percent of those with chest pain who had significant heart disease.

Ironically, there are some hints from a few small studies that people with these attacks of panic may be more at risk for certain diseases of the heart. For example, LIJ's Gorman has found that mitral valve prolapse (a condition in which one of the heart's four valves closes improperly, sending blood in the wrong direction down a one-way street) is twice as common among panic patients. Others have found a higher rate of stroke and cardiovascular death.

Dr. William Coryell, a psychiatrist at the University of Iowa, said that he believes that panic patients become more prone to heart illness because of the things they do—drink and smoke—and don't do—exercise—to avoid panicky feelings.

Joan K. describes her experience with the medical community in one word: exhausting. "I have been to internists, emergency rooms, two neurologists, orthopedists, and rheumatologists. I've had CT scans, MRIs, the works. I

> **Panic patients appear more prone than others to heart disease, perhaps because of the things they do—and don't do—to avoid panic.**

just kept thinking that doctors hadn't found what was wrong."

Pecere's monsters have become quiet since receiving behavioral treatment at the TERRAP center in Huntington. He relies on meditation and relaxation techniques to quell alarming thoughts. "Sometimes the what ifs pop into my head, but it doesn't stop me from doing something." □

For More Information

Anxiety Disorders Association of America, 6000 Executive Boulevard, Rockville, Md. 20852

OF CABBAGES AND KALE

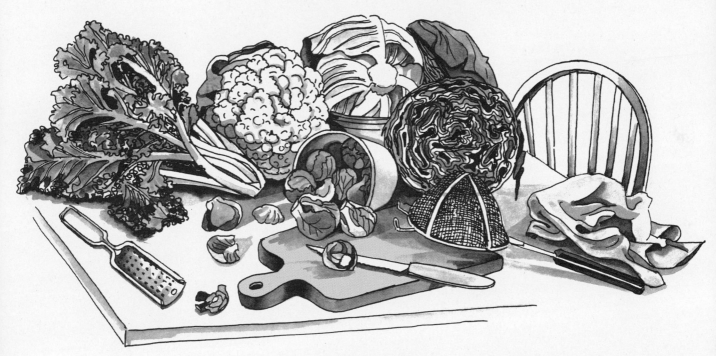

Louise Bloomfield

When was the last time that you were told to eat all you could of a certain food, instead of avoiding it as much as possible? Or that a real nutritional bargain, available fresh all year round, turned out to be equally easy on your pocket and your palate? If you thought healthful eating meant snapping up the latest exotic seaweed import at your local natural foods store, think again. Your best bet may be literally in your own backyard—in the cabbage patch, to be precise.

Cabbage—along with other so-called cruciferous vegetables— belongs to the biological genus *Brassica* of the plant family Cruciferae. There are dozens of *Brassica* species, and they vary so widely that no one would suspect they were related. Those commonly referred to as cruciferous vegetables include broccoli, brussels sprouts, cabbage, Chinese cabbage, bok choy, cauliflower, collard greens, kale, kohlrabi, mustard greens, rutabagas, and turnips. (As Mark Twain put it in *Pudd'nhead Wilson*, "cauliflower is nothing but cabbage with a college education.") The name "cruciferous," meaning cross-bearing, dates all the way back to the Middle Ages, when it was given to broccoli and cauliflower; these plants, along with their cruciferous relatives, have cross-shaped flowers.

Remedies Ancient and Modern

Cultivation of cruciferous vegetables began long before medieval times; in fact, it predates historical records. Cabbage is native to the Mediterranean region, yet it can also flourish in cold climates. It has been cultivated for more than 4,000 years; some other crucifers, such as broccoli and brussels sprouts, were later discoveries. Cabbage was brought to the western hemisphere by the French explorer Jacques Cartier in the 16th century.

The ancient Romans saw cabbage as something of a cure-all. More than 2,000 years ago the author Cato wrote that cabbage "would purge wounds full of pus and cancers . . . when no other treatment can accomplish it." Cato also advised eating cabbage before and after dinner because "it will make you feel as if you had not eaten, and you can drink as much as you like." As recently as the early 20th century, cabbage was recommended against scurvy, gout, rheumatism, asthma, tuberculosis, gangrene—and cancer, decades in advance of modern studies. Yet by the end of World War II its status had sunk to that of a homely, lower-class food.

A Nutritional Cornucopia

With the fruits of recent scientific research, the cabbage family has been rehabilitated. Many health professionals now regard cruciferous vegetables as both nutritional stars and possible protectors against devastating illness.

It's not just that crucifers are low or altogether lacking in some substances that can be notorious dietary hazards when consumed to excess—cholesterol, fat, and sodium. Many crucifers are rich in vitamins—chiefly vitamin C, vitamin E, and a substance from which the body produces vitamin A—as well as in such minerals as calcium, iron, and potassium. Moreover, a growing body of evidence suggests that some of their nutrients can be used by the body to fight the two leading killers: cancer and heart disease. Where science leads, tastes follow: in recent years U.S. consumption of broccoli and cauliflower has increased many times over. Even George Bush, whose aversion to broccoli became well known when he banned it from the presidential dinner table, admits to eating cabbage.

Cruciferous vegetables promote health in several ways. They are

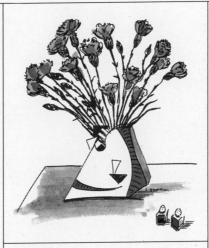

naturally low-calorie foods—a whole cup of shredded raw cabbage has only 15-20 calories; a cup of cooked broccoli, 45 calories. Many crucifers, including broccoli, cabbage, cauliflower, and kale, are high in fiber, an important part of any balanced diet. Fiber prevents constipation and the intestinal disorder diverticulosis, and some of the fiber in crucifers may protect against cancer of the digestive tract. Fiber also helps create a sense of satiety, or fullness, for the eater. High fiber and low calorie content make crucifers a boon to people who are concerned about excess weight; they can eat their fill of these vegetables without fear of tipping the scales at more than they would like.

Arsenals Against Cancer?

Broccoli and many other crucifers are a particularly good source of a class of nitrogen compounds called indoles. Indoles are thought to stimulate the production of enzymes that can neutralize carcinogens (cancer-causing substances) within the body, preventing them from initiating tumor formation. Indoles may have an additional role against breast cancer. Animal and human studies have found that they increase the rate at which the female hormone estrogen—which may promote the growth of breast tumors—is converted to an inactive form.

Other compounds found in cruciferous vegetables may also have an anticancer effect. Crucifers contain isothiocyanates, or mustard oils, volatile chemicals that are responsible for the pungency of mustard and cabbage. In studies with rats injected with carcinogens, isothiocyanates triggered the production of enzymes that slowed the growth of tumors, suggesting that crucifers might be useful in fighting existing cancers. Isothiocyanates may also act to prevent carcinogens from damaging cells. A study that was published in early 1992 indicated that sulforaphane, a mustard oil-type chemical that is found in broccoli and some other crucifers, might be especially protective against carcinogens.

Vitamin Virtuosos: Anticancer, Pro Heart?

You may have had a bellyful of Mom's urgings to eat your broccoli because it would give you vitamins and minerals, but even Mom probably didn't know just how sound her reasoning was. Broccoli, brussels sprouts, bok choy and other types of cabbage, cauliflower, collard greens, and kale are excellent sources of beta-carotene, an orange pigment that is converted into vitamin A in the intestinal wall. (Vitamin A itself, however, is found only in animal products.)

Beta-carotene is a potent antioxidant. In the body, antioxidants can help neutralize the unstable molecules known as free radicals, which are thought to injure cells. Free radicals are believed to cause tumors by damaging cells' DNA (the substance that carries the genetic blueprint of life). They are created as the body breaks down food (a process called metabolism), but they can also arise because of environmental factors such as cigarette smoke, ultraviolet light, and air pollution.

Recent studies have indicated that beta-carotene might protect against several types of cancers of

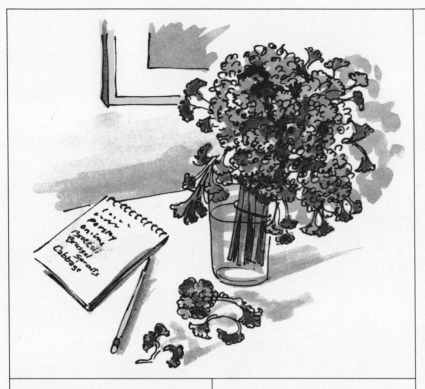

the lung, breast, throat, and bladder. There is also research suggesting that beta-carotene may be able to help fight existing epithelial cancers (tumors of the skin and lining tissues).

If the cancer findings aren't enough to persuade you to clean your plate, what about evidence that beta-carotene may help combat heart disease? An ongoing Harvard University study of 22,000 U.S. physicians found that those taking a beta-carotene supplement had only half the anticipated rate of cardiovascular events such as heart attacks and strokes. A study carried out at the University of Minnesota further found that adding cruciferous vegetables to a high-fat, high-cholesterol diet could serve to reduce blood cholesterol levels. (The buildup of cholesterol in arteries—cholesterol is a fatty substance manufactured by the body but also contained in animal foods—ranks as a major cause of heart disease.) Beta-carotene has one other advantage that is worth noting: unlike vitamin A, it is not toxic in large doses.

Research suggests that vitamins C and E may also protect against heart disease, as well as aiding in cancer prevention. Vitamin C, especially abundant in broccoli and brussels sprouts, may act to prevent skin cancer. It may also help ward off cancers of the bladder and esophagus by preventing the body from forming carcinogenic compounds known as nitrosamines. Nitrosamines result when the body metabolizes nitrites and nitrates, chemicals found especially in smoked, pickled, and cured foods like hot dogs and ham.

High blood levels of vitamin C have been correlated with high levels of so-called good cholesterol. This is cholesterol contained in "high-density lipoproteins" (HDL). HDL molecules carry cholesterol through the blood to the liver, where it can be eliminated from the body instead of being deposited along artery walls. This finding suggests one reason why vitamin C might be effective against heart disease. Furthermore, vitamins C and E both act as antioxidants, and there are indications that they can prevent the oxidative modification of "low-density lipoproteins" (LDL), which also carry cholesterol. Many scientists think that oxidation of LDL may begin a process ultimately leading to the formation of plaque in an artery wall. Vitamin E is thought to help prevent cancer largely because of its action as an antioxidant, forestalling the destructive effects of free radicals, but it also helps maintain healthy

Crucifer Tips

Cold storage: When buying fresh cruciferous vegetables, choose only those that are refrigerated or on ice, with firm stalks and no wilting of the leaves. Avoid cauliflower and broccoli whose florets are discolored.

At home, store fresh crucifers in a vegetable crisper at 32°F to prevent loss of moisture.

Some crucifers, including broccoli and cauliflower, can be bought frozen, with their nutrients largely intact. Frozen vegetables should not be thawed before they are cooked, to guard against spoilage.

Clean carefully: Wash crucifers thoroughly, just before use. Do not soak leafy vegetables; indoles and vitamin C may be lost in the water. Separate leafy greens, and slosh the leaves in tepid water to remove grit.

Crisp cooking: Crucifers cooked until they are just tender-crisp retain the most nutrients and flavor; cabbage, brussels sprouts, and cauliflower turn bitter if cooked too long. Cruciferous vegetables should not be cooked in aluminum-surfaced pots and pans, which affect both their color and their flavor. Cook stalks longer than florets, or cut gashes in broccoli stalks and brussels sprout bottoms to reduce cooking time. Use as little water as possible, to preserve indoles and vitamin C.

cells. Leafy cruciferous vegetables, chiefly collard greens, mustard greens, and turnip greens, are good sources of vitamin E (along with such foods as plant oils, nuts, and wheat germ).

Mineral Mainstays

Minerals, especially calcium, are another vital nutrient in the cruciferous repertoire. Some 99 percent of the body's calcium stores are used to develop and maintain teeth and bone, but calcium is also needed to regulate heartbeat, hormone and enzyme activity, transmission of nerve impulses, and muscle contraction. When the body does not obtain enough calcium from dietary sources, it takes what it needs from the bones. In the early decades of life new bone develops to replace tissue lost for this or other reasons, but in later years the rate of bone loss exceeds that of new bone formation. This can leave bones brittle and prone to fracture, a condition known as osteoporosis. For postmenopausal women, whose bone mass is less dense to begin with than that of men and whose bodies no longer produce in substantial amounts the estrogen that slows bone loss, this condition is especially hazardous and is responsible for many hip fractures and other serious injuries.

A number of crucifers—among them bok choy, turnip greens, mustard greens, and kale—are particularly rich in calcium; moreover, they contain it in a form that can be readily absorbed by the body, unlike the calcium in, say, spinach. One study even found that the calcium in kale was more readily absorbed by the body than that in milk. Like their vitamin E, crucifers' supply of calcium is concentrated in the leaves. Such leafy greens with absorbable calcium can supply all the body's calcium requirements, though dairy products are the primary calcium source in most Western diets. For vegans (vegetarians who consume no dairy products), cruciferous vegetables are especially important as calcium sources.

Calcium may be cruciferous vegetables' chief mineral contribution to the diet, but it is not the only one. Crucifers also supply significant amounts of iron (vital to regulating the oxygen content of the blood) and potassium.

Turning Over New Leaves

Most nutrition experts stress the value of making nutrient-rich foods such as cruciferous vegetables a mainstay of a balanced diet. This is more likely to foster good health than is taking megadoses of isolated chemicals in the form of supplements. Fortunately, the culinary uses of crucifers are as various as the vegetables themselves. (The many varieties of cabbage make it one of the most versatile members of the cruciferous family.) Some crucifers can be eaten raw: shredded cabbage is the basis for coleslaw, and broccoli and cauliflower are also delicious raw or only barely cooked. Turnips and rutabagas can be used in stews and soups. Leafy crucifers like kale can be cooked briefly and served as a side dish or in a stir fry.

Most health authorities say that a balanced diet should contain at least five servings of fruits and vegetables every day. (For broccoli or a leafy green vegetable, a serving would be half a cup.) Crucifers—easy to prepare and delightfully varied—are fine candidates for those vegetables. Keep in mind, however, that even the most nutritious foods are only as healthful as their preparation allows. When cauliflower is smothered in cheese sauce or broccoli swims in a lake of butter, what could have been a healthful side dish is weighed down with calories, fat, and cholesterol. The fact that a stir fry heavily salted or drenched in soy sauce started out with plenty of low-sodium cabbage won't help people watching their sodium intake one bit. But a mixture of nutritional common sense and some imagination is the best recipe for turning crucifers into real stars. □

Crucifers: An Epicure's Guide

Delicious recipes using cruciferous vegetables are easy to find. For those who prefer to experiment, following a few general guidelines will enhance flavor while preserving nutritional value:

broccoli—use in soups, stir fries, or casseroles; serve raw or lightly blanched in salads or with dips; steam or microwave, and serve as a side dish

brussels sprouts—serve as a side dish, lightly steamed, briefly boiled, or microwaved, and seasoned with lemon juice or a small amount of cheese

cabbage—shred into a slaw; bake with another vegetable or meat stuffing; stir-fry; use in soups

cauliflower—serve raw or lightly blanched in salads or with dips; use in soups, stir fries, or casseroles; when microwaved or steamed, can be a tasty side dish

collard greens—serve cooked in seasoned broth as a side dish

kale—stir-fry or serve lightly steamed (wilted) as a warm salad green or a side dish

kohlrabi—shred raw into a slaw or serve braised as a side dish

mustard greens—serve as a side dish, cooked in a seasoned broth

rutabaga—serve diced and braised as a side dish, or use in soups or stews

turnips—serve as a side dish or in soups or stews; the greens can be prepared like collard greens

Living With Cataracts—and Without Surgery

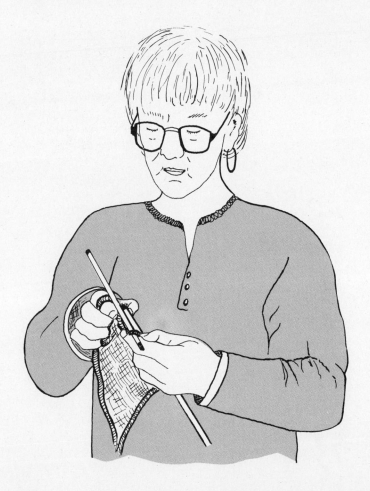

In some instances cataracts may progress rapidly, and early surgery may be recommended. In most cases, however, cataracts develop very slowly, and surgery may well be postponed, or never become necessary.

The first symptom of cataracts that most people notice is a definite, painless decrease in visual acuity. Everything becomes dimmer, as if your glasses were always in need of cleaning. Sometimes a difference in the degree of opacity in one part of the lens as compared to another causes rays of light entering the eye to split into different parts, resulting in double vision. Sometimes your vision of near objects will actually improve for a period of time, and you will be able to read without the aid of your bifocals. This is because a cataract in the center of your lens has caused the lens to thicken and thus become optically stronger. In time, however, this thickening of the lens will cause progressively more severe near-sightedness.

Paradoxically, your vision may be worse in very bright light, because light causes the pupil to contract and, since most cataracts are located in the center of the lens, the contraction of your pupil will restrict your vision to that portion of the lens most severely affected by the cataract.

Finally, as the cataract progresses, the nucleus of the lens becomes more and more yellow, which means it will absorb violet light rays and, later on, the blue light rays, causing the world to lose these colors and appear increasingly yellow.

Of course, if you have any such symptoms as these, you should consult your ophthalmologist, as you would with any visual problem. But if your physician diagnoses cataracts, you should not worry unduly: they are a ubiquitous and normal part of aging. Changing your glasses may help temporarily, and, in a very few patients, dilating drops have proved to be helpful.

In the United States half of the population over the age of 40 has some degree of visual impairment due to cataracts, an opacity or clouding of the eye's lens that progresses over time. And by the age of 60, 75 percent of Americans have cataracts, whether mild or severe. Currently, the only effective treatment for cataracts is surgery, but fewer than 15 percent of people with cataracts have visual impairment so severe as to require it.

If your cataracts progress to the point that they force you to give up something that is important to you—such as driving, reading, working, or watching television—you will want to consider surgery. There are a number of rare situations in which cataract surgery cannot be safely delayed. Your ophthalmologist will explain these to you. Otherwise, if you can

Half of all Americans over age 40 have some physical impairment due to cataracts; by the age of 60, three out of four Americans have cataracts.

still take part in your favored activities, it is usually fine to delay surgery indefinitely, as most people do—and learn a few tricks to make it easier to get along.

Ways to Enhance Your Vision

1. Either too much light or too little may cause vision problems if you have cataracts. When you are indoors, make certain you have plenty of light. And when you go out into the sunshine, wear sunglasses with yellow-tinted lenses. A yellow-tinted lens will absorb blue light, which is the light most readily scattered—and so transformed into glare—by incipient cataracts. Corning makes a lens called "glare control," which is a yellow-to-amber gradient lens (darker at the top than at the bottom); the lens is available as a clip-on, or it can be ground to your prescription. You might buy clip-on lenses to try them out and, if they work well for you, have prescription lenses made to order. Many cataract patients do not notice any benefit from wearing sunglasses, some of which can be quite expensive. You will need to experiment.

2. Outdoors, wear a large brim hat or a hat with a visor, or sit under an umbrella to minimize glare.
3. You may do better with outdoor activities if you can keep them in shady areas rather than out in the bright sun.
4. Indoors, incandescent light is generally better than fluorescent light if you have vision troubles.
5. Keep your light sources below your eye level (for example, table lamps may be better for you than ceiling fixtures).
6. Make sure you have good area lighting for stairs and entrances.
7. Install dimmer controls so you can get just the right level of light.
8. Install any mirrors you may have in your home in such a way as to minimize confusing, or multiple, reflections—especially if you are having trouble with double vision.
9. Large-print books and newspapers will help.
10. A magnifying glass may help you read some things, if the type is crisp and clear. But, if the type is indistinct around the edges, as newspaper type is, a magnifying glass will just give you a larger, but still blurred, image. And if the visual problem comes from a lack of contrast between the letters and the printed page—that is, if the letters are not good, dark

When your cataracts force you to give up an activity you cherish, it may be time to consider surgery. In other cases, surgery can often be delayed.

images against a white background—a magnifying glass won't help very much.
11. The best reading light is a desk or floor lamp with an adjustable arm and an opaque reflector shade. Have the light shine over

your shoulder onto the page of the reading matter. And make sure the lamp is close enough. Many floor lamps may be adequate when they are close to you, but quite inadequate if they are as much as six or eight feet away. Experiment with the placement of a floor lamp to get it at just the right distance for you.
12. If glare is troublesome when you read, try covering the half of the page you are not reading with a piece of black matte cardboard, which will reduce the glare from

Both too much light and too little can cause problems if you have cataracts. Better lighting indoors and sunglasses outdoors may help.

the page. In recent tests performed at The Lighthouse (a national organization founded to help people with visual impairments), it has been found that standard 60-watt to 100-watt light bulbs are often the best to use; if glare remains a problem, try a 50-watt indoor incandescent flood lamp with a metal shade.
13. Don't use a miniature clip-on light designed for reading in bed or a pinpoint halogen light. Such lights produce a bright spot of illumination that will cause your pupils to contract. You want a moderate, diffuse light.
14. When you watch television, don't have another light on in front of you; it will only produce a distracting glare.

For additional information on cataracts and on other visual problems as well, contact The Lighthouse at 111 East 59th Street, New York, N.Y. 10022, 212-355-2200. If you have vision problems resulting from cataracts, you should discuss them with your ophthalmologist. □

SINUS INFECTIONS

Sinuses, those eight hollow cavities at the front of the head, are better appreciated for the trouble they cause than for any good they do. In fact, no one really knows why the sinuses exist, but an estimated 31 million Americans have had sinus problems.

The symptoms are painfully unmistakable: stuffy nose, headaches, a seemingly never-ending drainage of yellowish-green mucus, the face perhaps tender to the touch. But all the torment can be tamed. Usually all it takes is a little preventive know-how or quick action once infection sets in. And for certain stubborn cases that occur over and over again, a relatively new procedure has made surgery an easy-to-face solution.

How Sinusitis Begins

The sinuses, which open and drain into the nose, normally contain air, which keeps the mucous membranes that line them in good health. Sinusitis, or inflammation of the sinuses, occurs when a blockage cuts off a sinus's access to air, explains allergist Dr. Gailen Marshall, assistant professor of medicine and director of allergy and clinical immunology at the University of Texas Medical School at Houston. A familiar type of blockage is the nasal congestion and swelling associated with colds and allergies.

When a sinus becomes blocked, the mucosal cells use up the remaining oxygen inside the cavity. This creates a vacuum that pulls on the mucous membrane, creating that sensation of pressure a person feels with a cold or allergy, Dr. Marshall says. The pulling on the membrane also causes inflammation, which can produce fluid inside the sinuses.

Sneezing, or blowing your nose, only worsens the situation. It forces open the blocked ducts, allowing the low-pressure atmosphere of the affected sinus to suck in even more mucus from the nose. As mucus thickens and

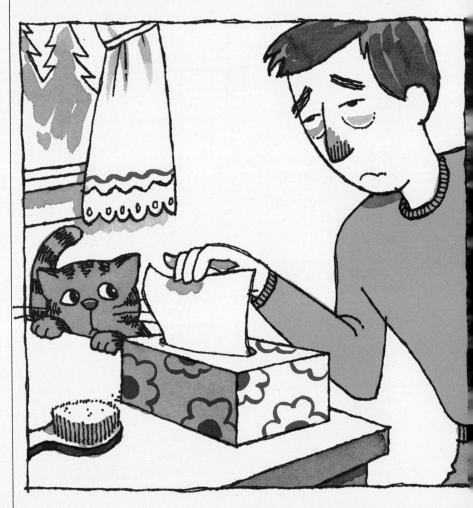

stagnates in the sinus, it becomes an excellent breeding ground for bacteria.

Usually sinusitis is associated with a bacterial infection preceded by a cold or allergy, says Dr. Marshall. But any number of other conditions can cause sinus problems, including viral or fungal infections, ruptured tooth abscesses, or injury to the face.

In the typical case, taking an over-the-counter decongestant at the first sign of nasal congestion is the best insurance against a case of sinusitis. "Any sinus blocked

234

long enough eventually will get infected," Dr. Marshall warns. When full-blown sinusitis develops, a trip to the doctor and antibiotics are in order. It's time to seek treatment when the thick, yellowish-green mucus continues to drain; the area of the face overlying the affected sinus perhaps feels tender to the touch or is swollen; and a low-grade fever develops.

A first-ever or occasional case of sinusitis usually responds to antibiotics, which should make you feel better within three to four days. But it takes them at least two weeks—and sometimes three weeks—to vanquish the bug. Failure to finish the prescribed course of drugs invites the infection to return. If an antibiotic doesn't begin to bring relief within three to four days, the involved bacteria probably are resistant to the drug. In that case, the doctor may prescribe a more powerful antibiotic.

Complications of sinusitis are rare but potentially dangerous. Because some of the sinuses are so close to the brain, infection can spread to the linings of the brain to cause meningitis. The eyes and nearby bones also are vulnerable to serious infection.

Chronic Sinusitis

A stubborn sinus infection that doesn't go away after two to three weeks of antibiotic treatment is considered chronic sinusitis. If an infection is the culprit, longer antibiotic therapy usually will be required.

But the most common underlying problem, says Dr. Marshall, is chronic recurrent allergic rhinitis—the stuffy nose and sneezing familiar to people with hay fever and other allergies. Other suspects include a tumor or an anatomic abnormality that restricts drainage and air flow. When sinus infections recur every two months or so, it may be time to consider consulting an ear, nose, and throat specialist for possible surgery.

Some 31 million Americans have had sinus problems. Luckily, there are ways to prevent them and also to tame them.

A procedure introduced in the late 1970s has made surgery less destructive, says Dr. Becky McGraw-Wall, an ear, nose, and throat specialist. Endoscopic sinus surgery can be used instead of conventional surgery in most people, says Dr. McGraw-Wall, an assistant professor of otolaryngology at the University of Texas Medical School at Houston.

The goal of surgery is to provide drainage for the obstructed sinus. Conventional surgery usually entails entering the sinus through an incision on the face or under the upper lip, chiseling out the bone at the front of the affected sinus to remove the infected contents and then creating an opening into the nose at the bottom of the cavity to allow the sinus to drain by gravity.

In contrast, endoscopic sinus surgery involves inserting a thin, telescopic tube through the nose. The endoscope magnifies the nose's anatomy as the surgeon uses tiny instruments to remove any obstructions of the sinus and to enlarge the opening. Retaining the normal sinus opening encourages proper drainage, because cilia—tiny hairlike structures on mucosal cells—continue to push secretions toward the normal sinus opening.

Conventional surgery may still be indicated to treat extensive disease or complications of sinusitis involving the eye. But for less extensive disease, endoscopic surgery may be preferable. The surgery is done as an outpatient procedure, it's less bloody and less destructive, and patients recover faster. Both types of sinus surgery carry some risks. But in experienced hands, sinus surgery is considered to be safe. And it's likely to bring an end to the vexing cases of sinusitis that won't yield to simpler solutions. □

SEVEN TIPS TO PREVENT SINUSITIS

The watchwords for avoiding sinusitis are "Keep the nose open." Houston allergist Dr. Gailen Marshall offers the following suggestions to help keep nasal passages open during a cold or an allergy attack:

- Take oral decongestants such as Sudafed or Afrin at the dosage recommended on the label. Use topical nasal decongestants no longer than five days. (People with high blood pressure, heart disease, or insomnia should check with their doctor before using nasal sprays.)
- Drink plenty of water. Fluids keep mucus thin, and thin mucus drains more easily than thick.
- Take medications such as Robitussin that contain an expectorant, or thinning agent, like guaifenesin.
- Avoid alcohol. Alcohol can cause congestion and it dehydrates the body, making mucus thicker.
- Try saline nasal sprays. They soothe by keeping the tissues moist. In a few people, however, they will actually cause congestion.
- Clear the nose by blowing gently, one nostril at a time. Loud, forceful blowing causes rebound congestion.
- Try breathing steam in a shower or leaning over a sink of hot water. Avoid using steam machines, which can burn the inflamed membranes. In low-humidity climates, humidifiers may help.

COUNTERING
SERIOUS SCARRING

Jane E. Brody

Even under the best of circumstances, injuries and operations are not readily forgotten. When they leave behind a scar that is disfiguring or that limits mobility, the legacy can be emotionally scarring as well.

In recent years plastic surgeons and dermatologists have devised promising preventives and treatments for these ugly and uncomfortable scars. In some cases the remedy can be successfully ap-

> **When an injury or operation leaves a disfiguring scar, the legacy can be emotionally scarring as well.**

plied even to scars that are years old, but most work best when a scar is just forming, so patients should tell their doctors about past scarring problems.

The Scarring Problem

Living tissues of all kinds form scars, which represent new cells laid down to close a gap in the skin, whether from a kitchen knife or surgeon's scalpel, a burn or blister, a scrape or a chemical. Whether the wound is superficial or deep, the process is basically the same.

After an injury, whether accidental or deliberate, the body musters an inflammatory response, bringing white blood cells and antibodies to the area to help de-

stroy or expel intruders like infectious organisms and dead cells. As the inflammation subsides, scar tissue begins to form. It includes tiny new blood vessels called capillaries to restore circulation. Then cells in the adjacent skin called fibroblasts start producing a fibrous connective tissue, collagen, similar to the tissue inside the end of the nose. Linkages form between the fibers, increasing the strength of the scar. The more fibers, the firmer and less flexible the scar.

For unknown reasons, in some people scar tissue grows far beyond the amount needed to heal a wound, forming a benign tumor-like growth called a keloid that is uncomfortable and unsightly. For a person who forms keloids, ear piercing can cause a scar the size of a golf ball. The tendency to form keloids is especially common among blacks and Asians, strongly suggesting a genetic factor. People who form keloids are usually advised to avoid cosmetic surgery.

In another more common type of abnormal scarring, called hypertrophic scars, the scar tissue overgrows but stays within the confines of the original wound. The raised portion may subside with time, but many of these scars remain an ugly problem, causing pain, itchiness, or irritation and sometimes interfering with body movements.

Far more troublesome are the big, angry-looking hypertrophic scars that can develop when extensive burns heal. These scars can impede movement, especially around a joint.

According to Dr. William W. Monafo, a professor of surgery at Washington University School of Medicine in St. Louis, hypertrophic scars are neither predictable nor preventable. They most often form in children, adults under 40, and dark-skinned people after deep wounds or incisions as well as burns.

Even people who do not scar abnormally often develop cosmetically undesirable scars after a deeply scraped knee or elbow. If the scrape bleeds, a scab will soon form to cover the wound. But when the scab falls off, the scar beneath it typically forms a depression and may remain indented indefinitely.

Getting Help

Let's start with the easy ones first. The trick to avoiding indented scars is to prevent scabbing. This can be done by covering the

> **Plastic surgeons and dermatologists have had success with treatments ranging from drug therapy to promising new surgical procedures.**

cleaned wound with a nonstick or other semipermeable bandage that keeps the wound warm and moist but allows air to penetrate.

Ordinary surgical scars can sometimes be removed by a popular technique called dermabrasion, often used to minimize acne scars. Dr. Bruce E. Katz and colleagues in the department of dermatology at Columbia University College of Physicians and Surgeons in New York recently reported good results from scarabrasion, as they call it. In a study of 48 patients, half the scars treated at eight weeks after injury disappeared.

Scarabrasion, which can be an outpatient procedure, involves numbing the area with an anesthetic spray, abrading the scar, applying an antibiotic ointment, and keeping it covered with gauze for about one week.

Hypertrophic scars are more challenging. Surgical remedies often leave a worse scar, although there has been some success with skin grafts, which have more stretch than the scar tissue.

More recently, Dr. Thomas A. Mustoe, a plastic surgeon at Washington University School of Medicine, in studies with Dr. Monafo and their colleagues, tested a treatment for hypertrophic scars that is moderately to greatly effective in two-thirds of patients. The treatment works best with scars that are a few months old, but even when the scars are a year to four years old, the St. Louis team has reported beneficial results in many patients.

The treatment involves placing a sheet of silicone gel over the scarred area for 12 or more hours a day over a period of several months. The area can be hidden by clothing; the gel is best left in place all day, except for brief daily cleaning.

In patients who are helped, the raised scars become flatter, lighter in color, and more flexible. Studies thus far indicate that the improvements last at least six months. A few patients successfully treated several years ago have thus far retained the improvements, Dr. Mustoe said. He added that ''you can tell within a month if the treatment is working,'' thus sparing patients who would not be helped the months of treatment.

Since the initial reports from the St. Louis team, there have been four other reports of success with the therapy from surgeons in other countries, and many physicians in burn centers in the United States have adopted the approach, Dr. Mustoe said. A self-adhering gel for large areas is now under development.

The most difficult scars to treat are keloids. While there have been a host of efforts, including the use of lasers to remove keloids, recurrences are extremely common. Patients who know they form keloid scars and are anticipating surgery should tell the surgeon in advance.

Treatment with antibiotics and corticosteroids either applied to the surface or injected into the scar as it forms can often inhibit keloid formation, reduce pain, and even cause a keloid to shrink, according to Dr. Ted Rosen, a dermatologist at Baylor College of Medicine in Houston. Some patients may benefit from repeated freezing of the scar with liquid nitrogen, followed by corticosteroid injections.

When all other methods fail and a keloid is disfiguring or debilitating, surgical removal may be attempted, followed by periodic corticosteroid injections as the wound heals. □

Anatomy of a Scar: When Healing Backfires

When the skin has been injured, cells adjacent to the injury produce collagen, a fibrous connective tissue. Sometimes far more new tissue grows than is needed to heal a wound. Tumorlike growths of excess tissue are called keloids. A more common condition, raised tissue within the confines of the original wound, is called a hypertrophic scar.

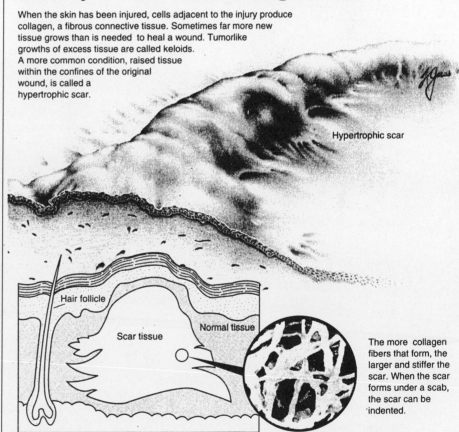

Hypertrophic scar

Hair follicle

Scar tissue

Normal tissue

The more collagen fibers that form, the larger and stiffer the scar. When the scar forms under a scab, the scar can be indented.

Sources: "Dermatology: A Medical Artist's Interpretation," Geras (Sandoz); "Your Skin," Haberman and Fortino (Playboy)
THE NEW YORK TIMES

237

MENACE OF THE MAT

Joseph Gustaitis

With all the training, exercise, and competition that high school and college wrestlers take part in, you'd think they would be in top-notch health. And they are, except for one thing. Why are so many being stricken with an illness that can cause rashes, cold sores, headaches, and fevers that can zoom to 105°F?

The answer is that many of them are falling victim to a condition called herpes gladiatorum, a form of herpes infection that strikes competitive wrestlers.

The Nature of Herpes

Herpes infections can take several forms. The ancient Greeks, who were renowned athletes in their day, recognized the symptoms, and the term "herpes" is derived from *herpein*, Greek for "to creep," a reference to the rash or sores that tend to creep across the skin of a victim. It wasn't, however, until the beginning of the 20th century and the discovery of viruses that scientists finally recognized the causes of the various herpes infections.

It turned out that there are five different herpesviruses that infect humans. (Dozens of others infect different kinds of animals). One causes chicken pox and shingles, a second causes infectious mononucleosis, and a third is responsible for an infant infection called cytomegalic inclusion disease.

The fourth one, known as herpes simplex virus, comes in two types, type I (HSV-1) and type 2 (HSV-2), and is the virus that causes the diseases most people think of when they hear the word "herpes."

These two familiar forms of herpes are oral and genital. The first, usually transmitted through kissing, normally takes the form of cold sores or fever blisters on the lips or face. Genital herpes, which is considered a sexually transmitted disease, also shows up in the forms of rashes and blisters, but these occur below the waist. For the most part (but not exclusively) oral herpes is caused by HSV-1 and genital herpes is caused by HSV-2.

The Wrestlers' Problem

Herpes gladiatorum is the fifth of the herpes viruses that infect humans. It is contracted through the rough-and-tumble contact that comes with grappling with an opponent in a wrestling match. The virus can travel from one contestant's rash or cold sore into a break in the other's skin, or it can be picked up directly from a contaminated mat. Whatever the avenue, after a two-day to seven-day incubation period, the virus causes its victim to break out in a rash or cold sore and perhaps also suffer such symptoms as headaches, fever, and chills. Like the other herpesviruses, it stays in the body for life and may cause recurrences, especially during times of stress (and, coaches point out, wrestling matches are preeminently stressful). Theoretically, the virus could be spread by an athlete in any sport, but in most other sports the players are protected by uniforms, pads, or helmets, and even in basketball or boxing, where much of the skin is exposed, there is little of the kind of constant body contact that occurs in wrestling.

A U.S.-wide study published in 1988 found that 7.6 percent of college wrestlers and 2.6 percent of high school wrestlers had herpes gladiatorum. That report was based on a survey taken during the 1984-1985 wrestling seasons; the numbers today are probably higher.

What Can Be Done?

The rules now state that wrestlers at all levels must have skin inspections before they compete, and at the college level, at least, trainers are careful to wash mats with a disinfectant, sometimes three times a day. Such heroic efforts are impractical at the high school level, however, where mats may be used for other sports besides wrestling and where physicians are usually unavailable to examine wrestlers and coaches are ill-prepared to distinguish herpes from, say, poison ivy. There is no vaccine that can prevent infection with the virus, and there is no real cure, although the drug acyclovir may help reduce the healing time of the rash or sores.

As a result, one of the world's oldest forms of athletic competition may be thrown into a high-tech future. Although not all coaches would necessarily agree, Bobby Douglas of Arizona State has even suggested that future grapplers may have to come to meets with a body suit, helmet, and mouth guard. "We need to get ready for the 21st century," he warns, "and stop thinking about what wrestling is like in the 20th."

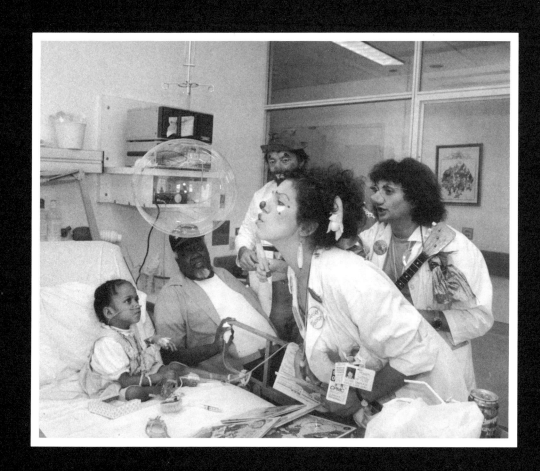

HEALTH &
MEDICAL NEWS

Contributors

Authors of articles in the Health & Medical News section

Boettcher, Iris F., M.D. Assistant Professor, Department of Medicine, Michigan State University; Director of Geriatrics, Butterworth Hospital; Medical Director, Grand Valley Health Center, Grand Rapids, Mich. AGING AND THE AGED.

Davis, Sharon Watkins, M.P.A. Director, Cancer Information Service, Fox Chase Cancer Center, Philadelphia. CANCER (coauthor).

Engstrom, Paul F., M.D. Vice President for Population Science, Fox Chase Cancer Center, Philadelphia; Professor of Medicine, Temple University School of Medicine. CANCER (coauthor).

Fisher, Jeffrey, M.D. Clinical Associate Professor of Medicine, Division of Cardiology, New York Hospital-Cornell Medical Center, New York City. HEART AND CIRCULATORY SYSTEM (coauthor).

Guze, Barry H., M.D. Assistant Professor of Psychiatry and Biobehavioral Sciences and Director, Ward 2-South, Neuropsychiatric Hospital, University of California at Los Angeles. MENTAL HEALTH.

Hager, Mary. Correspondent, Washington Bureau Staff, *Newsweek*. ENVIRONMENTAL AND OCCUPATIONAL HEALTH; GOVERNMENT POLICIES AND PROGRAMS: UNITED STATES.

Higgins, Linda. Free-lance health and medical writer; columnist, *Hippocrates* magazine. NUTRITION AND DIET; PUBLIC HEALTH.

Koren, Michael J., M.D. Medical Director, Cardiovascular Sonography Labora-

tory, Memorial Medical Center of Jacksonville; Clinical Assistant Professor of Medicine, University of Florida, Gainesville. HEART AND CIRCULATORY SYSTEM (coauthor).

Mandel, Irwin D., D.D.S. Associate Dean for Research, Columbia University School of Dental and Oral Surgery. TEETH AND GUMS.

McMillan, Julia A., M.D. Deputy Director and Residency Program Director, Department of Pediatrics, Johns Hopkins School of Medicine. PEDIATRICS.

Mickleburgh, Rod. Health Policy Reporter, Toronto *Globe and Mail*. GOVERNMENT POLICIES AND PROGRAMS: CANADA.

Pelot, Daniel, M.D. Clinical Professor, Division of Gastroenterology, Department of Medicine, University of California, Irvine. DIGESTIVE SYSTEM.

Ramos, Andrés A., M.D. Attending Physician and Director of Ambulatory Division, The Francis Scott Key Medical Center, Baltimore; Clinical Instructor, Johns Hopkins School of Medicine. OBSTETRICS AND GYNECOLOGY.

Travis, John. Free-lance science writer, contributor to *Science* magazine. GENETICS AND GENETIC ENGINEERING.

Zuckerman, Connie, J.D. Assistant Professor of Humanities in Medicine and Coordinator of Legal Studies, State University of New York Health Science Center, Brooklyn, N.Y. BIOETHICS.

AGING AND THE AGED

New Law Helps Enforce Patients' Treatment Preferences • Cataract Surgery Evaluated • Overcoming Incontinence • Alzheimer's Drug Update

Patient Treatment Preferences

A new federal law helps protect Americans' rights to decide what medical treatment they will accept in case of permanent unconsciousness or a condition where death is a likely outcome. The measure, known as the Patient Self-Determination Act, went into effect in December 1991. It requires all healthcare institutions that receive Medicare or Medicaid funds to provide adult patients with written information about their legal rights, under the law of the state where the institution is located, to stipulate in advance their wishes regarding life-sustaining medical care.

The new measure is the first federal law to focus on an individual's right to refuse treatment and on so-called advance directives. These may take the form of documents such as living wills, which spell out an individual's treatment preferences in the event of future incompetence. Or the directive could be a "durable power of attorney for healthcare" or similar document appointing someone as a proxy to speak for a person should he or she become incapable of declaring preferences. Individuals may file either a living will or a proxy appointment or both.

A goal of the new law is to educate members of the public on their rights, as well as on the benefits of advance directives—which can improve communication between doctor and patient, increase understanding of the patient's wishes, and help ensure that treatment is in accordance with a patient's values and preferences. Despite these benefits, it is estimated that fewer than one-fourth of Americans have filed advance directives. The new law is intended both to encourage filing and to ensure that healthcare professionals and institutions honor the directives. Most states have laws or judicial decisions that recognize treat-

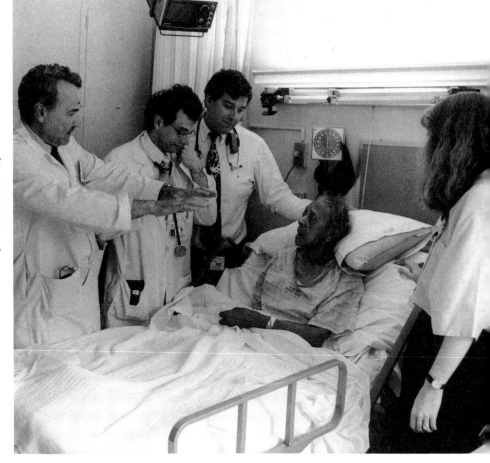

As the population of the United States gets older, the need for physicians with expertise in the care of the elderly grows. In this pilot program at the Mount Sinai Medical Center in New York City, some geriatrics training is given to physicians in other specialties.

ment directives, yet there is evidence that these are ignored or overridden a fourth of the time.

Institutions subject to the law include hospitals, nursing homes, hospices, home healthcare agencies, and health maintenance organizations (HMOs). They must provide patients with written information on state law covering advance decisions and refusal of treatment, as well as on their own institutional policies regarding these matters. Institutions are required to include any advance directives in the individual's medical record and must not in any way discriminate against patients on the basis of the presence or absence of an advance directive. The law also mandates that institutions keep their policies on self-determination up to date, have written procedures for implementing the policies, and provide staff and community education on advance directives.

Safety of Cataract Surgery

As people age they become more likely to develop a cataract, which is a clouding of the lens of the eye. The most frequently used method of removing a cataract is also the safest, according to a 1991 study that analyzed all Medicare patients who had cataract surgery in 1984.

Three procedures are currently used to remove cataracts. In the most common, called extracapsular cataract extraction (ECCE), only the cloudy lens is removed, while the transparent capsule surrounding the lens is left in place. A tiny piece of plastic is implanted to replace the part taken out. The study suggested that leaving the capsule intact may stabilize the internal structure of the eye and reduce the risk of a detached retina—that is, the separation of the delicate light-sensitive nerve layer from the back of the eye. Retinal detachment can lead to permanent blindness if untreated.

Another way of removing a cataract is known as intracapsular cataract extraction. In this procedure the lens and surrounding capsule are removed, and a larger piece of plastic is implanted in the front part of the eye between the iris—the pigmented muscle that gives the eye its color—and the cornea, the clear protective layer on the front of the eye. The researchers noted that this procedure can cause corneal swelling, inflammation, and glaucoma. They found that patients undergoing it were more likely than ECCE patients to suffer retinal detachment later.

The third procedure that is currently employed, phacoemulsification, is also the newest. It uses ultrasonic vibrations to fragment the lens. The study found that retinal detachment occurred more often after this procedure than after ECCE. Younger patients and white patients were more likely to suffer this complication.

Reducing Urinary Incontinence

Another 1991 study found that bladder training programs are effective in reducing or eliminating urinary incontinence in older women. Urinary incontinence—the inability to control the release of urine—occurs in up to 42 percent of older women. It can cause psychological problems, and coping with it can pose a financial burden.

The study involved more than 100 women aged 55 or older who were all functionally capable of using the bathroom but who all had at least one episode a week of urinary incontinence. About half of the women underwent a bladder training program, involving audiovisual, written, and oral instruction to help them keep to a set schedule of urination. Every week their progress was checked, and they were encouraged to continue following the schedule. The other women in the study formed a "control" group, which did not undergo the training program. When the two groups were compared after six weeks, the women in the training program had significantly fewer episodes of incontinence. More of them had regained continence, and the amount of urine they lost through incontinence was less.

The researchers concluded that since bladder training is less expensive and less risky than either surgery or medication, it may be the best way to begin treatment for incontinence, unless the presence of an underlying medical condition calls for a more drastic approach.

Tacrine and Alzheimer's Disease

The U.S. Food and Drug Administration declined in 1991 to approve the marketing of a controversial drug for the treatment of Alzheimer's disease, despite pressure from some researchers and the public for its release. The drug, which is known as tacrine, or tetrahydroaminoacridine (THA), had been used experimentally since the early 1980s to attempt to stay the progression of Alzheimer's disease, a gradual deterioration of intellectual abilities that may rank as the fourth leading cause of death in the United States, according to some experts' estimates. Preliminary findings suggesting tacrine could be a useful treatment for Alzheimer's were not borne out by subsequent researchers. The drug was found to cause liver damage and possibly other problems in the high doses originally given. Moreover, studies with lower doses failed to find substantial benefits from tacrine. New studies using larger doses are under way to evaluate both the drug's effectiveness and its safety. Late in 1991 the FDA agreed to expand the number of patients taking tacrine under its program for experimental drugs.   IRIS F. BOETTCHER, M.D.

BIOETHICS

Physician-assisted Suicide • Organ Transplants From Living Donors • Curbs on Free Speech in Family Planning Clinics • A Grandmother as Surrogate Mother

The Right to Die

The right to die and the involvement of doctors in patient suicides were focuses of wide debate among the American public in 1991, as several developments drew attention to the impact of a technologically sophisticated but sometimes inhumane healthcare system on people facing the end of life.

Physician-assisted Suicide. In a November 1991 referendum, voters in the state of Washington narrowly rejected a historic proposal to legalize a form of euthanasia, or mercy killing. The measure would have permitted doctors to administer lethal doses of medication to patients who had six months or less to live and had made a written request for suicide assistance. Early polls predicted strong voter support for the proposal, although many doctors believed the measure would require violating their Hippocratic Oath. The initiative's defeat was attributed largely to voter concern that the measure lacked sufficient safeguards. In particular, fears were voiced that vulnerable elderly patients might seek suicide assistance because of subtle pressure from family members or a reluctance to impose a burden on others.

In a March 1991 article in the *New England Journal of Medicine*, Dr. Timothy E. Quill of Rochester, N.Y., wrote about how he became involved in a patient's suicide even though he courted the risk of legal liability. His patient—a woman with acute leukemia—decided not to undergo grueling, experimental chemotherapy, which offered a 25 percent chance of survival. She chose to take medication only for relief of pain and to spend her remaining time at home with her family. The patient, however, requested that Quill prescribe enough medication to allow her to take her own life if her suffering became unbearable. Reluctantly, Quill agreed, and eventually the woman did commit suicide. A grand jury declined to indict Quill on criminal charges of aiding a suicide, and the New York State Health Department decided not to discipline him for professional misconduct. Given his thoughtful account of the case, his long-term relationship with the patient, and the safeguards he built into his decision (including careful discussion of her choice with her and her family), Quill's actions were greeted sympathetically, if not entirely supported, by other doctors and the public.

By contrast, Dr. Jack Kevorkian, a retired Michigan pathologist who had invented a "suicide machine," was widely condemned after he made public the device's availability and the machine was actually used in 1990. A local judge in 1991 barred Kevorkian from using the device again, but late in the year he helped two women—neither of whom he had treated previously—to take their own lives. His medical license was later revoked, and in early 1992 he was indicted on two counts of murder.

Suicide Manual. *Final Exit*, a "how-to" suicide manual, was a best-seller in 1991. Its author, Derek Humphry, was the founder of the Hemlock Society, an organization that supports suicide for the terminally ill. Many observers found the public's inordinate interest in this topic a sad commentary on the inadequacies of American society in providing support for

The surprising success of the best-selling Final Exit, *a "how-to" suicide manual by Derek Humphry, was a vivid indication of the wide public interest in the controversy over the right to die.*

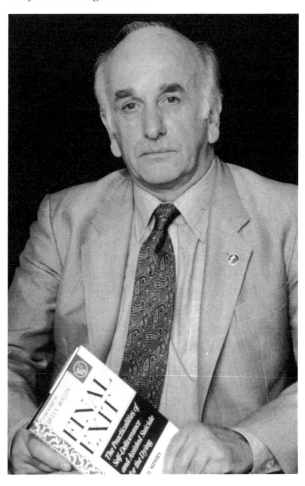

those in dire need. Others, however, praised the availability of such a manual, citing the right to commit suicide as the ultimate freedom in an era marked by a healthcare system whose technological sophistication often eclipses humane caring.

New Protection for Patients' Wishes. Federal legislation is now in place in the United States that obligates healthcare facilities receiving Medicare and Medicaid funding to educate patients about their rights regarding end-of-life decisions under the law of the state in which the facility is located. The Patient Self-Determination Act, which took effect on December 1, 1991, mandates that patients be alerted to the possibility of filling out an "advance directive," such as a living will or a "durable power of attorney for healthcare," which authorizes another person to make the patient's healthcare decisions if the patient should lose the capacity to make them. By taking advantage of these options, patients can ensure that their wishes regarding acceptance or refusal of medical treatment are respected, even if they are incapacitated at the time a treatment decision needs to be made. The use of advance directives can help patients have more control over their care while saving doctors from having to resolve difficult ethical dilemmas.

Debate Over Medical Futility. Doctors in a Minnesota hospital took the unprecedented step of seeking court approval to remove a permanently comatose woman from a life-support system even though her family refused to give its consent to the action. Helga Wanglie, an 87-year-old woman with severe brain damage, was in a vegetative state for over a year while her family and physicians attempted to reach agreement over her care. The doctors believed that keeping the woman alive by means of a respirator was medically futile, but her husband, with the concurrence of their children, wanted life-sustaining care to be maintained, asserting that both he and his wife believed in preserving life at all costs.

The court's decision, issued in early July 1991, sidestepped the substantive issue of what, if anything, constitutes "futile" care. Instead, the judge chose to affirm the role of the patient's husband as the appropriate surrogate decision maker for this incompetent patient and ordered the hospital to keep Mrs. Wanglie on the respirator. She died three days after the court ruling, however, leaving behind an increasingly necessary debate over the limits of a physician's obligations to provide care in cases of a hopeless prognosis.

Controversial Lung Transplant

The ever worsening shortage of donor organs in the United States, accompanied by increasingly sophisticated transplantation capabilities, has led healthcare providers, patients, and families to seek alternative, at times controversial, methods for helping people in desperate need of new organs.

In Minnesota, nine-year-old Alyssa Plum was in dire need of a lung transplant after a rare virus virtually destroyed her own lungs' ability to function. Her situation became so grave, and the lack of a suitable donor so critical, that doctors took the unusual step of transplanting a small portion of her father's lung in an effort to save her life. The operation was not successful, and her mother then volunteered to be an addi-

---

Instant Information

The length of time between the completion and review of a medical research paper and its actual publication in a journal can run anywhere from eight weeks to three years. In a more leisurely era that sort of time frame may have been acceptable, but nowadays the pace of research has become so rapid that protracted delays in publication can mean that valuable new findings go unreported much too long—and when the information is potentially lifesaving, the delay becomes unconscionable.

For this reason, the American Association for the Advancement of Science, in conjunction with the Ohio-based Online Computer Library Center, has launched a venture that promises to bring the medical journal into the computer age. It is a publication called *The Online Journal of Current Clinical Trials*, and it is accessed "online," that is, through a computer over telephone lines.

Submissions (which can also be sent in electronically) undergo a peer review process, just like articles in print journals, but once they are accepted they are available to subscribers within 24 hours. Taking advantage of current computers' abilities, the electronic journal carries not only text, but also sophisticated graphics in the form of tables, charts, graphs, and equations. The cost is in line with the price of print journals.

Dr. Edward J. Huth, the editor, says that the new publication was designed "precisely because patients could benefit if research findings were made available sooner" and asserted that it is "the first journal to make available immediately findings that could affect the lives of Americans."

tional donor. Unfortunately, Alyssa died during the course of the second transplant operation.

The use of donor organs from living people is highly unusual. In Alyssa Plum's case the situation was complicated by the enormous pressures on the donors. Critics argued that it was virtually impossible for the parents to render voluntary, informed consent. Concern for their daughter's well-being left them unable to weigh objectively and reasonably the risks that the procedure posed for their own health. Many commentators suggested that this was a situation where what is technically feasible may not be ethically defensible in actual medical practice.

HIV-infected Healthcare Workers

The plight of 23-year-old Kimberly Bergalis, who died of AIDS in December 1991, sparked a fierce national debate concerning the risk to patients from doctors and other healthcare workers infected with the human immunodeficiency virus (HIV), the virus that causes AIDS. Bergalis, along with four other individuals, had apparently become infected during dental procedures performed by Dr. David Acer, a Florida dentist who subsequently died of AIDS in 1990. Before Bergalis died, she aggressively lobbied for federal legislation to require mandatory testing of healthcare workers for HIV infection and to prohibit those infected from performing invasive procedures.

The U.S. Centers for Disease Control entered the debate, asking organizations of healthcare professionals in mid-1991 to draw up lists of "risk-prone" procedures from which infected health workers should be barred. Almost all professional organizations refused to cooperate, citing the lack of scientific evidence that, if they followed proper infection-control procedures, infected health workers posed any significant risk to their patients. (It is believed that Dr. Acer did not follow infection-control guidelines already set by the CDC.) The CDC ultimately agreed that closer attention to infection-control measures and individual monitoring of the fitness of infected health workers were sufficient to ensure patient safety.

Abortion and Free Speech

The U.S. Supreme Court in May 1991 upheld federal regulations barring employees of family planning clinics that receive federal funds from discussing the option of abortion with clinic patients. Although most such patients have a legal right to abortion, the government ordered that clinics receiving federal financial support not promote abortion in any way. In supporting the government's position in the case (*Rust v. Sullivan*), the Supreme Court said that such patients were no worse off than they would be if no federal money were available.

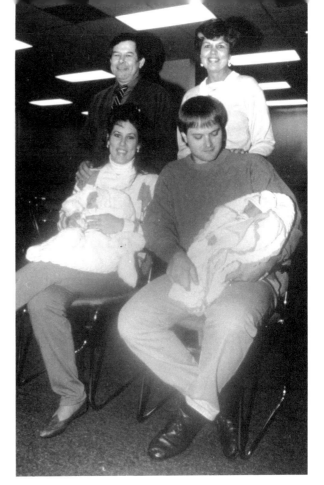

The issue of surrogate motherhood took an unusual twist when Arlette Schweitzer (top right, with her husband, Dan) became pregnant with her own twin grandchildren. She served as a surrogate mother for her daughter, Christa Uchytil, and her husband, Kevin (in front with the twins).

Critics of the decision, including major medical organizations, saw it as a governmental intrusion into the doctor-patient relationship and the process of informed consent. Critics also said that the regulations imposed an inequity on poor women, who are often members of minority groups and who may have nowhere else to turn. In March 1992 the government announced it would not enforce the counseling ban against doctors. This position was criticized on the grounds that without new regulations it had no legal standing, that it would make no difference to most patients because doctors do very little of the abortion counseling in clinics anyway, and that there were still limits on what doctors could tell their patients about abortion.

Unusual Surrogate Mother

The continuing controversy over surrogate motherhood took on a new twist in 1991, as 42-year-old Arlette Schweitzer gave birth on October 12 to twins whose biological mother was Schweitzer's daughter.

245

Schweitzer was the first woman in the United States known to have given birth to her own grandchildren. Her daughter, 22-year-old Christa Uchytil, had been born without a uterus and thus could not herself become pregnant. Eggs taken from Uchytil's ovaries had been fertilized in the laboratory with her husband's sperm and subsequently implanted in her mother's uterus.

The surrogate mother arrangement has always been subject to the criticism that it constitutes nothing more than a technologically sophisticated form of baby selling. Sizable amounts of money are often paid to surrogate mothers. The opportunity for financial gain, many observers fear, may cause poor women to ignore the risks involved—not only the physical risks associated with a pregnancy but also the psychological risks associated with subsequently giving up the child. In fact, several cases of surrogate motherhood in recent years led to custody battles between the surrogate and the couple arranging for the services. These disagreements have arisen both where the surrogate is the biological mother of the resulting child and in the more controversial arrangement where the surrogate merely "houses" an embryo produced by another woman and her spouse.

Nevertheless, many commentators found Arlette Schweitzer's decision to become a surrogate above reproach, as she acted solely for altruistic reasons. There was no prospect of financial gain to influence her, and the two children she bore would not be ensnared by custody battles. Yet some found her seemingly beneficent gesture highly disturbing. What, they wondered, would be the psychological consequences for the children when they learned of their grandmother's role in their birth. Since such consequences are unknown at present, and perhaps ultimately unpredictable, this may be yet another case where technological achievement is complicated by moral uncertainty. CONNIE ZUCKERMAN, J.D.

CANCER

Cancer Survival Rates Improve • Risks of Radon Exposure Debated • Coupling Breast Cancer Surgery With Chemotherapy or Hormone Therapy • Advances in Treatment for Leukemia • Gene Therapy and "Vaccines" for Cancer

Survival Rates Up

Advances in diagnosis and treatment over the past couple of decades have added years to the lives of people who get cancer. Data published in 1991 showed that significant improvement had been made in the United States since 1971 in five-year survival rates—the percentage of patients still alive five years after diagnosis—for testicular cancer, Hodgkin's disease, and childhood malignancies; smaller improvements were seen for most major cancers. In addition, deaths from every major childhood cancer have declined significantly, in spite of a small increase in the number of children diagnosed with cancer. Earlier detection has pushed down the death rate for urinary bladder and cervical cancers.

However, the overall five-year cancer survival rate for blacks in the United States is about 14 percentage points lower than that for whites. According to a

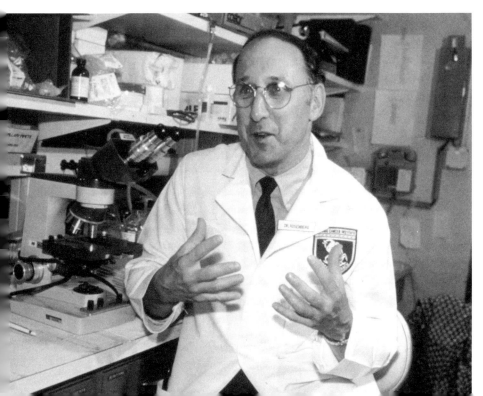

An experimental attempt to "immunize the patient against his own cancer" was launched by Dr. Steven Rosenberg of the National Cancer Institute. The radical new process involves extracting some of the patient's tumor cells, genetically altering them, and reintroducing them in the hopes that the altered cells will bolster the body's immune system in its fight against the disease.

study published in April 1991 by the National Cancer Institute, poverty and, to some extent, cultural differences are to blame. There is no indication that the racial differences in cancer incidence or survival are genetically caused. Rather, Americans who are poor tend to have low educational levels, substandard living conditions and nutrition, and a lack of medical insurance and access to opportunities for early detection. When they develop cancer, they may delay seeking medical care until the tumor is too far advanced for effective treatment.

Prevention and Early Detection

Lung Cancer. A New York University study that was made public in March 1991 found that the U.S. Environmental Protection Agency had overestimated the risk of exposure to radon in American homes. The findings bolstered a February report by the National Academy of Sciences that reached the same conclusion. Radon is a colorless, odorless, radioactive gas produced by the naturally occurring decay of uranium, found in certain rock formations. Seepage from underlying rocks is a common way for it to enter a house. The gas is thought by some experts to be the second-leading cause of lung cancer in the United States, after cigarette smoking, and the EPA in 1988 urged that radon testing be done in all American homes. Much of the concern over the potential hazards of radon, however, is based on data for uranium miners. It has been suggested that studies identifying radon in homes as a significant cause of lung cancer are actually measuring the interactive effect of smoking and radon exposure. Many scientists who support this point of view say that campaigns for preventing lung cancer should still place their major focus on getting people to quit smoking, rather than on ridding such homes of radon.

Lung cancer is now the leading cause of smoking-related deaths among smokers in the United States, ahead of coronary artery disease. Smokers can lower their risk of coronary artery disease by about half during the first year after they give up smoking, but the risk of lung cancer remains high even a decade after quitting. The National Cancer Institute estimated that cigarettes caused more than 127,000 deaths from lung cancer in 1991 and were associated with about 29,000 deaths from other types of cancer, including cancers of the mouth, bladder, and kidney. Smokers can get free help from the Cancer Information Service by dialing 1-800-4-CANCER.

Breast Cancer. Women who undergo surgery for breast cancer that is at an early stage can significantly increase their chances of survival by subsequently receiving additional treatment, such as chemotherapy or hormone therapy, according to a report published in early 1992. This finding, based on an analysis of data from 133 studies involving 75,000 women, provided support for the National Cancer Institute's 1988 recommendation that all breast cancer patients, even those with a very early stage of cancer, receive hormone therapy or chemotherapy following surgery.

The 1992 report confirmed that hormone therapy with the drug tamoxifen was an effective treatment after surgery. Tamoxifen seems to block the action of the female hormone estrogen, which can foster the growth of some breast tumors. The drug is currently being tested as a means of prevention for women with a high risk of developing breast cancer, and a large, nationwide study was to be launched in 1992. Because tamoxifen works by blocking hormones rather than by killing cells, there are few side effects associated with it. (Among the potential side effects are menopausal symptoms like hot flashes and sweaty palms, and the drug may increase the chance of developing cancer of the lining of the uterus.)

Prostate Cancer. Early detection of cancer of the prostate gland may become easier and more reliable if doctors use a certain blood test, according to a study published in April 1991. The test measures blood levels of prostate-specific antigen (PSA), a protein produced solely by the prostate and present at higher than normal levels in men with prostate cancer and other prostate diseases. The test is more accurate than the standard method of examination—palpating the prostate from inside the rectum—but it is not perfect. The study found that the test missed some cases of cancer and indicated a high PSA level in some men who did not have cancer. The study authors said that a combination of the blood test and a rectal examination, with the addition of an ultrasound exam in men with abnormal findings, was a better approach to detecting prostate cancer than any one of the three methods alone.

There is some disagreement among researchers about whether it is helpful to try to detect prostate cancer early. In many men the disease grows so slowly that they die from other causes before it can become fatal. However, because the cancer develops quickly in some men, the American Cancer Society recommends annual rectal exams for all men aged 40 and older. Prostate cancer is the number two cancer killer of U.S. men, after lung cancer.

New Role for Aspirin? An aspirin a day not only may decrease the risk of having a heart attack or stroke, it also appears to reduce the chances of developing cancer of the colon or rectum. In a study of over 6,000 people, men and women who took aspirin or other "nonsteroidal anti-inflammatory drugs" (such as ibuprofen) four or more times weekly for at least three months cut their risk of colorectal cancer in half.

Researchers cautioned, however, that more studies were needed to confirm the findings.

Reducing Dietary Fat. Increasing evidence has indicated that a low-fat, high-fiber diet may help prevent colon and breast cancer. A high-fat diet has been linked to damage to DNA (the substance in cells that carries the genetic blueprint of life), which in turn has been associated with tumor production. However, a 17-year study of the link between diet and cancer showed that modest reductions in fat intake will not reduce a person's risk of cancer. Fat intake must be below 30 percent of total calories to have an effect.

Advances in Treatment

Taxol. The most exciting development in the treatment of cancer of the ovaries in recent years was the discovery of the usefulness of the drug taxol, made from the bark of Pacific yew trees. Taxol has been shown to reduce the size of tumors where other forms of chemotherapy have failed. There are also indications that the drug may be effective against advanced cancers of the breast and lung. Reports about taxol's anticancer activity have set off a dispute between medical researchers and environmentalists who fear endangering yew trees in old-growth forests in the Pacific Northwest. It can take six 100-year-old Pacific yews to treat one patient. Efforts to make the drug from the needles of Pacific yew trees or to produce it synthetically are under way.

Bone Marrow Transplants. Bone marrow transplants are the only effective treatment for people with some types of leukemia or other blood diseases. The difficult process of finding an acceptable bone marrow donor has recently become a little easier, as bone marrow registries, which began in patchwork fashion, have grown larger and better coordinated. A new drug that can help speed the recovery process after a bone marrow transplant gained approval by the U.S. Food and Drug Administration in 1991. Known as GM-CSF or sargramostim (trade names, Leukine, Prokine), it is a genetically engineered version of one of a group of naturally occurring hormones called colony-stimulating factors that promote the production of blood cells. The FDA also approved another genetically engineered colony-stimulating factor, known as G-CSF or filgrastim (Neupogen), which can help prevent the life-threatening infections patients may develop when taking cancer-fighting drugs that deplete the immune system.

Retinoic Acid. Researchers have reported successfully using a drug that is a type of retinoic acid, a derivative of vitamin A, to induce complete remission in a number of patients with a form of leukemia called acute promyelocytic leukemia. In leukemia, immature white blood cells multiply uncontrollably, crowding out normal blood cells and performing no specific function. Unlike conventional cancer drugs, which kill cancer cells, retinoic acid spurs cells to mature, or differentiate, into normal adult cells, which do not divide. Treatment with retinoic acid has had few side effects. However, no one knows how long remission can be maintained with the drug. Such "differentiation therapy" is now being studied in other types of cancer.

The discovery that the drug taxol, made from the bark of Pacific yew trees, may be able to shrink certain cancer tumors was good news for patients but bad news for the trees. Their numbers already reduced by loggers, who considered the trees weeds and burned them, Pacific yews are now the targets of poachers. Here, Officer Terry Bertsch examines yews in Oregon that have been almost completely stripped of their bark.

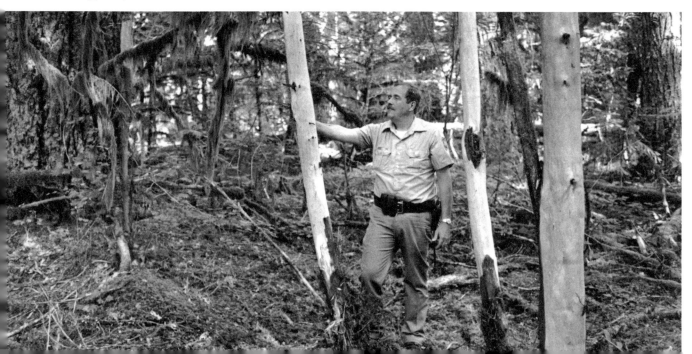

"Vaccination" With Tumor Cells. Dr. Steven A. Rosenberg of the National Cancer Institute continued to lead the way in gene therapy for cancer. In October 1991 he began a study in which cancer patients are injected with experimental doses of their own tumor cells, genetically altered in such a way as to bolster the patients' immune systems. Genes for a natural, cancer-killing substance called tumor necrosis factor (TNF) were added to the cells. The TNF was expected to stimulate the white blood cells known as lymphocytes to attack the altered tumor cells, as well as enhancing the immune system's ability to recognize and kill off other tumor cells. Three months after the initial injection, Rosenberg planned to remove some lymphocytes, which would be used to grow many more for administration to the patients.

"Vaccinating" patients with deactivated tumor cells is also being widely tested, especially for colon and kidney cancer and the type of skin cancer called melanoma. Researchers are currently working on vaccines for lung, cervix, and breast cancer. Cancer vaccines are intended to do two things: push the immune system into responding and tell the immune system what to attack.

Unorthodox Treatment

Some cancer patients turn to unorthodox treatments to prolong their lives, believing that traditional medicine has nothing to offer them or that the side effects of traditional medicine would be too difficult to bear. A 1991 study showed that while traditional treatments may not do better than a well-known and popular set of unorthodox treatments in prolonging the lives of terminal cancer patients, they can make possible a significantly better quality of life. Patients reported more side effects from the unorthodox treatments, which included a vegetarian diet, enemas, and a vaccine that purports to energize the immune system. Those receiving conventional therapy consistently reported a more satisfactory existence.

SHARON WATKINS DAVIS, M.P.A.
PAUL F. ENGSTROM, M.D.

DIGESTIVE SYSTEM

*Gene for Colon Cancer Discovered •
Removing Polyps Cuts Cancer Risk •
Smoking and Pancreatic Cancer • Stomach
Cancer Linked to Bacterial Infection*

Colon Cancer Gene Discovered

Japanese, U.S., and French researchers reported in August that they had discovered a gene that, when

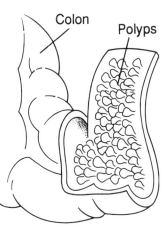
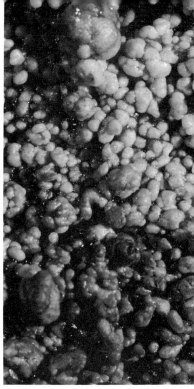

By studying a disease that causes the growth of thousands of tiny polyps (right) inside the colon, as shown above, researchers discovered a gene that, when defective, can cause cells lining the colon to become cancerous.

defective, causes the cells lining the colon and rectum (large intestine) to form polyps that may become cancerous. The scientists believe the proteins made by this gene, called the adenomatous polyposis coli (APC) gene, and several other genes normally control the growth of cells lining the colon and rectum. Defects in the genes may result in uncontrolled cell growth, eventually leading to cancer.

Colorectal cancer is the third most common cause of cancer deaths in the United States, resulting in over 60,000 deaths annually. Most colorectal cancers appear to arise from adenomatous polyps—benign, mushroom-shaped growths in the lining of the colon and rectum.

Researchers discovered the APC gene by looking at genetic information in people afflicted by a rare inherited disease called familial adenomatous polyposis (FAP). In this condition the defective gene causes the growth of thousands of tiny adenomatous polyps, which are very likely to develop into cancers. The researchers also detected the gene in the cells of tumors in people with the more common form of colorectal cancer, which is not inherited.

Environmental factors—particularly a diet high in fat and low in fiber—are also thought to play a role in the development of most colorectal polyps and cancers. It is believed that there is an interaction between the gene or genes and the environmental factors. While genetic factors may determine relative susceptibility, environmental factors determine which genetically susceptible people develop cancers.

The discovery of the APC gene is expected to lead to the development of a screening test to identify individuals who may be at risk for developing precancerous colorectal polyps and should improve scientists' understanding of all types of colorectal cancer.

Removal of Precancerous Polyps

Researchers reported in May 1991 that detection and removal of polyps in the large intestine significantly decreases the incidence of colorectal cancer. The National Polyp Study, from which these results came, is an ongoing clinical study that was begun in 1980. The study enrolls patients with at least one adenomatous polyp who have not had colorectal polyps removed prior to entering the study and who have no history of colorectal cancer. All polyps are removed at the be-

Art for the Blind

A blind person studying the history of art? It sounds like a contradiction in terms.

Yet an innovative new program is making that improbable scenario a reality. The people at Art Education for the Blind (AEB), headquartered in Manhattan's Whitney Museum of American Art, one of AEB's collaborators, believe that art can indeed be made accessible to the blind and the visually impaired, and to prove it they have developed an array of strategies and devices that have been employed with great success.

The most significant "hands-on" tools are computer generated raised-line drawings that allow the student to get the feel of paintings, sculptures, and architecture. These are supplemented with two types of audiotapes. One contains descriptions of the art objects and information on their place in art history. The second is a more unconventional "non-narrative" tape developed by a sound artist to create a sense of movement, space, composition, and emotional content. To describe a cathedral interior, for example, the tape would capture its acoustics and convey its size with the sound of footsteps and the bang of a stick at each column.

The learning system is designed to do more than give blind persons a "feel" for art. Art Education for the Blind is also developing a package that college students can use in conjunction with an art history textbook. Each of the package's 22 sections is accompanied by 11 raised-line drawings, with the appropriate audio accompaniment.

ginning of the study, and patients subsequently are offered follow-up colonoscopy and X-ray examinations to detect the growth of additional polyps and of cancers. Through 1991, more than 3,500 people had enrolled in the study, and more than 1,400 had returned for follow-up examinations. Four years after the removal of all polyps, significantly fewer patients than predicted by study researchers had developed colorectal cancers, and those cancers were also less advanced than expected. In prior studies of patients who were found to have colorectal polyps but who refused to have them removed, the incidence of colorectal cancer has been reported to be between 12 and 37 per 1,000 people.

To detect polyps early and prevent the onset of colorectal cancer, the American Cancer Society recommends that beginning at age 50 everyone should have a test called flexible sigmoidoscopy, in which a physician examines the lining of the last 2 feet of the large intestine with a lighted tube. If polyps are detected during this examination an additional test, called colonoscopy, should be performed to view directly the lining of the entire large intestine. All polyps detected during this examination should be removed. The ACS also recommends that the colonoscopic examination be repeated every 3 to 5 years for detection and removal of any additional polyps that may develop.

Smoking Linked to Pancreatic Cancer

In a study published in May 1991, Canadian researchers implicated cigarette smoking as a risk factor for developing cancer of the pancreas. The incidence of and death rate from pancreatic cancer has increased during the past few decades. Several surveys have suggested a number of causative factors for this form of cancer, including alcohol, coffee, and tobacco. Cigarette smoking, however, has shown the strongest positive association as a risk factor.

The Canadian study involved 179 patients with pancreatic cancer and 239 control subjects without cancer. The researchers studied the possible role of tobacco, alcohol, and coffee as causes for pancreatic cancer. There was about a fourfold increased risk of pancreatic cancer among heavy cigarette smokers compared with nonsmokers. No significant association was found between pancreatic cancer and the use of tobacco in forms other than cigarettes. Former cigarette smokers had a lower risk as compared with current smokers. These results confirmed findings of an earlier study about pancreatic cancer and smoking.

The new study also found that alcohol drinkers had a lower risk of developing pancreatic cancer than nondrinkers. Coffee drinkers were also found to be at a lower risk than nondrinkers, especially when coffee was consumed with meals.

Stomach Cancer an Infectious Disease?

Investigators in Hawaii and California reported in October that past infection with *Helicobacter pylori*, a bacterium, is associated with a significant increase in the risk of developing stomach cancer. Stomach cancer is estimated to be the world's second most common cancer. Although there has been a marked decrease in the incidence of this cancer in the United States and Western Europe during the past 50 years, the incidence of the disease remains very high in Latin America and Asia.

In the Hawaii study 94 percent of the patients with stomach cancer had been infected with *H. pylori*, while 76 percent of the healthy control subjects revealed evidence of infection. In the California study 84 percent of the patients had been infected, as compared with 61 percent of the healthy control subjects. Data from the latter study suggested that 60 percent of stomach cancers may be caused by infection with *H. pylori*. *H. pylori* causes stomach inflammation, and chronic stomach inflammation is associated with stomach cancer. Since most people infected with the organism do not develop stomach cancer, however, there must be other factors involved. Studies in the future will attempt to identify these other factors that increase the risk of stomach cancer among people with *H. pylori* infection.   DANIEL PELOT, M.D.

ENVIRONMENTAL AND OCCUPATIONAL HEALTH

Healthcare Workers and the Risk of AIDS • Hazards of Asbestos Again Debated • New Light on Mercury Contamination • Danger Level for Lead in Children's Blood Revised • Irregular Work Schedule May Pose Safety Threat

AIDS Rules for Health Workers

A growing focus of public attention in 1991 was the possibility of contracting AIDS from doctors or other healthcare workers infected with the human immunodeficiency virus, or HIV, which causes the disease. Concern was sparked by reports that at least five people infected with the virus (one of whom died in 1991) had been treated by a Florida dentist who died of AIDS the previous year. According to researchers, however, patients of HIV-infected doctors were at very low risk, and healthcare workers faced a far greater chance of getting AIDS from infected patients.

Nonetheless, the U.S. Centers for Disease Control in July announced a plan to publish a list of "invasive" procedures (which involve work within the body and thus increase the risk of exposure to infection) that healthcare workers infected with HIV should not perform. But the plan was eventually dropped after many medical and dental groups refused to help formulate the list of high-risk procedures on the ground that there was no scientific basis for it. The CDC instead proposed that local panels determine on a case-by-case basis what procedures HIV-infected health workers could perform, depending on such factors as the nature of the procedure, whether the worker meets standards of infection control, and the medical condition of the worker.

In December the U.S. Occupational Safety and Health Administration (OSHA) issued long-delayed rules for protecting healthcare workers from AIDS, hepatitis, and other blood-borne diseases. The new rules applied to an estimated 5.6 million American workers and were intended to prevent the 9,200 infections and 200 deaths that occur each year from exposure to human blood and other potentially infectious materials. The rules gave the force of law to certain "universal precautions" that had been recommended by the CDC, such as the use of protective clothing, gloves, and masks and recapping or removing needles with a mechanical device or a one-handed technique. Employers were required to provide protective equipment and to offer hepatitis B vaccine at no cost to employees. The rules, which were to go into effect in early 1992, also required health facilities to submit infection exposure control plans and provide employee education and training.

Asbestos Risks

A controversial study commissioned by the U.S. Congress added one more chapter in 1991 to the continuing, often bitter, debate over the hazards of asbestos. The report from the study, which involved a review of the scientific literature, cautioned against overgeneralizing about asbestos as if all the hazards it presented were the same. The review supported the views of those who argue that well-maintained asbestos in public buildings poses little health risk to office workers and other building occupants. Performed by a panel of scientists set up by the nonprofit Health Effects Institute-Asbestos Research organization, the study found that the levels of asbestos inside well-maintained buildings are virtually the same as outdoor levels. Nonetheless, the report recommended providing adequate protection for janitors who might disturb the asbestos in the course of their work and workers involved in renovation, maintenance, and asbestos removal.

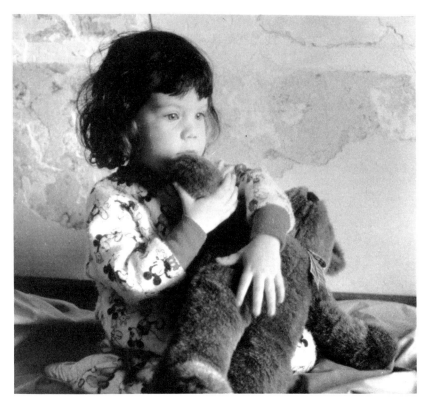

Calling lead the biggest environmental threat to young children, the U.S. government sharply reduced the acceptable blood level of lead. Youngsters often ingest lead by eating paint that flakes off walls, such as the one behind this little girl.

The reviewers found strong evidence that longer asbestos fibers play a role in causing mesothelioma, a rare but deadly form of cancer, but left open the highly contentious issue of whether short fibers from chrysotile, the type of asbestos most widely used in the United States, play the same role. In a letter appended to the report, Dr. Arthur Upton, a New York University pathologist and environmental health scientist who chaired the panel, said that the issue could not be resolved with certainty from the available data. While one side in the controversy criticized the report for failing to absolve chrysotile asbestos completely, the other attacked it for downplaying health risks associated with very short fibers. The report was also faulted for failing to recommend to the U.S. Environmental Protection Agency such policy changes as requiring asbestos monitoring in public buildings.

In October a federal appeals court struck down major provisions of an EPA ban on asbestos products, saying the agency had not provided sufficient evidence to justify a total ban. The EPA had ordered a gradual phaseout of asbestos products in 1989 after studies linked prolonged exposure to asbestos with lung cancer and other respiratory diseases. The court ruling let stand the first stage of the ban, which took effect in 1990, prohibiting the use of asbestos in cloth-

ing and interior building materials. It threw out provisions that would have barred the use of asbestos in automobile components, roofing material, and water pipes by 1997. The EPA later announced that it would not appeal the decision.

Airborne Contaminants Feed Mercury Pollution

Though the outright dumping of mercury into U.S. waterways has long been banned, significant levels of the metal recently have been detected in lakes throughout the northeastern and north central United States as well as in Canada. A three-year study by the Center for Clean Air Policy, founded in 1985 by a group of state governors, suggested that the high water level of mercury was caused, in part, by the movement of airborne mercury over long distances. Unlike most metals, mercury emitted from power plants and incinerators is a gas, which is carried hundreds of miles downwind and, via precipitation, eventually ends up in lakes and rivers.

The study found that coal-burning power plants accounted for one-third of atmospheric mercury, while incineration of household batteries and evaporation from paints were responsible for most of the rest. Even though recent action to phase out mercury in paints and reduce the amount used in batteries would cut emissions by 25 percent in the next decade, even greater reductions could be made by the utility industry, the study authors said.

The study report faulted the EPA for looking only at risks from mercury to people in the immediate vicinity of power plants and failing to consider risks from long-range atmospheric transport and bioaccumulation through the food chain. The study concluded that although residents of the immediate vicinity of a power plant are not likely to be at risk from mercury emissions, people and animals that consume large quantities of mercury-contaminated fish probably are at risk.

The authors called upon the EPA to do more scientific research on emission levels and on human exposure through the food chain. Excessive mercury exposure can affect fetal development and cause permanent damage to the nervous system. Such effects may already be occurring, the report suggested, citing evidence of mercury-linked problems involving the nervous system or physical movement that studies had found in such population groups as Quebec's Cree Indians, who consume large quantities of fish.

New Lead Standards

Calling lead "the most common and societally devastating environmental disease of young children," the federal government in October 1991 reduced the danger level for lead in children's blood to 10 micrograms per deciliter. The old threshold of concern had been 25 micrograms. The new threshold, set by the Centers for Disease Control, meant that between 10 and 15 percent of U.S. preschoolers—about 3 million children—had unacceptable blood lead levels, placing them at risk for the intellectual impairment and health problems associated with lead poisoning. Some experts, however, called the new level unrealistically low and criticized the studies underpinning the new standard, pointing out that with the elimination of lead from gasoline and from new household paint, sources of lead had been dramatically reduced.

The EPA in May 1991 set new standards to reduce exposure to lead from another source—tap water provided by community water supplies. The old standards for U.S. drinking water allowed an average lead level of 50 parts per billion. The new rules, to begin taking effect in 1992 and 1993, required municipal water suppliers to test lead levels at customer faucets, with tap water lead values eventually not to exceed 15 parts per billion in at least 90 percent of households monitored.

While lead in water, in food, and in dust and chips from old paint accounts for much of Americans' current lead exposure, a study by some of the leading U.S.

environmental groups in conjunction with the Hazardous Waste Treatment Council, a trade organization, censured the EPA for permitting more than 500,000 pounds of lead to be released into the air each year through the widespread burning of used motor oil. Despite its lead content, used motor oil is not considered a hazardous waste in the United States, except in California.

According to the EPA's own estimates, more than 90 percent of "recycled" used oil is burned for fuel. Despite the phaseout of lead-containing gasoline in the United States, oil still has high levels of lead—about 100 parts per million. The burning of this oil releases more lead into the air than any other industrial source, the study showed. In addition, the study alleged that unregulated school, apartment building, and industrial boilers are allowed to emit higher amounts of airborne lead than facilities that have permits to burn hazardous waste. Urban residents are also exposed to lead through the burning of some 86 million gallons of contaminated oil in private homes each year.

The study groups called upon Congress to declare used oil a hazardous waste once it is picked up for recycling and disposal. Such a move would eliminate uncontrolled burning of contaminated fuel. Enactment of proposals to require that new motor oil contain a certain percentage of recycled and rerefined oil would help eliminate the burning of unsafe oil.

Employee Burnout

A virtual epidemic in job-related stress is leading to lower productivity, higher absenteeism, greater job turnover, and frequent health problems, according to a 1991 survey of workers that was sponsored by the Northwestern National Life Insurance Company. The firm undertook the study because of a dramatic twofold increase in stress-related disability claims over the preceding decade. On average, stress-related disability payments cost $73,270 per case when the problem was not resolved, compared with $1,925 for rehabilitating an employee.

The survey found that one in three employees seriously thought about quitting because of job stress and that one in three anticipated burnout on the job. Moreover, seven in ten said job stress caused frequent health problems, and the same proportion said stress made them less productive on the job. Forty-six percent considered their jobs "highly stressful," and 17 percent reported stress-related absenteeism. The employees tended to blame their problems on too much work.

The study found no relationship between burnout and geographic region, size of company, type of job, or worker age. It did find, however, that significant burnout occurred in companies where employees frequently worked overtime or where major changes had taken place—such as a change in ownership, reductions in employee benefits, and layoffs. Employees did relatively well at firms that had supportive work and family policies, provided coverage for mental illness and treatment of addiction to drugs or alcohol, and offered flexible work hours. Companies of this type had almost half the burnout rate of those that failed to provide such programs.

Biorhythms and Work Schedules

Shift workers have a nonstandard work schedule that upsets the body's inner biological rhythms, and this can affect worker health, safety, and job performance, according to a 1991 report by the congressional Office of Technology Assessment. Researchers have found that such difficulties are experienced by one in five Americans—some 20 million people—who work at night, for noncontinuous hours, or for extended periods. The OTA, however, declared U.S. research in understanding human biological rhythms to be "minimal and uncoordinated" and said that collection of statistical data on shift work by the federal government "has been inconsistent, precluding any accurate,

thorough measurement of the scope, nature, and impact of shift work in this country."

The data that are available suggest, though, that people vary greatly in their ability to adjust to shift work. Some have few problems, while others are unable to tolerate certain work schedules. In some workers shift work produces chronic malaise and may be a risk factor for other health problems. Moreover, fatigue and sleep loss may compound disturbances in biological rhythms, potentially endangering the safety of the worker and, in some occupations, that of the public as well.

Contract Workers and Oil Industry Accidents

A new study provided fresh evidence that the use of contract workers has contributed to a spate of recent accidents in the petrochemical industry. The study was done for the U.S. Labor Department by the John Grey Institute of Lamar University in Texas and released in 1991. It showed that about one-third of work during regular operations, and more than half when equipment is being repaired or upgraded, was being performed by outside, contract workers who were often poorly educated, inadequately trained, and

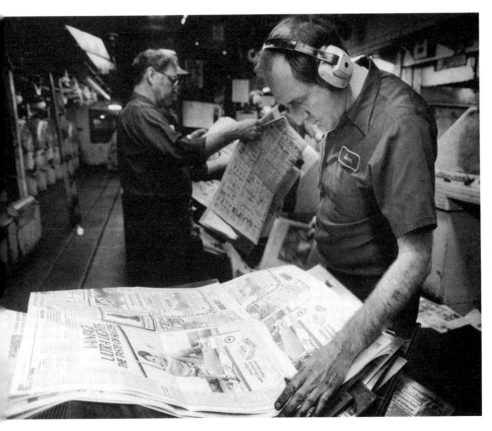

A new U.S. government report found that employees who work shifts outside of normal daytime hours, such as newspaper printers, can experience a disturbance of the body's normal biological rhythms that can lead to problems with health, safety, and job performance.

not prepared for emergencies that might arise in a chemical plant.

Industry representatives told researchers that the use of outside workers helped control costs and gave managers flexibility to meet staffing needs during slack and peak production periods, while maintaining a steady force of full-time workers. However, reviews by safety experts suggested that mistakes by outside workers may be implicated in some of the explosions that have beset the industry since 1987, killing more than 80 people, injuring nearly 1,000, and accounting for some $2 billion in damage. Precise death and injury figures are not available, since U.S. law requires reporting only when regular workers are involved.

Fatal Fire Spurs Safety Concerns

After a fire killed 25 workers in a North Carolina poultry plant in September, OSHA took over much of the responsibility for enforcement in the state's occupational health and safety program. The unprecedented action gave the agency authority to investigate all of the state's workplace fatalities, as well as complaints from workers who say they are being retaliated against for whistle-blowing and complaints about the way the state administers the safety program. Federal law allows states to administer and enforce their own programs as long as the programs meet federal regulations and have been approved by the federal government. North Carolina was one of 23 states that had been enforcing OSHA regulations under an approved state plan. Investigation showed that the poultry-processing plant had never been inspected by the state during its 11 years of operation. The fatalities were attributed to locked or blocked fire exits, but the plant also lacked automatic heat-detection sprinkler systems, its fire doors did not meet national safety standards, it had only one fire extinguisher, and it lacked an evacuation plan.

"Fetal Protection" Policy Banned

The U.S. Supreme Court ruled in 1991 that employers may not exclude women from jobs in which exposure to toxic substances could harm a developing fetus. The decision was a victory for the labor unions and women's groups that had challenged the "fetal protection" policy at Johnson Controls, the largest manufacturer of automobile batteries in the United States. The policy had been adopted in 1982 to prevent female employees from being exposed to lead. It applied to all women, regardless of plans for childbearing, except those who could show medical proof of sterility. All nine justices agreed that the policy violated the federal Civil Rights Act of 1964, which prohibits sex discrimination in employment.

MARY HAGER

GENETICS AND GENETIC ENGINEERING

Gene Therapy Experiment Fights Cancer With Cancer • Gene Found for Alzheimer's Disease • New Knowledge About a Cause of Mental Retardation Syndrome • Research on Genetic Aspects of Cancer

Gene Therapy Update

The most dramatic development in gene therapy in 1991 was an attempt at the U.S. National Institutes of Health to immunize terminally ill cancer patients with their own cancer cells. In this experiment, which got under way in October, researchers surgically extracted tumor cells from the patients, added to the extracted cells the gene for tumor necrosis factor, an immunity-stimulating protein that kills cancer, and then injected the cancer cells back into the patients. Experiments in animals had suggested that such modified cancer cells would stimulate the immune system to attack any new tumor formation.

Even as human trials of gene therapy proceeded, researchers were exploring better ways of introducing new genes into the body and were seeking to determine which diseases could be combated in this way. French and U.S. researchers developed genetically engineered cold viruses that can deliver therapeutic genes into genetically defective lung tissue via a simple nasal spray. (The cold viruses are rendered incapable of causing disease.) Such a nasal spray may prove an effective treatment for genetically caused emphysema, cystic fibrosis, or other inherited diseases affecting the lungs.

Alzheimer's Disease

Researchers in 1991 reported the identification of genetic defects that appear to cause some cases of the debilitating neurological disorder known as Alzheimer's disease. The findings helped shed light on a key question centering on the protein deposits, called plaques, that are found in the brains of Alzheimer's patients during autopsy: Are these unusual deposits, which consist of the protein known as beta-amyloid, a cause of Alzheimer's or a result of the disease?

In February, British researchers associated a genetic defect, located on chromosome 21, with an inherited form of Alzheimer's. The defect causes cells to create a flawed version of amyloid precursor protein, a substance that can break down into beta-amyloid. The defective amyloid precursor protein appears to give rise to unusually large amounts of beta-amyloid.

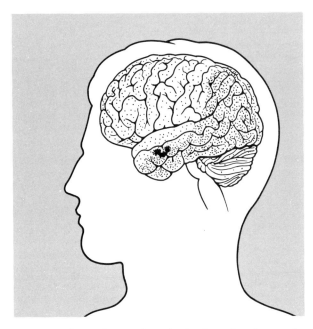

Autopsies have shown that the brains of patients who had Alzheimer's disease contain numerous protein deposits called plaques (seen here as small dark dots). Now researchers have identified, in people with one type of Alzheimer's, a defect in a gene that helps produce that protein. This and other discoveries may make it possible to create new drugs to fight the illness.

The British discovery suggested that beta-amyloid is indeed responsible for the disorder and not a result of it. Later in the year researchers discovered additional genetic defects at the same location that appear to cause Alzheimer's.

Meanwhile, experiments with animals—including one in which beta-amyloid was injected into the brains of mice and others in which genes for beta-amyloid were inserted into mouse embryos—produced Alzheimer's-like symptoms and the telltale plaques, convincing many researchers that beta-amyloid is the guilty party. Scientists hope that such mice models for the study of Alzheimer's will speed the discovery of drugs to fight the disease.

Mental Retardation

U.S. and Dutch researchers revealed in May 1991 that they had identified the gene that causes fragile X syndrome, the most common form of inherited mental retardation. Fragile X syndrome draws its name from a weak spot on the X chromosome. Doctors diagnose the syndrome by putting sample cells from the patient under a microscope and looking for the chromosome weak spot. However, this method of detection reveals only about three-quarters of those affected, who include healthy individuals not retarded themselves but capable of passing the disorder on to their children or grandchildren.

Although the researchers did not know the normal function of the responsible gene, dubbed FMR-1, they found that, in healthy persons who are carriers of fragile X syndrome, the gene repeats a section of DNA (deoxyribonucleic acid, the substance that carries the genetic blueprint of life) for a long stretch. In people with the disorder, the repetitive area is significantly longer, and the researchers believe that this inactivates the gene and causes the retardation.

In December scientists in France and Australia announced the developement of screening tests for prospective parents to determine whether they carry the FMR-1 gene.

Genes and Cancer

Breast Cancer. University of North Carolina researchers reported in December that medical X rays increase the risk of breast cancer by over fivefold in women who inherit the so-called A-T gene from one parent. The risk of any cancer is 3.5 times normal for women carrying such a "single copy" of the gene and 3.8 times normal for men with a single copy. It was already well established that people who carry two copies of the A-T gene—one from each parent—face nearly 100 times the normal cancer risk and will develop ataxia-telangiectasia, a progressive nerve and immune system disorder. Two to three million Americans, however, are believed to carry just a single copy of the gene, and the researchers said that these people, especially women who get regular mammograms, should limit their exposure to X rays. No screening test for the gene now exists, but a person closely related to someone with ataxia-telangiectasia is a likely carrier of the A-T gene.

Skin Cancer. In November a team of scientists led by researchers at Yale University clearly linked ultraviolet radiation from the sun to the development of tumor cells in a type of skin cancer. It was the first time a genetic mutation causing cancer had been directly attributed to a specific carcinogen.

The defect—located in the p53 gene, which regulates cell division—could have been caused only by the penetrating ultraviolet-B waves of the sun. Cells with the defective p53 gene were found to lack normal restrictions on their growth—leading to a form of skin cancer known as squamous-cell carcinoma. This cancer is usually curable—only a few percent of those afflicted die from the disease—but it can be fatal if untreated. Doctors are seeing growing numbers of the cancer in younger patients and have attributed it to the popularity of sunbathing, a cause now confirmed by this discovery.

Colon Cancer. Researchers from Japan, France, and the United States, in two separate efforts, identified the gene responsible for familial adenomatous polyposis, an inherited form of colon cancer striking 1 in 5,000 people in the United States and 1 in 17,000 in Japan. When the gene, called the APC gene (for adenomatous polyposis coli), is defective, cells within the large intestine form polyps that usually become cancerous. The researchers suggested that a second, still unknown, genetic defect is required in order for the polyps to be converted to cancer. They voiced hope that their findings would help in the screening of individuals for colon cancer.

Rare Skin Disorder

Three American research groups isolated genetic defects responsible for the skin disease epidermolysis bullosa, and their findings may reveal important clues about the structure of skin itself. For those suffering from this rare disorder, which affects an estimated 50,000 people in the United States, the slightest touch on the skin produces painful blisters. Some infants with the disease die right after birth because they are so severely blistered by the trauma of being born. In one form of epidermolysis bullosa, gene mutations were found that lead to defective keratin, a protein crucial to the structure of skin. In a second form of the disease, the culprit was a broken gene for collagen, a protein that helps hold skin layers together.

Key Brain Receptor

Researchers from Japan and the University of Kansas independently claimed in November that they had cloned the gene responsible for production of a vital brain protein that may play a role in learning and memory but also seems to be involved in neurological damage caused by stroke, epilepsy, or head injuries. The protein, known as the NMDA receptor, is found on the surface of nerve cells. It responds to glutamate, one of the substances called neurotransmitters that carry "messages" between nerve cells. When brain cells are injured, they appear to release large amounts of glutamate, which binds to NMDA receptors in additional brain cells, overexciting and killing the cells.

Some scientists believe that most of the cell death that follows a brain injury may be due to overstimulation of cells that have NMDA receptors rather than to oxygen deprivation (or a combination of oxygen deprivation and cell overstimulation), as is commonly thought. If this is true, a drug that blocked the NMDA receptors' activity could presumably preserve much brain tissue. Cloning the NMDA gene would be expected to aid in developing such drugs, as well as in increasing scientists' understanding of the compli-

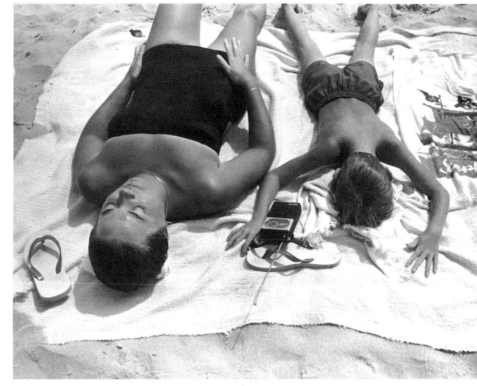

Why is too much sunbathing associated with skin cancer? One newly discovered reason is that ultraviolet radiation from the sun produces mutations in a gene that regulates skin cell growth—causing the cells to grow out of control and form tumors. The finding marks the first time a genetic mutation has been directly attributed to a specific carcinogen.

cated receptor. However, the genes found by the two research teams were different, so it remained to be seen which group was on the right track.

JOHN TRAVIS

GOVERNMENT POLICIES AND PROGRAMS

United States

Reforming the U.S. Healthcare System • Changes in Medicare Reimbursement • Physician Investments in Healthcare Facilities • Breast Implant Safety Investigated • Research on Women's Health Planned

Healthcare System Changes Proposed

Concerns about the soaring costs of healthcare and the growing ranks of Americans with either no insurance (an estimated 31 to 37 million people) or inadequate

Voters in Pennsylvania sent a strong message that healthcare costs and insurance have become a major public concern when they gave Harris Wofford a stunning upset victory in a November 1991 senatorial election. Wofford, a Democrat, had made a call for national health insurance a centerpiece of his campaign.

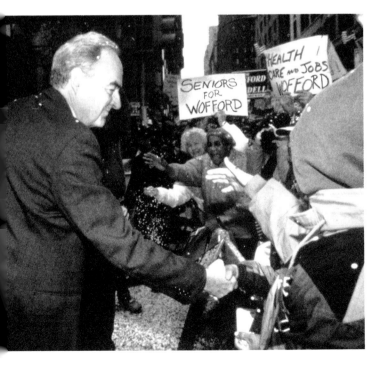

coverage led members of Congress to offer more than 30 legislative proposals in 1991 for changes ranging from malpractice insurance reform to a Canadian-style national healthcare system. Democratic presidential hopefuls made healthcare a priority issue, and little-known Harris Wofford, campaigning on economic and health cost issues, defeated Richard Thornburgh, former Pennsylvania governor and former U.S. attorney general, in the November Pennsylvania senatorial election. Sensing the growing political importance of the problem, President George Bush made a general commitment to reform the healthcare system in his January 1992 State of the Union message. In one effort to control costs, Health and Human Services Secretary Louis Sullivan convened a summit of insurance experts to examine ways to cut administrative costs. It is estimated that administrative costs account for anywhere from 13 to 33 percent of the United States total health bill. Options considered included simplifying and cutting down on the number of different forms used by insurers, processing claim forms electronically, and computerizing patient records.

The 1991 Advisory Council on Social Security calculated that, if current growth patterns were not checked, healthcare could consume 31 percent of the gross national product by 2020, a prospect that would not only destroy the economy but throw the nation into bankruptcy. Among its recommendations to reverse the trends, the council called for an immediate $3 billion investment in school area clinics for children under 12, school based insurance for children and youth up to age 22, the establishment of 250 new community health centers, and a doubling of the National Health Service Corps to get doctors and other health professionals to underserved rural and inner-city areas. The group suggested that another $3 billion be spent to test on a small scale such reform proposals as greater use of managed care and tax incentives, to evaluate how well they work. Recommendations made by past advisory councils have led to major policy changes.

Medicare Payment Reform

The Department of Health and Human Services put into place the most significant revision in the 25-year history of Medicare of the way in which physicians are paid. The system sets fixed payments to doctors for approximately 7,000 medical services. The payments are based on assigned numerical "values" for all services that take into account the time, effort, overhead, and malpractice expenses required to provide a given service. HHS Secretary Sullivan said the changes would create a fairer and more rational physician payment system, by bringing greater predictability, equity, and consistency to payments. The goal of the new fee schedule was not to reduce total spending on Medicare but to reapportion the money spent. Primary care physicians were expected to benefit most under the new system at the expense of some surgical specialties.

When the initial proposal was unveiled in May 1991, however, doctors were outraged by significant fee reductions for some procedures that would have cut about $7 billion in payments to doctors over five years. In setting the fees the Health Care Financing Administration had assumed that doctors would compensate for smaller fees by performing more procedures, an assumption the American Medical Association (AMA) said was unfounded.

Lobbying by doctors and protests from Congress caused the HCFA to amend the rules, and the original

plan not to cut total payments was restored. During the five years it was expected to take to move fully to the new payment system, the HCFA calculated, spending for covered services would increase by 74 percent, from $27.3 billion to $47.5 billion.

Despite the changes doctors were still uncomfortable with the proposals. At a December 1991 meeting AMA members vowed to continue efforts to change the "current flawed data" used to adjust for geographic differences in the costs of practice and to determine whether payment rates were accurately calculated. AMA leaders reminded members the group had supported the change in the interests of "simplicity, rationality, and fairness to our undercompensated primary care physicians and rural colleagues." Rather than continuing to battle the inevitable, they suggested resources should be turned to helping physi-

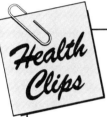

Eat for Heat

Up in Alberta, Canada, where winter's long reign brings the coyote's howl, the snowmobile's roar, and subzero temperatures, the folks know a lot about frigid weather. Thus it stands to reason that a scientist at the University of Alberta in Edmonton has developed a new kind of snack to prevent hypothermia—the dangerous drop in body temperature that can result when the body's heat-producing ability fails to keep pace with the heat loss that occurs in very cold conditions.

This ingenious foodstuff is called the Canadian Cold Buster, and it's very much like a chocolate bar, except your average slab of candy is not the result of 15 years of physiological research and over Can$1 million in funding from such sources as the Canadian National Defence Department and the Canadian Medical Research Council. The Cold Buster contains cocoa powder, skim milk protein, honey, and other natural ingredients, all formulated according to a process that its developer, Lawrence Wang, is not about to reveal—at least not as long as its patent is pending. The reason is that the bar is designed actually to alter the body's responses to cold exposure.

When the mercury nosedives, the body copes by burning more fuel, chiefly fat. This burning process, however, is accompanied by the production of adenosine, a substance that interferes with the conversion of fat into fuel. The Cana-

dian Cold Buster, asserts its inventor, inhibits the effect of adenosine, thus promoting better fuel utilization—hence, toastier tootsies.

Wang tested the bar on rats and on lightly clad volunteers who were placed in a climatic chamber at a temperature of around 16°F for three to six hours. The body temperature of those subjects who ate the Canadian Cold Buster dropped about one degree; the others went down about two degrees. That 50 percent improvement in cold tolerance, says Wang, gives a person stranded in a snowstorm twice as much time to find shelter.

The bar was launched in early December 1991 with great success. Soaring sales, however, were soon crimped by a bizarre episode. Because of Wang's animal testing, unknown persons claiming to represent an animal rights group threatened to poison random samples on store shelves. Two weeks later the perpetrators revealed that the whole thing was a hoax, but not before all the Cold Buster bars had been recalled. The flap proved minor, however, as even real animal rights activists denounced the hoax. Ironically, the incident brought the product to the attention of many who hadn't known about it.

Of course, Wang points out, you don't have to be lost in a blizzard to appreciate his invention's warming effects—a frosty football stadium will do. Who knows? The Cold Buster could even replace the hip flask.

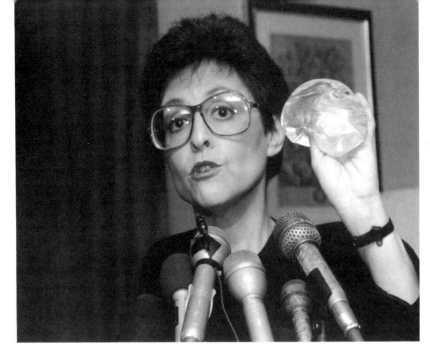

An ongoing debate on the safety of silicone-based breast implants led to a recommendation by an advisory panel of the U.S. Food and Drug Administration that the use of the devices be restricted. One of those who testified in support of the implants was Karen Berger, author of a book on the subject, who is seen here holding one at a press conference.

cians understand the changes that are "lumbering toward them." The amended rules went into effect on January 1, 1992.

Self-referral Rules

After a 1991 state-sponsored study found that at least 40 percent of Florida's physicians had financial stakes in clinical laboratories, diagnostic imaging centers, and physical therapy facilities to which they referred patients, physicians were under increasing pressure from both the government and medical societies to abandon so-called self-referrals. The study showed that doctor-owned facilities had both higher utilization rates and higher revenues per patient than those without physician investment, though study directors emphasized it was not clear the high rate indicated any wrongdoing. A 1989 study by the AMA had concluded that less than 10 percent of practicing physicians had such investments.

Because of growing conflict-of-interest concerns, Representative Pete Stark (D, Calif.), chairman of the House subcommittee that oversees Medicare, pushed for a ban on physician-owned facilities for Medicare referrals. In 1989, Congress had approved a Stark proposal that bans physicians from referring Medicare patients to clinical laboratories in which they have a financial interest; the law was to take effect on January 1, 1992. Hospital-based radiologists and physical therapists backed an expanded ban, while opponents argued that such an expansion would limit competition, giving hospital facilities a virtual monopoly, and limit the availability of new technology.

Stepping into the debate, the Department of Health and Human Services set forth stringent guidelines to provide "safe harbors" for physicians with joint venture investments. As defined by the Medicare pro-

gram in July 1991, the safe harbor regulation allows up to 40 percent of the investing partners in a facility to be physicians who refer to that facility, as long as they account for no more than 40 percent of patient procedures at the facility. In December 1991 the AMA adopted a policy saying that in general, physicians should not refer patients to healthcare facilities in which they have invested. The association warned entrepreneurs to look beyond medical practitioners for potential investors in medical facilities.

Breast Implants

In February 1992 a U.S. Food and Drug Administration advisory panel recommended placing substantial restrictions on the use of silicone-based breast implants. The recommendation followed FDA Commissioner Dr. David Kessler's January 1992 call for a voluntary, 45-day moratorium on the use of silicone breast implants because he did not feel he could assure patients about their safety. His concern was based on statements and data, not previously reviewed, found in internal documents from Dow Corning Wright, the leading manufacturer of the implants, and on an informal survey of rheumatologists that suggested an abnormally high rate of connective tissue and autoimmune diseases in women who had received implants. The breast implants are used both by women who have had breasts removed because of cancer and by those who wish to enhance their breasts for cosmetic reasons.

Silicone breast implants have been in use since the 1960s, long before legislation was enacted that would have required them to be evaluated for long-term safety. The FDA was prompted to evaluate the devices by continuing reports of health problems linked to leakage from the implants as well as persistent concerns about their long-term safety. In November, an FDA advisory panel rejected manufacturers' safety data as inadequate, but recommended that implants remain in use pending further study, as long as a registry of recipients was developed and women were fully informed of safety concerns.

When the panel reconvened in February 1992, it advised making all new implants part of a large, nation-wide medical experiment to determine whether the implants are linked to autoimmune diseases. The panel said that all women having reconstruction after surgery for breast cancer would be eligible to participate in the experiment. Women wanting breast enlargement would have to apply to doctors conducting the experiment.

The panel also issued several statements of advice and information for women who already have implants or are considering them. It said that women should expect to have the implants replaced several times over the course of a lifetime, that the implants leak a certain amount of silicone into the body even when not ruptured, that the frequency of rupture is unknown, and that implants can interfere with mammograms, necessitating a more complicated series of X rays to check for breast cancer.

Before the moratorium, about 10,000 silicone breast implants were performed each month, about one-fifth of them following breast cancer surgery, the rest for cosmetic reasons.

Women's Health Initiative

Women's health research got a major boost in April when new National Institutes of Health Director Dr. Bernadine Healy announced a major ten-year study to redress past neglect.

The $500 million study, involving more than 140,000 postmenopausal women, will have three major components. One will evaluate the effectiveness of hormone replacement therapy, diet modification, and vitamin supplements in preventing cancer, heart disease, and osteoporosis in 70,000 women. The second will look for effective ways to promote healthy behavior in local communities. And the third will involve at least 70,000 women over the age of 50 and screen them for signs of progressive diseases and any predictors of future disease problems.

Experts disagreed on whether the massive effort was workable as designed and on whether it would provide clear answers to the questions being raised. Some expressed concern that women would drop out of the hormone replacement study because of side effects, others doubted that thousands of women would agree to stay on hormone therapy, modify their diets, and take vitamin supplements simultaneously for a ten-year period. Some suggested the effects of simple

exercise would be far easier to study. Even with such questions still up in the air, Congress provided first-year funding of $25 million to get the initiative under way.   MARY HAGER

CANADA

New Federal Policy to Cut Healthcare Costs • AIDS Initiatives • Controversy Over Reproductive Technology Commission

Controlling Federal Spending

The major issue in healthcare policy in Canada in 1991 was the federal government's decision to restrict the cash transfer payments to the ten provinces that were part of its share of funding Medicare, the country's universal healthcare system. Under a complicated funding formula passed during the year, the federal government froze payments to the provinces at the 1990 level, and extended the freeze until 1995. The provinces received an estimated $3.3 billion less than they expected for fiscal year 1991, causing thousands of layoffs and hospital bed closures throughout the country. (Canadian dollars used here and throughout.) There was also a growing concern among healthcare groups that the future of Medicare was being imperiled by the federal cutbacks, predicted to total almost $30 billion by the end of 1995. By year's end, however, despite the drop in hospital bed numbers, there was little evidence of a decline in the quality of care. Indeed, many argued that the system was actually becoming more efficient under the cost crunch.

AIDS Initiatives

Condoms were made available to prisoners in federal jails as a way of preventing the spread of the human immunodeficiency virus (HIV) that causes AIDS. The federal government also eased restrictions on visitors to Canada who are HIV-positive. Ontario endorsed anonymous testing for the AIDS virus, setting up 13 clinics across the province where individuals may be tested without their identities being known. The federal Health Protection Branch approved the anti-AIDS drug DDI.

Patent Protection for Drugs

Early in 1992, Canada announced it would increase the patent protection available for brand name prescription drugs, a move expected to seriously restrict the country's thriving generic drug industry. Consumer groups predicted that the loss of competition from cheaper, generic products would cause the price of prescription drugs to rise.

261

Nurses' Settlement

After an 11-day walkout in May hospital nurses in Saskatchewan settled for a 9 percent pay raise over two years rather than the 19 percent they had sought, but the largest nurses' settlement of the year was achieved in March in Ontario without a work stoppage. There, senior nurses won a raise of nearly 30 percent over two years, making them the highest-paid nurses in Canada at $52,000 a year.

Healthcare Reform in British Columbia

In November 1991, British Columbia's Royal Commission recommended reforms aimed at maintaining the quality of healthcare without dramatically increasing costs. The commission proposed cutting the number of acute-care hospital beds by 25 percent, decentralizing healthcare decision-making, and restricting the income of doctors.

Reproductive Technology Controversy

The Royal Commission on New Reproductive Technologies, set up in December 1989 to investigate and make recommendations on the many sensitive and controversial issues arising from new reproductive technologies—such as surrogate motherhood and embryo research—became the center of a major controversy. Disagreements over the direction of this $25 million federal inquiry resulted in the government's firing of four of the nine commissioners, a legal challenge to the authority of the chair, Dr. Patricia Baird, and calls from many women's groups for the commission to be disbanded. Baird stated, however, that the commission would meet the planned October 1992 deadline for its final recommendations.

Provincial Healthcare Management

In January 1992, Canada's provincial health ministers agreed on an unprecedented national strategy to manage doctors and healthcare costs in the 1990s. The first step was an agreement to cut by 10 percent the number of students entering Canadian medical schools in the fall of 1993. The ministers also approved the establishment of national clinical guidelines to reduce unnecessary medical services, place more doctors on salary, reduce doctor monopolies in certain procedures such as baby delivery, and emphasize community-based care over institutional healthcare.

Sexual Misconduct Task Force

In Ontario a controversial task force on sexual abuse of patients by physicians recommended a minimum license suspension of five years and fines up to $20,000 for any doctor found guilty of sexual misconduct with a patient.

The recommendations, believed to be the toughest suggested anywhere in North America, were accepted in principle by the province's College of Physicians and Surgeons, which established the task force. Doctors found guilty of sexual abuse would only get their licenses back by proving they were no longer a threat to patients, a condition considered so difficult to meet that many observers regarded the proposed penalty as, effectively, a lifetime ban on practicing medicine.   Rod Mickleburgh

Nurses in Saskatoon, Saskatchewan, walk the picket line in front of St. Paul's Hospital in May. They staged an 11-day walkout demanding a 19 percent pay raise.

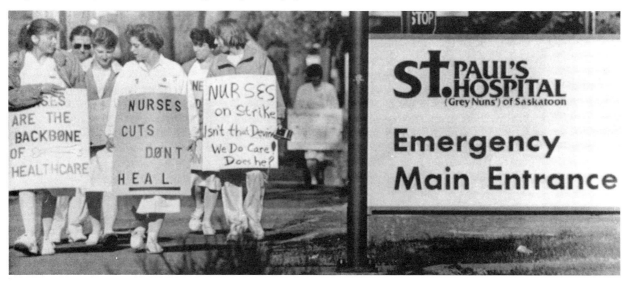

HEART AND CIRCULATORY SYSTEM

Treating Heart Disease in Women • Alcohol and the Heart • Artificial Hearts • Treating High Blood Pressure

Women and Heart Disease

A study published in July 1991 found that men were up to 45 percent more likely than women to be referred for coronary artery bypass surgery and angioplasty (a surgical procedure in which a tiny balloon is used to widen blocked arteries), despite similar heart disease mortality rates for both sexes. Furthermore, women who undergo open-heart surgery are two to five times more likely to suffer complications, including death.

This discrepancy in access to and results following cardiac procedures probably has several explanations. Heart operations, like many other medical procedures, are more risky as patients get older. Women, who on average develop heart disease at a later age than men, are older when they require cardiac procedures, their physicians are less likely to refer them for surgery because they are leery of the risks involved, and, if they do have surgery, they have higher rates of complications during operations. In addition, women's smaller heart and blood vessel size compounds the technical difficulties and risks involved in cardiac procedures.

Women's health advocates argue that the less favorable statistics for women with heart disease may also be due to biased decision making in the male-dominated medical specialties of cardiology and cardiothoracic surgery—that male doctors are less likely to recognize and aggressively treat early stages of heart disease in women. Of the patients with newly diagnosed heart disease whose records were analyzed for the 1991 study, men underwent diagnostic angiography (heart catheterization) and cardiac procedures to reestablish blood flow 15 percent to 45 percent more often than women. In other research, women were found to require emergency heart operations more frequently than men, presumably due to delayed diagnosis or treatment. Because emergency surgery is riskier than elective operations and often precludes the use of the most sophisticated new technologies, women are more likely to have a poor outcome.

The problem of underrecognition of heart disease in women may also stem from the reduced accuracy of routine diagnostic tests for coronary artery disease in female patients. For example, the standard treadmill stress test, which assesses the heart's response to exer-

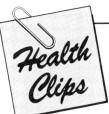
Health Clips

Covering the Rear

Going into the hospital is depressing enough. But when you are ordered to strip and don one of those open-back gowns that leaves much of your rear on display, it's adding insult to injury.

But help may be on the way—in the form of what its inventors aptly call the No Moon gown. The traditional hospital gown, with its string-type closures in the rear, leaves the patient exposed from the mid-back on down—and feeling, well, a bit cheeky. The No Moon, however, is longer and has an overlapping back with Velcro fasteners—hence its name.

The restoration of dignity is not all the No Moon offers; it was designed to meet serious medical needs. The sleeves can be opened for examination of the torso and easy insertion of intravenous tubes; the V neck is more comfortable than the old gown's choking high neckline and also accommodates tracheostomy care; inside loops can carry a drainage bag; and the garment comes with two pockets that can hold monitoring devices—or just a couple of tissues.

The No Moon sells for almost twice the price of the most expensive conventional gown, which goes for around $9. However, Anita Chaffee, the company's co-owner, argues that No Moon's more durable fabric lasts longer and that harried nurses in emergency situations will not cut knotted strings or slit the cloth, which they often do with the traditional gown. "If one looks at the cost of this gown in proportion to the cost of other items involved in a hospital stay, it certainly is minor," she adds. Indeed, it might also be pointed out that consumers have long known that it's worth paying the price for effective medical coverage.

cise, is often falsely positive in women, perhaps because of hormonal factors. Thallium testing, in which a radioactive isotope is injected into the bloodstream and followed by a scanner, is also less reliable in women, since the strength of the radioactive signal may be reduced by breast tissue. Newer testing methods, such as stress echocardiography (sound-wave imaging of the heart) and positron emission tomogra-

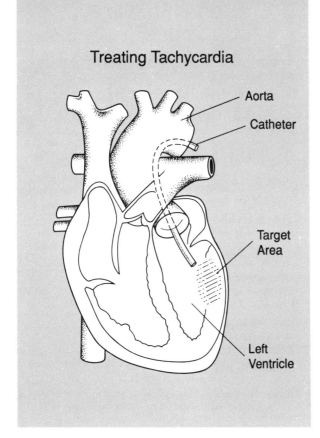

Treating Tachycardia

Aorta

Catheter

Target Area

Left Ventricle

A new procedure to treat certain types of tachycardia (rapid heartbeat) was shown in several reports to be safe and effective—and is less invasive than open-heart surgery. In the procedure a catheter is threaded through the circulatory system and the aorta to a target area of heart muscle. Radiofrequency energy is then delivered to the target area, disrupting the abnormal electrical circuits that cause the problem.

phy (PET scanning), which in cardiology is used to assess the metabolic function of the heart, may in the future become important tools for diagnosing coronary artery disease in women.

Alcohol and Heart Disease

A large, well-controlled study of more than 44,000 male healthcare professionals published in August 1991 confirmed a long-held but much debated hypothesis that moderate consumption of alcohol reduces the likelihood of coronary artery disease. Men who drank two or three alcoholic beverages each day were less likely to have heart attacks than those averaging one alcoholic drink or less per day. Twenty-three percent of the subjects reported never drinking alcohol, and these subjects had the highest rate of heart attacks in the study, even after other factors such as diet and overall health were taken into account. The effect of heavy drinking could not be assessed, since only 3.5 percent of subjects reported consuming four or more alcoholic drinks each day. However, other studies have shown that heavy alcohol consumption is associ-

ated with the development of heart failure and damage to other vital organs.

The reason for the beneficial effects of modest alcohol intake has not yet been clearly established. However, it is known that alcohol can raise the blood level of high density lipoproteins (HDL, the so-called good cholesterol). HDL molecules carry cholesterol (a waxy fat substance) through the blood to the liver, preventing it from building up along artery walls. Many investigators believe this may account for the reduced rate of heart attacks associated with moderate drinking.

Researchers have begun studying the population of France, which has a relatively low incidence of heart disease compared with the United States, despite a high consumption of fat and cholesterol, to better understand the relationship between alcohol, dietary patterns, and cardiovascular disease. Some scientists have postulated that the French custom of drinking wine with meals may be an important factor in reducing heart disease. Others believe that the relatively recent shift toward a high-fat diet in France may result in increased heart disease rates in the future.

Artificial Heart Update

In a review published in 1991 the National Academy of Sciences strongly endorsed a U.S. federal program to develop artificial hearts and mechanical assist devices. The review was begun in 1988 after Congress overruled a decision by the National Heart, Lung, and Blood Institute to stop the artificial heart program.

Earlier in the year the first fully portable long-term mechanical assist device—a ventricular assist device, or VAD—had been implanted in a critically ill patient, whose heart was failing, in the hope that it would keep him alive until a heart donor could be found. The man died within two weeks, of causes unrelated to the implant. A second patient, Michael Templeton, received an implant of the same kind of VAD in the fall and early in 1992 was leading a relatively normal life while awaiting a transplant. The first clinical trials of a new type of VAD were expected to begin in 1992.

VADs are not intended to replace the failing heart. Rather, they divert a large portion of the blood supply to a mechanical pump, which greatly reduces the cardiac work load. Meanwhile, efforts to develop a total artificial heart are continuing.

Devices previously available were impractical for long-term use because they required large external power sources and their reliability was poor. The new VADs and artificial hearts would be powered by electricity transmitted across the skin from rechargeable batteries worn by the patient.

The development of an artificial heart could benefit

thousands of Americans each year. Current medical treatment of advanced heart failure is often inadequate, and human heart transplantation, while successful in over 70 percent of patients, is limited by the scarcity of donor hearts (about 2,000 in 1990) and complications of organ rejection and drugs used to suppress the immune system.

Although the technological challenges of mechanical heart devices are being overcome, issues regarding the cost of and access to this therapy may prove more difficult to resolve. The devices are likely to cost between $50,000 and $100,000, with hospitalization and physician fees adding another $100,000.

New Tachycardia Treatment

Several recent reports have demonstrated the safety and effectiveness of a new procedure used to treat certain types of tachycardia (rapid heartbeat). The procedure, called radiofrequency catheter ablation, involves identifying abnormal electrical circuits in the heart and disrupting them by applying radiofrequency energy delivered through special catheters (tubes). The procedure is an important medical advance since it is less invasive than the surgical treatment previously available, open-heart surgery. It uses a catheter inserted into a vein in the groin and threaded into the heart.

Clinical research teams from Oklahoma and Michigan published their experiences with the new procedure in June 1991. Collectively, the studies involved 272 patients. Most of the patients had a condition called Wolff-Parkinson-White Syndrome, which causes tachycardia and is associated with one or more extra circuits of electrically active tissue in the heart. The researchers showed that the extra circuits could be destroyed by radiofrequency energy in most cases (a 92-99 percent success rate) and that complications, none of them resulting in death, developed in less than 2 percent of patients. Most cardiologists agree that the catheter procedure will soon replace the open-heart operations currently performed for certain arrhythmias, or heart rhythm abnormalities, and will offer a new mode of treatment for patients with tachycardia who respond poorly to medication.

Electrocardiograms

In 1991 it was announced that as of January 1992, Medicare, the U.S. health insurance program for elderly Americans, would no longer reimburse physicians for interpreting electrocardiograms (ECGs). Electrocardiography, developed more than a century ago, is the oldest technological means in modern use for cardiac diagnosis and is still the first and most common test ordered by cardiologists for the evaluation of heart disease. The change in payment policy,

which is expected to save the federal government several billion dollars each year, was challenged by cardiologists.

Part of the rationale for the change in reimbursement policy is the proliferation of computer programs that interpret ECGs immediately after they are done. In the United States alone, more than 50 million ECGs are read by computer each year. Ironically, the first major scientific study comparing computerized interpretations of electrocardiograms to readings by cardiologists was published in December 1991, long after the change in U.S. reimbursement policy was decided. The study showed a great variability in the diagnostic accuracy of computer programs, with most programs performing less well than cardiologists.

Yo-Yo Dieting Could Harm the Heart

Large or frequent fluctuations in body weight, a common result of "yo-yo" dieting (repeated attempts at weight loss), may increase the risk of heart attack and coronary disease, according to a study that appeared in 1991. The report analyzed the records of more than 3,000 men and women who participated in the Framingham Heart Study. That study, begun in 1948, follows the medical history of more than 5,000 residents of Framingham, Mass., to determine trends in heart disease.

The new study found higher rates of death and coronary heart disease among people whose weight varied often or by large amounts than among individuals whose weight remained stable. The authors calculated that some risks associated with extreme variations in body weight are as great as those faced by people who remain obese (more than 20 percent overweight). Among adults in the United States, roughly 50 percent of all women and 25 percent of men are dieting at any given time, yet a very high proportion of diets prove unsuccessful in the long term. In pointing to possible hazards of yo-yo dieting, the 1991 study highlighted the importance of maintaining a healthful weight loss.

The Syndromes X

The term "Syndromes X" may sound more fitting in a spy novel than a medical textbook, but it is used by physicians referring to two different medical mysteries. The first of these involves the frequent coexistence in a patient of obesity, diabetes, high blood levels of the body fats known as triglycerides, and hypertension (high blood pressure). For years scientists and clinicians have wondered whether the association of these conditions was caused by a common underlying factor. Recent scientific data suggest one possible biological link, the phenomenon of insulin resistance. Insulin resistance occurs when various tissues of the body do not respond appropriately to insulin, a hormone whose function is to regulate the level of sugar in the blood. A study published in 1991 found that nearly all patients classified as having this first kind of Syndrome X demonstrated some degree of insulin resistance in laboratory analyses. Insulin resistance may explain why some patients with normal or even above normal levels of insulin in the blood nonetheless develop diabetes.

A second condition, also called Syndrome X, refers to patients who suffer from angina or heart attacks but who in diagnostic tests are found to have normal coronary arteries without significant blockages. Although the cause of heart attack and angina under these circumstances is not fully understood, two possible explanations are offered by cardiologists. One is that obstructions in cardiac blood vessels too small to be assessed by angiography may cause symptoms. The other is that coronary arteries can contract due to spasms, at times even in the absence of coronary blockages. Thus, the arteries of patients prone to coronary spasm might only appear abnormal when a spasm was taking place.

Treatment of Hypertension in the Elderly

The results of a large controlled study of treatment for elevated blood pressure in patients aged 60 or over provide new insights into the benefit of blood pressure medication.

Blood pressure levels, especially systolic blood pressure (the higher of the two blood pressure values) tend to increase with age, and for many years physicians have debated whether treatment guidelines for older patients should be the same as those used for younger hypertensives. In particular, the benefit of treating patients with elevated systolic blood pressure when the diastolic pressure was normal was unknown.

The final results of the Systolic Hypertension in the Elderly Program (SHEP), a study begun in 1984, were published in June 1991. Patients in this program, who had elevated systolic levels but normal diastolic levels, were treated with either a placebo or with one of two antihypertensive medications (chlorthalidone, a diuretic, or atenolol, a beta blocker). During five years of follow-up, it was found that individuals taking one of the medications had 36 percent fewer strokes and 27 percent fewer nonfatal heart attacks and coronary heart disease deaths than did patients receiving placebos. These results will undoubtedly alter the treatment practice of many physicians who previously focused on elevations of diastolic blood pressure alone.   JEFFREY FISHER, M.D.
MICHAEL J. KOREN, M.D.

MENTAL HEALTH

New Light on Suicide Among Youth • Research on Schizophrenia • Improving the Outcome of Psychotherapy • Prozac Fears Allayed • Halcion Attacked for Psychiatric Side Effects

Suicide

Suicide and attempts at suicide are a major public health concern in the United States. Particularly worrisome is the fact that the suicide rate for individuals between the ages of 15 and 24 has risen markedly in recent decades. U.S. government data indicate that suicide in this age group is currently the third-leading cause of death, after accidents and homicide (coupled with "legal intervention"). According to a national survey released by the U.S. Centers for Disease Control in the fall of 1991, about 1 in 12 U.S. high school students attempted suicide in the year preceding the survey. The number of suicide prevention programs for high school students in the United States has been increasing rapidly. Most teenagers and adults believe that reporting a suicidal act by a peer is a caring, not a betraying, act that can help the individual get proper mental care.

A 1991 study by researchers at the National Institute of Mental Health suggested that teenagers seriously considering suicide can best be spotted by asking them directly about feelings of hopelessness and thoughts about suicide. In their responses to a standard questionnaire, teenagers who had recently attempted suicide stood out in two ways from healthy teens and from teens who were regarded as at risk of attempting suicide because of sexual abuse, drug abuse, or severe depression: one was that the suicide attempters revealed more hopelessness, and the other was that they more often reported feeling life was not worth living and said they had contemplated suicide as a way out.

New Findings on Schizophrenia

Some recent research on possible links between schizophrenia and abnormalities in specific parts of the brain has focused on the temporal lobe. Schizophrenia is a long-lasting illness that impairs a person's ability to function in daily life; symptoms may include delusions, hallucinations, illogical thinking, and a seeming lack of emotion. The temporal lobe is one of four lobes into which each half, or hemisphere, of the main part of the brain (the cerebrum) is divided.

In some schizophrenics the left temporal lobe appears to be reduced in size, and its surface, the cortex, seems to show atrophy, or wasting. These abnormalities have been found to correlate with the severity of schizophrenic symptoms. In particular, there is a relationship between changes in the size of the temporal lobe and the presence of hallucinations; the changes are more likely to be found in chronic schizophrenics, as opposed to new cases. Evidence of changes in the functioning of this brain structure has also been found—such as a reduction in the amount of small proteins called neuropeptides, which play an important role in nerve activity. Parts of the temporal lobe are involved in memory, and certain types of memory problems have been observed in schizophrenic patients. Researchers have also noted that the form of epilepsy that has its origin in the temporal lobe (called temporal lobe epilepsy) often shows schizophrenia-like symptoms.

One of the areas being explored by scientists trying to uncover the causes of schizophrenia is possible damage—caused, say, by a viral infection—to the fetus's developing brain. A 1991 study found new evidence suggesting that people born immediately after influenza epidemics may be at a significantly higher risk of developing schizophrenia as adults than are people born in years without high flu rates. The researchers discovered that the rate of schizophrenia among people born in England and Wales in early 1958, following a late 1957 flu epidemic in the region, was 88 percent higher than the rate among people born two years earlier and two years later, when there was not a high incidence of influenza. Although the scientists did not know if the mothers of the schizophrenics were actually infected with the flu virus during their pregnancy, the findings corroborated the results of an earlier study done in Finland.

The Outcome of Psychotherapy

Researchers have found that a characteristic known as psychological mindedness can be used to help predict which patients will benefit most from psychotherapy. Psychological mindedness is the ability to see relationships between thoughts, feelings, and actions and to understand the causes of behavior and their meanings. A high degree of psychological mindedness suggests a successful outcome for a broad range of psychotherapy techniques, including individual treatment, group treatment, family therapy, and marital therapy. It results in improved social functioning and reduced symptoms after treatment.

A 1991 research report suggested that psychotherapy for depression may be more successful over the long term when the therapist and patient focus consistently on improving the patient's social skills and relations with others. The researchers said that if this focus on interpersonal issues is confirmed to be beneficial by other studies, it could be a viable alternative to long-term drug therapy, which some people cannot or will not tolerate.

With suicide standing as a leading cause of death among people age 15 to 24 in the United States, the number of high school suicide prevention programs, which often include counseling services, has increased rapidly.

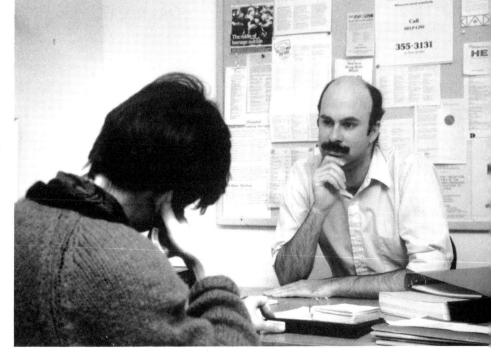

267

Prozac and Suicidal Thoughts

Since it was approved for marketing by the U.S. Food and Drug Administration in 1987, the antidepressant drug Prozac (fluoxetine) has received a large amount of media scrutiny because of claims that its use produces an increase in suicidal and violent behavior. But in September 1991 an FDA advisory committee concluded that there is no solid scientific evidence proving that Prozac (or other antidepressant drugs) causes suicidal or violent behavior among users.

There have been roughly 500 reports of suicide attempts among Americans taking Prozac. It is not uncommon for depressed people, including those being treated with an antidepressant drug, to have suicidal thoughts, and the existence of such thoughts does not necessarily mean that the drug caused them. The FDA advisory committee voted down a call to strengthen the side-effect warnings on Prozac's package labeling, but it did urge that more research be carried out on antidepressant medications.

Currently, approximately 2.5 million Americans take Prozac regularly. Sales for 1991 were estimated to total as much as $1 billion. Prozac is effective for patients suffering from a variety of types of depression and can be helpful in other psychiatric conditions such as obsessive-compulsive disorder and eating disorders like bulimia.

Halcion Under Fire

The popular sleeping pill Halcion (triazolam) was much in the news in 1991 as allegations were made that it produced more adverse psychiatric side effects than expected. Instances of such reactions as anxiety, rebound insomnia, amnesia, confusion, hallucinations, hyperexcitability, and uncharacteristic violent behavior have been reported over the years since the drug first came on the market in Belgium and the Netherlands in the late 1970s. (It entered the Canadian market in 1978 and gained FDA approval for marketing in the United States in 1982.)

In 1989, Halcion's maker, the Upjohn Company, was sued for negligence by a woman who claimed that the effects of the drug had caused her to kill her mother. (The case was settled out of court in 1991.) In preparing documents requested by the woman's lawyers regarding Halcion testing, Upjohn reportedly discovered that some data on side effects had been mistakenly left out of the summary report of a study used in its U.S. licensing application. The company alerted various regulatory agencies to the oversight. After reviewing the previously undisclosed data and additional evidence, Great Britain banned the sale of Halcion in October 1991, saying the drug was more likely to cause such side effects as memory loss and depression than were other sleeping medications. Upjohn appealed the ban.

Halcion's defenders argued that it was a beneficial and safe drug if used properly and that most of the reported adverse reactions, if true, could be attributed to patients taking the drug for too long or in too large doses. In November 1991, following discussions with the FDA, Upjohn said it would repackage the drug in the United States, selling it in ten-tablet amounts (instead of the previous 30 or 100) and including inserts explaining to patients the drug's risks and benefits. The package labeling for doctors was to be changed to emphasize that Halcion is intended for short-term treatment of insomnia. Meanwhile, the FDA was reviewing the scientific data reported on the drug.

Cost Issues in Mental Health

Having to close sizable budget gaps, many states in 1991 cut spending on mental hospitals, claiming that the facilities were underused and expensive and that more patients could be treated at less expense in community-based centers. In an October report, however, the inspector general of the U.S. Department of Health and Human Services asserted that nearly half of community mental health centers required to provide basic services under federal contracts had failed to do so. Since the 1960s some 600 community mental health centers had received several hundred million dollars in construction money from the federal government, in return for which they agreed to supply basic mental health services within their communities, including emergency treatment, outpatient services, inpatient care for the seriously ill, and educational services. Some of the care was to be free or at very low cost. Officials of the National Institute of Mental Health, which is in charge of the community mental health program, acknowledged that 10 to 15 percent of the centers were not providing basic care and that overall the community-based centers had not succeeded in adequately serving people who were released from institutions or very seriously ill.

Statistics show that mental illness is more prevalent among lower socioeconomic groups. People who meet U.S. government guidelines for poverty face a twofold increase in risk for psychiatric disorders. Although the percentage of Americans living in poverty has not changed significantly since 1980, the availability of state-financed mental health services for the poor has been greatly reduced. Statistics also indicate that people who do not have any form of health insurance—up to 13 percent or more of the U.S. population—are at greater risk for mental illness than those who have private insurance and have less access to care than individuals who have Medicaid or private insurance.

BARRY H. GUZE, M.D.

NEWSMAKERS

FRANCES CONLEY

After 25 years of building a reputation as a skilled neurosurgeon at Stanford University, tenured professor Frances Conley had had enough—not of the delicate and time-consuming brain surgery that is her specialty, but of the pervasive sexism she had encountered throughout her years at Stanford. On May 23, 1991, she submitted a letter of resignation. The decision to resign was sparked by the proposed promotion, to chair of the neurosurgery department, of fellow surgeon Gerald Silverberg, who, she felt, treated her in a sexist, demeaning manner. Promoting him, as she saw it, sent a message that sexist behavior is acceptable.

Originally, Conley meant to keep her resignation quiet, but the day after submitting it she attended a student-faculty senate meeting at which students described instructors using *Playboy* centerfolds to "spice up" lectures and acting in other ways that students found offensive and inappropriate. Until then, Conley said, she hadn't realized that sexism was so widespread, and she was appalled that medical students were encountering it "in their learning place, where they are supposed to be free to learn and to train to become professionals." Feeling the need to speak out, Conley wrote an op-ed piece for the San Francisco *Chronicle* recounting her reasons for leaving Stanford; the story was quickly picked up by the national media, and Conley was news.

Conley refrained from calling her experiences sexual harassment, preferring to speak of gender insensitivity, or just plain sexism. She said that when she was younger other doctors frequently publicly invited her to have sex with them, and she described instances of male doctors running their hands up her leg, or calling her "difficult" and suggesting that her disagreeing with them must

be related to her menstrual cycle. Although not physically harmful, this kind of treatment, she said, was a constant reminder that in the field of medicine, and particularly surgery, women are seen as inferior, and are expected to remain so.

When asked why she had put up with such treatment for so long, Conley said she did it to advance professionally, believing that if she made an issue of it, she could ruin her career. She described the world of surgery as a sort of old boys' club; for a female to be trained and get cases, she had to be accepted as a member of the club, which meant putting up with sexist attitudes.

At Stanford, however, Conley's resignation and complaints from female students appeared to have opened some eyes. The medical school put in place a series of programs to address concerns about sexism, and a committee was assigned to review the allegations against Silverberg. (After the committee made its report, early in 1992, Silverberg was removed as acting chair of the neurosurgery department and told he was not in the running for the permanent position.) As a result of the university's efforts to combat sexism, Conley agreed in September 1991 to rejoin the faculty, saying that further changes were more apt to happen if she were there than if she were not. However, she noted, her reception by colleagues was chilly upon her return.

Conley, whose husband, Phil, is an investment adviser, was born on August 12, 1940, in Palo Alto, Calif. She received her M.D. from Stanford in 1966. After her internship and residency at Stanford Hospital, she joined the staff in 1975, simultaneously joining the staff at the Palo Alto Veterans Administration Hospital, which is associated with Stanford. In 1981 she became an associate professor of surgery at Stanford. She was one of the first female neurosurgeons in the United States.

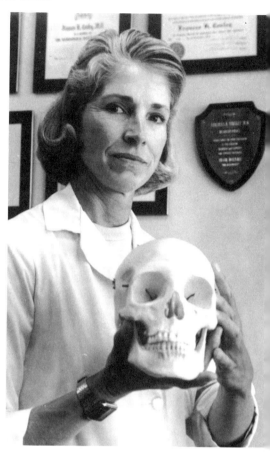

Frances Conley

In January 1992, Conley was honored by the Feminist Majority Foundation in Arlington, Va., along with 18 other women, for what were described as "extraordinary personal sacrifices for women's rights."

EARVIN "MAGIC" JOHNSON

Not many people could announce to the world that they were infected with HIV—the virus that causes AIDS—and come out smiling. But that's what 32-year-old basketball star Earvin "Magic" Johnson did on November 7, 1991, in a press conference at the Great Western Forum in Inglewood, Calif., where he had starred with the Los Angeles Lakers for 12 seasons, leading them to five

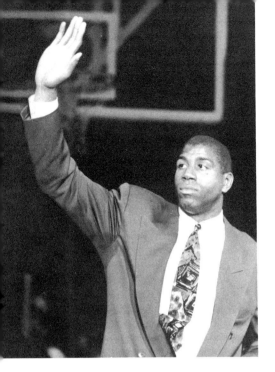

Earvin "Magic" Johnson

National Basketball Association championships and winning the league's Most Valuable Player award three times. Johnson said he was retiring from pro basketball but that he still felt well and did not yet have any AIDS symptoms. He pledged to become a spokesperson for AIDS prevention. "Life is going to go on for me," Johnson declared, "and I'm going to be a happy man."

Johnson's willingness to be so open about his condition was widely praised, since his celebrity gave the public a much-needed jolt of awareness that AIDS infection is not limited to homosexuals and intravenous drug users, the two groups hit hardest so far in the United States. While no one could escape the uncomfortable reality that Johnson's promiscuity—to which he candidly admitted—had promoted his tragedy, public health officials anticipated that his willingness to speak out on AIDS would, more than anything else, get the message out not only to the general public but especially to millions of young black men who might have a false sense of security about their chances of getting the disease. Johnson put it plainly: "Like most other blacks, I was denying that AIDS was spreading throughout our community

like wildfire while we ignored the flames." As he stated at the press conference, "It can happen to anybody, even me, Magic Johnson."

The impact of the announcement was quick and huge. Johnson was gratified to hear reports that people were pouring into hospitals and clinics seeking AIDS testing. Within less than a week, he received nearly 1,000 requests from AIDS groups for help and had to organize a committee of advisers so he could sort them out. One invitation that Johnson did accept quickly came from President George Bush, who asked him to join the National Commission on AIDS, a federal agency organized to formulate a national strategy for dealing with the disease. The commission's cochairman, Dr. David Rogers, verified the effect of Johnson's disclosure: "I can't tell you how many calls I've had from teachers saying, 'this is all my kids want to talk about.'" Johnson met with the president in January 1992 and said afterward that Bush "needs to do a lot" about AIDS, adding, "he is going to do his homework, and I am going to do mine."

One bright note was that Johnson's pregnant wife (he had married his longtime sweetheart, Earletha "Cookie" Kelly, on September 14, 1991) tested negative for HIV. Johnson himself began taking medication to delay the disease, and laboratory tests in February 1992 showed no evidence that his immune system was deteriorating. He not only played in the NBA All-Star game that month, he dominated it, scoring a game-high 25 points and winning the MVP trophy. He acknowledged that it might be his last game, but he had his sights set on the upcoming Summer Olympics in Barcelona. Since the average time between infection with HIV and the development of AIDS is 10 years, Johnson most likely has several years of health before him—years which he vowed he would live with the same desire to excel that had made him such a sen-

sation on the basketball court. As he wrote in an article published in *Sports Illustrated*, "Maybe one day I'll be able to help us get this thing under control, and then I can become an example to young people in a different way. Not as Magic Johnson dealing assists on the fast break, but as Earvin Johnson dealing with life—dealing with AIDS."

YUET WAI KAN

Sometimes it seems that hardly a week goes by without the media announcing that diligent medical researchers have found yet another gene responsible for one of the 3,000 or so health disorders caused by genetic defects. Indeed, the dramatic acceleration in knowledge of the relationship between defective genes and human disease has led some to predict that the 1990s will be "the decade of genetics."

In 1991 the Albert and Mary Lasker Foundation awarded its Clinical Medical Research Award—an honor regarded as second only to the Nobel Prize in prestige—to one of the most diligent of those researchers, Dr.

Yuet Wai Kan

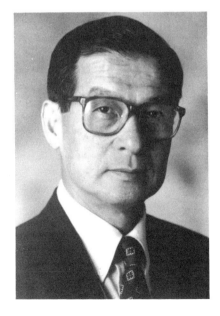

Yuet Wai Kan, head of molecular medicine and diagnostics at the University of California at San Francisco. His work has been pivotal in the study of the role of genes in inborn diseases, the development of prenatal tests to detect them, and the search for ways to treat them.

Kan, who was born in Hong Kong on June 11, 1936, and educated there, came to the United States in 1960, where he married his wife, Alvera, four years later (they now live in San Francisco and have two daughters). After a brief stint as an assistant professor of pediatrics at Harvard Medical School, he came to San Francisco in 1972, where he pursued his interest in the causes of inherited blood disorders.

His first breakthrough came in 1975, when he was studying the group of diseases known as the thalassemias, hereditary anemias found most commonly in people of Mediterranean, African, or Southeast Asian stock. Kan discovered that one of them, the type known as alpha-thalassemia, results from the absence of a part of a gene that makes hemoglobin, the molecule that carries oxygen through the bloodstream. This was the first documentation that gene deletion can cause human disease. Armed with this knowledge, Kan was able to develop a prenatal test for alpha-thalassemia, based on analysis of DNA, the substance that carries an individual's genetic blueprint. He then, in 1978, discovered a distinctive DNA pattern characteristic of sickle-cell anemia, a disease most prevalent in blacks. This work also made possible a screening test.

The methods pioneered by Kan led to many other tests by which researchers can detect inborn disorders through analysis of fetal cells obtained by amniocentesis, a procedure in which a needle is inserted into the uterus of a pregnant woman to draw off a little of the amniotic fluid (in which fetal cells are floating) that surrounds the fetus.

A notable practical payoff from genetic research by Kan and others has come in certain Mediterranean countries, where, he notes, genetic counseling and prenatal diagnosis have reduced the incidence of thalassemia considerably. Effective new drugs and genetic therapy for thalassemia and related disorders may eventually be another payoff. Kan today is trying to learn which gene regulates the hemoglobin molecule—that will be a crucial phase in developing treatments for inherited blood disorders involving hemoglobin. He has no doubt that the 1990s will see the introduction of successful genetic therapy, though he cannot predict which diseases will prove most treatable. "There are many genetic disorders," he points out, "and I think most people are thinking along the same lines."

That they are thinking along these lines, of course, has a lot to do with the work that Kan began some two decades ago.

DAVID KESSLER

The U.S. marshals made their move on the evening of April 24, 1991. They swooped down on a warehouse in Hopkins, Minn., found 2,000 cases of the stuff, and hauled it away. The raid was swift, sure, and unexpected.

What were they after? Contraband? Hijacked goods? Drugs? None of the above. The illicit booty was orange juice. Citrus Hill Fresh Choice orange juice, to be specific. The raiders were acting on behalf of the U.S. Food and Drug Administration, the federal agency responsible for overseeing the safety of new drugs and protecting much of the food supply of the United States. The FDA's objection was to the use of the word "fresh," when the juice was actually made from concentrate. Within two days, the product's maker, Procter & Gamble, agreed to drop the offending word.

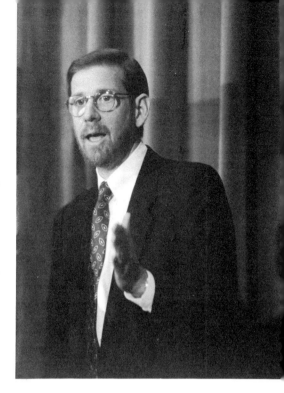

David Kessler

This high-profile, no-nonsense, quick-action event would scarcely have occurred in the FDA of the 1980s, a time when the agency was beset by tightened budgets, low morale, heavy criticism for its sluggishness, and, to top everything, a bribery scandal. But after Dr. David Kessler was sworn in as the agency's new commissioner in February 1991, the organization, the oldest federal consumer protection agency in the United States, began creating a new image—tougher, more credible, more activist.

When Kessler was named to head the FDA, a lawyer who served as an agency consultant summed up his prospects for reforming the organization by saying, "If he can't do it, no one can." Indeed, Kessler's whole career since he graduated from Amherst in 1973 seemed to be pointed toward the job. It is an indication of his energy and zeal that he earned a medical degree and a law degree simultaneously (the law degree from the University of Chicago in 1978, the M.D. from Harvard a year later). While training as a pediatrician in Baltimore, he helped a Senate committee draft new food safety legislation, and while serving as medical director of the hospital of Albert Einstein College of Medicine in New York City, he taught courses in food-and-drug law at Columbia Law School. As a result, he had the perfect résumé for the FDA job, and expectations were high when he agreed to take it.

He moved quickly. The great orange juice raid was only one of the more flamboyant of his moves. In his first year on the job, he

• reduced from 15 to 5 the number of review stages an FDA inspector's report had to clear before the agency could have a questionable product seized;

• forced a pharmaceutical company to stop distributing a promotional booklet trumped up to look like a medical journal;

• announced a policy of prosecuting drug companies that promote the use of drugs to treat conditions other than ones for which they have been approved (one example cited was the use of an antidepressant drug to combat obesity);

• ordered the seizure of more than $5 million worth of collagen (a substance injected under the skin to remove wrinkles and other deformities) from its principal manufacturer because labels carried inadequate warnings about possible harmful side effects;

• announced sweeping new food label regulations—to go into effect by May 1993—affecting virtually all foods sold in U.S. groceries;

• restricted the use of silicone-based breast implants because of concerns over their safety.

All in all, it was a barrage of activity that got Americans' attention and served notice that the FDA did, indeed, have a new profile. Kessler, who now lives in Washington with his wife, Paulette, and their children, Elise and Benjamin, says that he knew the FDA "had hit the big time" when comedian Jay Leno complained in his *Tonight* show monologue that his Bumble Bee tuna had no bumblebees in it.

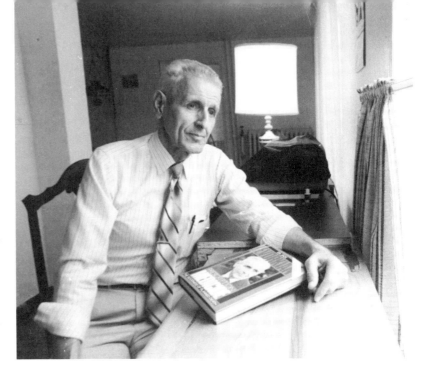

Jack Kevorkian

JACK KEVORKIAN

Neither woman was terminally ill, but neither wanted to live. So on October 23, 1991, they went to a cabin overlooking Tamarack Lake in Michigan and died—one by lethal injection, one by inhaling carbon monoxide. And once again, Dr. Jack Kevorkian, the man his critics labeled "Dr. Death," was in the headlines.

Kevorkian, a retired pathologist who had earned his M.D. at the University of Michigan and practiced in Pontiac, Mich., had become famous in June 1990 when he helped Janet Adkins, a 54-year-old Alzheimer's victim, end her life by hooking her up to a "suicide device"—he called it a "Mercitron"—set up in the rear of his 1968 camper. Adkins pushed a button that caused her to be injected with two chemicals; one rendered her unconscious, the other then stopped her heart.

The ensuing publicity, as Kevorkian promoted his belief in euthanasia (mercy killing) on talk shows and news programs, stirred a debate across the United States on the right of people with painful or terminal illnesses to have medical assistance in ending their lives. Although polls taken after Adkins's death indicated support for the notions that incurably ill people have the right to end their lives and that it is proper for physicians to help them, Kevorkian was eventually indicted for murder. The charges were later dismissed by a judge who ruled that Michigan had no law against assisted suicide, but Kevorkian was forbidden to use the machine again—a ban he lost little time in defying.

In 1991, Kevorkian published a book, *Prescription: Medicide*, in which he explained his passionate—some would say obsessive—advocacy of euthanasia. He recalled that as an intern he saw a woman ravaged by terminal cancer, her body deformed and discolored. "Out of sheer empathy alone," he wrote, "I could have helped her die with satisfaction. From that moment on, I was sure that doctor-assisted euthanasia and suicide are and always were ethical. . . ." Yet much of his subsequent career was devoted to a different, though related, field: the rights of condemned prisoners to have a humane, physician-assisted execution and to designate their bodies for organ transplantation or medical experimentation. In 1987, however, he visited the Netherlands, where euthanasia was gaining acceptance in the medical community, and upon his return to Michigan, as he wrote, "I decided to take the risky step of assisting terminal patients in committing suicide." He placed advertisements for "death counseling" in newspapers, and in 1989 his story began to be picked up by the local press and television. The publicity led to an item in *Newsweek* that was seen by Janet Adkins's husband.

The women who died at Tamarack Lake were Marjorie Wantz, 58, victim of an agonizing pelvic disease, and Sherry Miller, 43, a multiple sclerosis patient. Although Kevorkian had taken care that both women themselves activated the devices that killed them, the county medical examiner ruled the deaths homicides. Indicted on February 5, 1992, on two counts of murder and one count of delivery of a controlled substance, the 63-year-old Kevorkian was later ordered to stand trial on the murder charges.

Shortly after Kevorkian's indictment it was revealed that in July 1990, he had mailed instructions on building a Mercitron to a cancer-stricken California dentist and had counseled him by phone. The dentist had constructed the machine and used it to end his life on March 4, 1991.

Some who were inclined to agree with Kevorkian that physician-assisted suicide might be right in some instances tended to see him as a maverick, on the fringe of the debate and engaged in a tasteless pursuit of publicity. Nevertheless, his eagerness to make his case in such a dramatic way, and to flout the law by doing so, seemed certain to place him in the center of the euthanasia controversy for some time to come.

BURTON LEE

When Dr. Burton Lee has to make a house call, he doesn't have far to go—the building that contains his office is also his patient's home. On the other hand, a house call from Lee can cause press conferences to be held, stock markets to react, and headline writers to boot up their word processors.

That's because Burton Lee is President George Bush's personal physician. All in all, he would doubtlessly prefer it if his name never had to make the news, but inevitably it does—especially recently.

It began in April 1990, when Lee accompanied the president to Bethesda Naval Hospital for his annual checkup. Lee himself does not conduct the exam; he selects several specialists to do it. "Then we go over all the material together and see if there's a problem," he says. This time there was one. Bush was found to have early glaucoma in his left eye. Glaucoma can lead to blindness if not attended to but is easily treated with eyedrops.

The next medical event was not so benign. While jogging at Camp David, the presidential country retreat, in May 1991, Bush experienced an irregular and rapid heart beat (a condition called atrial fibrillation). The potentially dire event, however, turned out to have a cause

Burton Lee

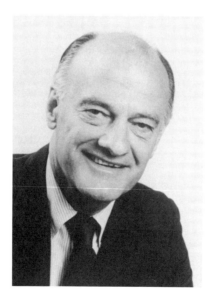

that was not so serious. Lee found that Bush had an overactive thyroid gland caused by the immune system disorder called Graves' disease; the president drank a concoction of radioactive iodine that killed off most of the thyroid's hormone-producing cells, and his condition returned to normal.

Oddly, however, Bush's wife, Barbara, had been diagnosed with Graves' a year and a half before. This puzzled Lee, because the odds of a husband and wife both contracting the illness seemed astronomically high. (An even stranger sidelight was that Millie, the First Dog, had developed lupus, another immune system disorder). In search of an explanation, Lee ordered tests of the water at the White House, at the Bushes' Kennebunkport, Me., estate, at the vice president's mansion (where the Bushes had lived during the Reagan presidency), and at Camp David—but the investigation came up dry.

In early January 1992, Bush vomited and collapsed at a formal dinner in Tokyo, and the disturbing sight of a prostrate, ashen president, his head being cradled by the Japanese prime minister, was replayed ad infinitum on national television. Lee, who was at the dinner, determined that the cause was a bout of gastroenteritis—commonly known as intestinal flu. He administered an antinausea drug, and Bush soon resumed his schedule. The matter would probably have ended there, but it came out that the president had been taking the sedative Halcion, a drug that had been banned in Britain a few months before and that, critics charged, could have serious psychiatric side effects such as amnesia, paranoia, depression, and hallucinations. The controversy focused on Lee as the president's doctor. Although he said that he prescribed Halcion to Bush "rarely" and that the president did not use the drug on a daily basis, Lee clearly felt the sting of the criticism: a month later he said he would try to avoid prescribing it again.

NEWSMAKERS

Dr. Burton James Lee III was born in New York City on March 28, 1930, and educated at Yale and Columbia. In 1960 he joined the staff at the prestigious Memorial Sloan-Kettering Cancer Center in New York City. It was in New York that he met George Bush's brother Jonathan, who in turn introduced him to the budding politician. Lee and George Bush, it turned out, had both gone to Andover and Yale, and they had mutual friends from both schools. The two men both had roots in Greenwich, Conn., and their daughters later roomed together in college. So although Lee was not Bush's doctor, Bush appointed his friend physician to the president (the official title) when he moved into the White House.

Although keeping an eye on the president's health is Lee's most prominent task, most of his time is spent supervising what is known as the White House Medical Unit, a staff of 19 people, including nurses, clerical help, physician assistants, and four other physicians. It is their job to provide healthcare to people in and around the White House, including cabinet members and their families. The unit also can care for visiting foreign dignitaries who may need medical attention while in Washington. Whenever Bush travels abroad, Lee goes along, but unlike previous White House physicians he does not accompany Bush on every domestic trip. He likes to give other staff members a chance to go instead, he says, because "they enjoy it." Of course, Lee is always available, and if the president were to have a medical emergency, he says, the extensive White House communications system would very quickly get in touch with him.

While 30 years as a cancer specialist may not be directly related to the kind of medicine he practices now, Lee argues that in one respect his previous work was good training. Numbered among his patients, he points out, were many of the rich

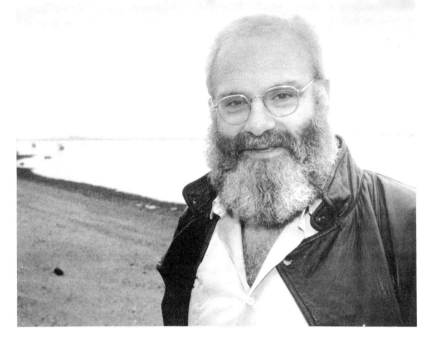

Oliver Sacks

and powerful, and that taught him about what he calls "VIP medicine." These people, he complains, often "try to call their own shots," as, for example, Bush did when he ignored Lee's advice to skip the dinner in Tokyo. No matter whom one is caring for, Lee says, "you have to do what you have to do."

OLIVER SACKS

Reflective, eccentric, often lonely, and shy to an extent that he himself calls neurotic, Dr. Oliver Sacks is not the kind of person on whom fame easily sits. Like Dr. Malcolm Sayer, his alter ego in the film *Awakenings*, one of his favorite activities is to walk and sit quietly among the plants at the New York Botanical Garden in the Bronx, the New York City borough in which he has made his home since 1965.

Yet fame has come his way. With the release in December 1990 of the highly praised *Awakenings* (based on Sacks's book of the same name), which starred Robin Williams as Malcolm Sayer and Robert De Niro as a patient whom Sacks awoke from 20 years of catatonia, Sacks's fascinating inquiries as a neurological researcher became known to millions who were unfamiliar with his ac-

claimed writings on the subject, including *Awakenings* (1973) and *The Man Who Mistook His Wife for a Hat* (1985).

Ironically, just as he was earning wider recognition for his work, Sacks became a victim of the fiscal crisis facing so many U.S. states and localities. In February 1991 he lost his job at the Bronx Psychiatric Center, one of 1,280 healthcare workers to receive pink slips in New York as the state, fighting an uphill battle to balance its budget in recessionary times, cut back its public health services.

Oliver Sacks was born in London on July 9, 1933. He studied at Oxford, earned his M.D. at London's Middlesex Hospital, and came to the United States in 1960. After postgraduate study in neurology in Los Angeles, Sacks moved to New York City, and in 1966 he began working at the Beth Abraham Home for the Incurable. There he encountered 80 survivors of the encephalitis epidemic of 1916-1929 who had become "living statues," virtually immobile or in comas so deep they could not be revived. At first, his attempts to help them with the new drug L-dopa were remarkably successful. The patients awoke, Rip Van Winkle-like, after decades of slumber. But the drug's effects didn't last, and nearly all relapsed into their previous state. The reception given to *Awakenings*, Sacks's book about the experience, was equally mixed. While no less a critic than the great British poet W. H. Auden called it "a masterpiece," it was years before the medical community as a whole accepted Sacks's research as legitimate.

After being laid off, Sacks refused to exercise his option to take a younger doctor's place at another hospital, and with his *Awakenings* book riding the film's success onto the best-seller lists, his income as an author seemed sure to satisfy his modest needs (Sacks, a bachelor, lives in a red-shingled house surrounded by a white picket fence on City Island, a part of the Bronx which lies in Long Island Sound.) After cleaning out his desk, he headed off for a European lecture tour. He will not lack patients, as the lost job was part time (although he does worry about finding *interesting* ones). He still works part time at Beth Abraham, visits patients in nursing homes, and teaches at Albert Einstein College of Medicine. He has become interested in music therapy and has begun research on his next book, which will be on Tourette's syndrome, a disorder characterized by involuntary tics and vocal sounds.

But for others, he warns, the impact of the budget cuts might not be so harmless. "All psychiatric care in the United States is being dangerously cut back now," he says. "I am deeply concerned, even fearful, for our patients."

MICHAEL TEMPLETON

Houston, being the home of NASA's Johnson Space Center, is usually associated with pioneers of spaceflight. But it is also home to pioneers of a different kind—the physicians, researchers, and patients of the world-famous Texas Heart Institute who explore the frontiers of the treatment of heart disease. And one of the enterprise's most gallant trailblazers is

Michael Templeton, a Houston area resident who in 1991 became the first person successfully to use a fully portable battery-powered pump to assist his failing heart.

Templeton, an electronics technician and father of three young children, had been diagnosed with cardiomyopathy, which eventually leads to heart failure. The precise cause of the problem was unknown, but Dr. Oscar H. ("Bud") Frazier, the surgeon who implanted the pump in September, suspected that it resulted from a viral infection. Before the device was installed, the 33-year-old Templeton was bedridden and constantly short of breath. Just a few weeks after the operation the changes in his condition were stunning. He was able to exercise on a treadmill and felt great; now, he told an interviewer, he "can breathe deep" and "eat the things I like."

The device is named the HeartMate and was developed by Thermo Cardiosystems in Woburn, Mass. Called a ventricular-assist device (VAD), it is capable of pumping 5 liters (over 5 quarts) of blood a minute and is surgically implanted in the patient's abdominal cavity, just below the diaphragm. The HeartMate's inlet tube is connected to the left ventricle, the part of the heart that ordinarily provides most of pumping action. Blood drains from the left ventricle into the device's pumping chamber. A flexible diaphragm then propels the blood through an outlet tube into the aorta, the main artery leaving the heart and carrying blood out to the body.

The HeartMate is set to pump a certain number of times a minute (in Templeton's case, 70), but it monitors the patient's activity and raises the rate when necessary. The pump is driven by a miniature electric motor powered by a battery that the patient carries in a shoulder holster, and the power is transmitted through a wire that pierces the skin. Thus, the HeartMate is not a totally implanted device, nor does it replace

the patient's ailing heart. But because it not only helps the patient to survive but permits greater freedom of movement than previous experimental VADs, it is considered a major technological breakthrough toward a true artificial heart.

The first implant of a HeartMate took place in May 1991, but the patient died a couple of weeks later from complications unrelated to the device. It was Templeton's case that provided researchers the first opportunity to see the HeartMate in operation for a lengthy period. He was slated to remain on the device only until a donor could be found for a heart transplant. But as a 210-pounder requiring a large heart, he was expected to have to wait longer than usual for a suitable donor. The HeartMate's success in keeping him going in the meantime offered hope to thousands of other heart patients, many of whom might die before donor hearts can be found. Frazier

Michael Templeton

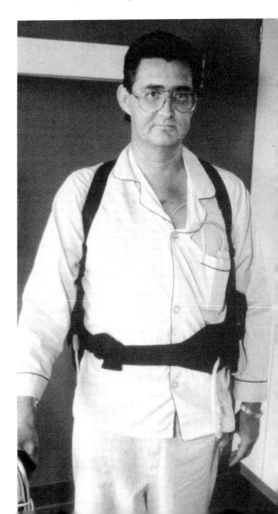

says, however, that the HeartMate's potential may lead to even more dramatic results: "We hope eventually the results will be so good that certain patients will be able to be supported with these devices and not require transplantation."

As Templeton awaited his new heart, his implanted pump was making it more likely that a transplant would succeed, because the better the patient's condition, the better the prospects. Since the HeartMate permitted Templeton to exercise and lead a relatively active life, some of the damage that his heart and other organs suffered was reversed. How fit was he? As Frazier put it, "It's a little embarrassing, but he's in a lot better shape than I am."

SIDNEY M. WOLFE

Toward the end of 1991, American television viewers following the debate over the safety of silicone gel breast implants were more than likely to encounter the image of Dr. Sidney M. Wolfe, who emerged as one of the most articulate and impassioned

Sidney M. Wolfe

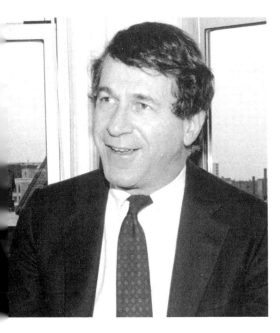

critics of the disputed devices. Chances are it was not the first time they had seen him on their TV screens. For two decades, whenever a controversy over healthcare, medical devices, or drugs has arisen in the United States, Wolfe has usually found himself involved. He has testified well over 100 times on health matters before Congress and other federal agencies, and he has contributed editorials, as well as letters to the editor, to the leading U.S. newspapers and medical journals. Among the issues that have caught his attention over the years are ineffective or dangerous drugs, unnecessary cesareans, physicians' competence, unnecessary surgery, pharmaceutical advertising, cosmetic safety, workplace hazards, and carcinogenic food additives and other chemicals.

The reason that Wolfe is so often engaged in the discussions of these subjects is that he has, since 1972, been the director of the Washington-based Health Research Group (HRG), which is the medical division of Ralph Nader's well-known consumer advocacy group, Public Citizen. Born on June 12, 1937, Wolfe received his undergraduate and his medical degrees from Western Reserve University in Cleveland. In 1966 he began working at the National Institutes of Health, conducting research on blood clotting and on alcoholism. It was at a meeting of the American Patients Association in Washington that he met Nader, who was then in the early stages of forging his reputation as a leader of the U.S. consumer protection movement. Wolfe began advising Nader on health issues, and shortly after the founding of Public Citizen in 1971, the two of them, realizing that the consumer health field was vast enough to require a separate entity, created the HRG. (Wolfe also served as president of Public Citizen from 1980 to 1982).

One of the first efforts put forth by Wolfe and his team was to seek a ban on Red Dye No. 2, an additive

widely used in processed foods—as well as in drugs and cosmetics—that was a suspected cancer-causing agent. After four years of HRG lobbying, the U.S. Food and Drug Administration banned the substance in January 1976. A similar success was achieved with the banning of the pesticide DBCP by the Environmental Protection Agency in 1979.

Among the projects pursued by the HRG in 1991 were an initiative to stop a Bush administration plan to speed the drug approval process at the FDA; challenges to several drugs, including the sleeping pill Halcion (which was banned in Britain in October); and the publication of the book *9,479 Questionable Doctors*, a 1,300-page volume listing doctors disciplined by state medical licensing boards and federal agencies. It was the controversy over silicone gel breast implants, however, that garnered the most public attention. The HRG had first raised questions about the implants' safety in 1988, arguing that they posed a cancer threat. Other fears are that they might cause infection or might rupture or leak, leading to immune system problems. The issue came to a head late in 1991, when the FDA convened an advisory panel to investigate. Testifying before the panel, Wolfe charged that an estimated 155,000 out of the approximately 2 million women who had received the implants may have suffered complications and that some 50,000 women may have had to undergo surgery to have the implants removed. In January 1992 the FDA called for a voluntary moratorium on the use of silicone gel implants, and in February the advisory committee recommended that their use be sharply curtailed.

It was a partial victory for the HRG, but while the organization pledged to continue pressing for a ban, it was already plunging ahead into another hot issue. As 1992 opened, Wolfe and the HRG were in the front lines of those calling for national health insurance.

NUTRITION AND DIET

Making Food Labels More Useful • Truth in Advertising • New Food Chart Withdrawn • More Fat Substitutes Introduced • Low-fat Diets and Life Expectancy

Food Labeling Reform

In November 1991 the U.S. Food and Drug Administration and the U.S. Department of Agriculture announced proposals for new food labeling regulations that would affect virtually all foods. The proposals covered most of the changes required by the 1990 Nutrition Labeling and Education Act. In response to an internal Department of Agriculture decision, they also covered raw and processed meats and poultry, which the act had exempted.

Under the proposed rules most processed foods on grocery store shelves would carry more accurate information on nutritional content. The required list of nutrients would emphasize those that have a significant effect on consumers' health, such as cholesterol, fat, and dietary fiber. Nutrition information would be presented in quantitative amounts—the number of grams, for example—or as a percentage of recommended daily allowances. Labels would also include consistent serving sizes, set by the FDA, in easily understandable measurements for most food categories. Currently, nutrition labeling for processed foods is voluntary for the most part. The new plan also included a voluntary nutrition labeling program for raw fruits, vegetables, and fish, as well as for raw, single-ingredient meat and poultry products.

In addition the FDA proposed to restrict disease-prevention claims on labels to those that have been scientifically proven. The FDA said the only claims that would be allowed initially would be those referring to links between calcium and osteoporosis, sodium and hypertension, fat and cardiovascular disease, and fat and cancer. The agency planned to continue studying the relationship between fiber and heart disease and between fiber and cancer before deciding whether to allow health claims for fiber.

A key portion of the plan dealt with terms such as "less sodium" and "reduced fat," which imply that a product promotes good health or is different from competitive brands. The agency proposed that "less" fat (or sodium, or calories, or cholesterol) would mean a reduction of at least 25 percent when the product is compared with the company's original products or an industrywide norm; "reduced" fat would mean a reduction of at least 50 percent. In February 1992, however, the agency offered alternative proposals that

would eliminate these percentages. To reduce confusion, the agency said, "less" and "reduced" would be synonymous. Furthermore, less stringent criteria would have to be met before such labels could be used. Critics charged that the FDA was caving in to outside pressures. In March the Department of Agriculture announced that it was postponing for one year implementation of both its required and its voluntary labeling programs. Under the terms of the 1990 act, final regulations were supposed to be completed by November 1992, and new labels were to start appearing in 1993.

Enforcing the Existing Law

In 1991 the FDA was already cracking down on misleading food labels under a law that predated the one passed in 1990. In April the agency seized 2,000 cases of Citrus Hill Fresh Choice orange juice, saying the word "fresh" was misleading because the juice was made from concentrate. The existing FDA policy states that the word "fresh" should not be used when foods have been subjected to any form of heat or chemical processing. The manufacturer of the orange juice, Procter & Gamble, subsequently agreed to change the label. In May the FDA forced three companies to drop "no cholesterol" claims on certain oils. According to the agency, the statement of no cholesterol wrapped around a picture of a heart on CPC International's Mazola Corn Oil, for example, implied that the product helps prevent or treat heart disease,

Start at the Bottom and Eat Up

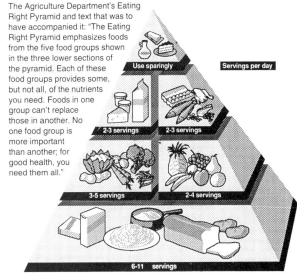

The Agriculture Department's Eating Right Pyramid and text that was to have accompanied it: "The Eating Right Pyramid emphasizes foods from the five food groups shown in the three lower sections of the pyramid. Each of these food groups provides some, but not all, of the nutrients you need. Foods in one group can't replace those in another. No one food group is more important than another; for good health, you need them all."

Source: U.S. Department of Agriculture

N.Y. Times News Service

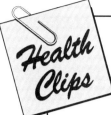

Do Kids Know What to Eat?

"Clean your plate."
"No cookies before dinner."
"No dessert till you finish your broccoli."

Parents have been launching these or similar admonitions at their children since—well, probably the Stone Age. Wouldn't it be nice if children possessed some kind of built-in regulator that instinctively prodded them to eat the right foods in the right amounts?

Parents, take heart. A study published in the January 24, 1991, *New England Journal of Medicine* strongly indicates that youngsters quite possibly *do* have such an inherent mechanism. Researchers at the University of Illinois at Urbana-Champaign studied 15 children aged two to five. Cooperating with the parents, they measured the kids' 24-hour food intake on six different days. All the children were offered the same menu and were allowed to eat as much or as little as desired. The foods were sensible, although such items as cookies, brownies, and corn chips were included.

The results showed, not surprisingly, that the amounts of food consumed varied widely from meal to meal. One child, for example, loved Wednesday's dinner entree of macaroni and cheese and gobbled it up. And yet, a remarkably consistent pattern emerged—while meal sizes varied greatly, the amount of food consumed over the course of the entire day varied little. As the researchers put it, "there was evidence that high energy intake at one meal was often compensated for by low energy intake at the next, and vice versa." And although the kids were allowed to eat all they wanted, none of them ate too much.

In light of this evidence, the authors discussed earlier studies showing that many parents, assuming that kids are unable to regulate their food intake by themselves, try to force them to eat—a strategy that often leads to obesity. Instead, the researchers argued, "the successful feeding of children is best accomplished by providing them with a variety of healthful foods and allowing them to eat what they wish."

If only it worked that way for grown-ups.

when in fact the oil is high in fat, which increases the likelihood of heart disease, cancer, and obesity. The no-cholesterol claim is further misleading, the FDA said, because all vegetable oils are free of cholesterol.

Convenience Food Advertising

Kentucky Fried Chicken, Dunkin' Donuts, and Nestle agreed with the New York State attorney general's office in October to stop using advertising and labeling claims that falsely suggested certain products were healthful. Under the agreement, Kentucky Fried Chicken changed the name of a new product, Lite'n Crispy chicken, to Skinfree Crispy. According to the attorney general, the percentage of calories from fat in Lite'n Crispy was the same as that in the company's Original Recipe product. Kentucky Fried Chicken also agreed to stop saying things that implied that the skin-free selection was more healthful.

Dunkin' Donuts promised to stop advertising that its doughnuts were free of cholesterol and more than 90 percent free of saturated fat. In the average doughnut, said the attorney general, 46 percent of the calories come from fat of some kind. Nestle agreed to stop suggesting that its nondairy creamer, Carnation Coffee-mate Liquid, was low in fat; it actually contains more than double the amount of fat in an equal portion of whole milk. Although the investigations leading to the agreements were done in New York, the settlements affected national advertising.

Meanwhile, Burger King, the nation's second largest hamburger chain, reached an agreement with New York City's Department of Consumer Affairs requiring Burger King restaurants in the city to display large posters showing, in readily understandable form, the calorie, fat, and sodium content of popular meals. Other chains, like McDonalds, offer nutrition information in booklets and posters, but critics have called them confusing and meaningless. Burger King said that use of the posters in restaurants outside the city would be optional.

Nutrition Guide Controversy

In what quickly became a controversial move, the Department of Agriculture indefinitely delayed publication of a new depiction of the four basic food groups. Called the Eating Right Pyramid, it was developed to clarify nutritional guidelines and would have replaced the food-wheel chart used by nutrition educators since the 1950s. The four-level pyramid represented food groups according to the number of daily servings recommended. Grains and cereals, with the most number of servings, were shown at the base of the pyramid, fruits and vegetables on the next level, meat and dairy products on the next, and fats, oils, and sweets at the tip.

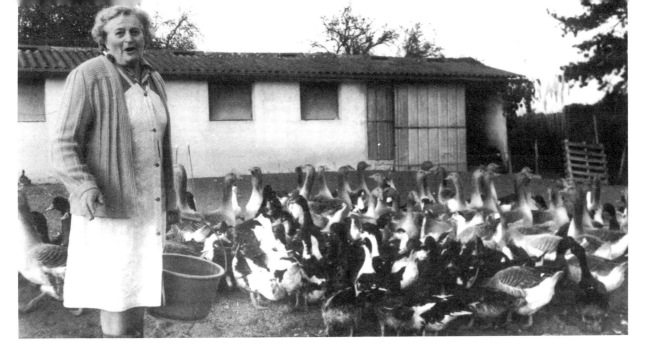

A French scientist reported that people in the Gascony region of France, despite eating huge amounts of the high-fat French delicacy foie gras, made from the fattened livers of ducks and geese, actually have relatively low heart attack rates. The study was good news to farmers like Lucette Baron, who tends her flock in the southern French town of Auch.

In April 1991, just before a pamphlet on the pyramid was to be published and distributed, the beef and dairy industries complained that the pyramid representation suggested that their products were less important than grains, fruits, and vegetables. Following the complaints, the Department of Agriculture postponed publication of the pamphlets. Critics, including federal officials and health professionals, charged that the department was bowing to pressure from the meat and dairy industries. Secretary of Agriculture Edward R. Madigan denied this, saying he wanted to test the pyramid to determine how it would be interpreted by children before disseminating it.

Also in April, an activist group urged the Department of Agriculture to drop meat and dairy products altogether from the basic food groups. Saying that the current food groups promote a high-fat, low-fiber diet that has created an epidemic of chronic diseases, the Physicians Committee for Responsible Medicine proposed replacing the current four food groups with whole grains, legumes, fruits, and vegetables. The American Medical Association denounced the group's proposal, saying that eliminating meat and dairy products would deprive Americans of important sources of minerals and vitamins.

Foie Gras Puzzle

If fat is detrimental to health, how do people in the Gascony region of southwest France get away with eating 50 times more fat-laden foie gras (fattened goose and duck livers) than Americans do and still have one-quarter the rate of fatal heart attacks? The

phenomenon, reported by a French scientist in the spring of 1991, is a mystery.

Dr. Serge Renaud, director of research at the National Institute of Health and Medical Research in Lyon, France, said findings of a ten-year study indicate that Gascons eat a diet higher in saturated fat than any other group of people in the industrialized world. Indeed, goose and duck fat as well as foie gras are dietary staples for people in the Gascony region. They eat twice as much foie gras as other French people. Yet they have the lowest rate of death from cardiovascular disease in France, according to findings of a World Health Organization study. In the city of Toulouse and a surrounding area that includes much of Gascony, 80 per 100,000 middle-aged men die of heart attacks each year, compared with 174 for all middle-aged Frenchmen in general and 315 for middle-aged American men.

Renaud claimed that goose and duck fat are closer in composition to olive oil than to butter or lard, and that olive oil does not increase blood cholesterol levels dramatically and may actually improve cardiovascular health. Other French people, capitalizing on previous publicity about heart disease rates in France, have attributed the comparatively low rate of heart disease in their country to wide consumption of French red wines. American nutritionists are quick to warn, however, that adding foie gras and red wine to the U.S. diet is not the answer. Numerous differences between the U.S. and French diets, many of them now under study, could contribute to the lower heart disease rates in France. And besides, although the

279

French rates are lower, heart disease is still the leading cause of death in France.

New Fat Substitutes

The quest for more palatable and more versatile fat substitutes turned up several new products in 1991. In February, Pfizer introduced Litesse, a fat substitute and bulking agent made of polydextrose (a combination of citric acid and dextrose sorbitol). The FDA approved polydextrose in 1981. At one calorie per gram (compared with nine for fat) Litesse is being promoted for use in frozen desserts, certain types of candy, yogurt, baked goods, and icings.

A product called Stellar, based on corn starch and made by A. E. Staley, was announced in June. It contains about one calorie per gram. Stellar is less likely to curdle than fat substitutes made from cellulose gel and is better tasting, the maker said. Staley said the product could be used to replace up to 75 percent of the fat in margarine, up to 96 percent of the fat in baked goods, and up to 100 percent of the fat in salad dressings. It cannot be used for fried foods. Because Stellar is made of modified corn starch, it did not require FDA clearance.

In August the FDA approved a new version of Simplesse, a fat substitute previously used only in frozen desserts. The new version, made from a whey protein found in milk, allows use of Simplesse in cheese spreads, butter, salad dressings, and baked goods. The older version, which was approved in 1990, is based on a protein found in eggs and cannot be used in cooking.

Slendid, a fat replacement made by Hercules, became available in September. It is made from pectin taken from citrus peels and did not require FDA approval. According to the maker, Slendid can replace up to 100 percent of the fat in a variety of processed food while adding virtually no calories. Suggested uses for Slendid include frozen desserts, dressings, soups, and baked goods. It cannot be used for frying.

Fat and Life Expectancy

What if Americans ate less fat? Researchers at the University of California at San Francisco asked that question and found that not much would change, at least in terms of average life expectancy. In a report published in June, the researchers calculated that if all Americans lowered their fat intake from 37 percent (the current average intake) to no more than 30 percent of their total calories, as recommended by federal agencies and health organizations, the change in diet would add only three to four months to average life expectancy. The study authors pointed out that since most deaths from fat-related diseases now occur in men over 60 and women over 70, these populations

would benefit the most from reductions in dietary fat. They also said that while the average increase in longevity would be only several months, for some individuals the increase could be as much as several years.

The report, which was widely publicized, dismayed many Americans struggling to cut down on fat intake. But critics rushed to the defense of a low-fat diet, reiterating that some individuals would benefit more than others from lowering their fat intake. For example, people with multiple risk factors for developing coronary heart disease might significantly slow down the progression of the disease by consuming a low-fat diet. Also, experts noted, the ultimate goal in eating a healthful diet is not necessarily to prolong life, but rather to improve the quality of life by preventing disease and enfeeblement. LINDA HIGGINS

OBSTETRICS AND GYNECOLOGY

Problems of Multiple Pregnancies • Estrogen and Heart Disease

Terminating Fetuses in a Multiple Pregnancy

Sometimes physicians advise the removal of one or more fetuses in a multiple pregnancy to improve the chances that the remaining fetuses will result in healthy births. This procedure is fraught with controversy: it carries inherent risks, and it raises moral and ethical questions. Yet, as the technology becomes more advanced and physicians gain familiarity with the procedure, it will become more readily available. A handful of institutions have developed techniques for the purpose, with mixed results.

It is very unusual for pregnancies to result in four or more fetuses unless fertility drugs were used to induce ovulation (release of eggs) or the eggs were fertilized in the laboratory before being placed in the uterus. These pregnancies are at a high risk for extremely premature delivery of the fetuses, jeopardizing their chances of survival after birth. In multifetal pregnancy reduction, as the procedure is called, one or more of the fetuses is terminated. This can be done under ultrasound guidance by extracting the fetus using a procedure called vacuum aspiration, or by means of an injection administered to the fetus through the mother's abdomen.

Multifetal pregnancy reduction can be carried out as early as seven or eight weeks into the pregnancy, though delaying it until a later stage would allow any fetuses that were destined to spontaneously miscarry to do so and might also allow detection of any fetal abnormalities. However, in the overwhelming majority of cases, no detailed genetic information about the fetuses is available. Consequently, it is not possible to select fetuses to be removed on the basis of abnormalities or gender. Decisions on which fetus to terminate are made on the basis of accessibility.

Potential complications of pregnancy reduction include bleeding, infection, and miscarriage of the entire pregnancy. There is also a risk of damaging the remaining fetuses, especially in cases of multiple pregnancies from one fertilized egg (such as produce identical twins), where there is no membrane separating the fetuses.

Tagging the Patients

These days we're all pretty used to having a plastic antitheft tag snipped off a piece of clothing before we take it home from the store. Soon, however, it may be just as routine to have a similar tag removed from a newborn baby before you take it home from the hospital.

Hospital security and safety experts have recently begun using electronic sensors on patients both large and small. These devices, just like the ones used in retail stores, set off an alarm when they pass a wired exit. They are especially useful on newborns. Between 1983 and 1990, 61 infants were kidnapped from U.S. hospitals, and while that number is minuscule compared to the approximately 30 million babies born in that period, new mothers welcome the sense of security that comes with their child's electronic bracelet. As one safety director put it, "We have never had a baby taken from this hospital. But mothers should not have to worry about whether their child is safe here."

Another application is with psychiatric and Alzheimer's patients, who may become disoriented, wander away, and put themselves at risk. At one Massachusetts nursing care center, where all the Alzheimer's patients now wear sensor bracelets, it once could take an hour to find a straying patient. Now, however, an alarm goes off immediately when a person leaves the ward. This leads, said the center's administrator, to "peace of mind" for both staff and families.

The ethical and moral issues raised by the possibility of terminating one or more fetuses are considerable, and both maternal and fetal interests need to be considered. It is unfortunate that the prospects for survival of four or more fetuses in a multiple pregnancy are so poor. In situations where the probability that all the fetuses would survive beyond delivery is very small, it may be argued that selective pregnancy termination may do more good than harm. These are complex matters that create very difficult decisions for the prospective parents.

Heart Benefits of Estrogen Therapy

The largest study of estrogen replacement therapy to date, published in the *New England Journal of Medicine* in September 1991, concluded that taking replacement estrogen after menopause (change of life) reduced by about half the risk of heart disease for postmenopausal women. Heart disease is the leading cause of death for women, especially after menopause, when their bodies stop producing estrogen naturally. (A postmenopausal woman's risk of dying from heart disease is estimated at 31 percent.) Estrogen, a female hormone, has been known for some time to protect against osteoporosis (thinning of the bones), thereby decreasing the risk of hip fracture and other serious or fatal injuries in elderly women. It has also been found effective in relieving menopausal symptoms such as hot flashes and vaginal dryness.

The new study, from Boston's Brigham and Women's Hospital, followed nearly 49,000 women who participated in the Nurses' Health Study for a period of ten years. The researchers found that women taking synthetic estrogen after menopause had just about half as many heart attacks or deaths from cardiovascular disease as those who did not take the hormone. Earlier studies had indicated a possible association between estrogen replacement therapy and increased risk of one form of cardiovascular disease, stroke. But the new study found no difference in the incidence of strokes between the women who took replacement estrogen and those who did not.

Estrogen replacement therapy had also been associated in some previous studies with a slight increase in the risk of breast cancer and a sixfold increase in the risk of endometrial cancer (cancer of the lining of the uterus). However, the links between the replacement therapy and the two cancers have come into question. It is generally held now that estrogen replacement in appropriate doses does not increase a woman's breast cancer risk. It is also believed that as estrogen is currently given in combination with the hormone progestin, rather than alone as used to be the case, the endometrial cancer risk is greatly reduced and may even be nullified.

ANDRÉS A. RAMOS, M.D.

281

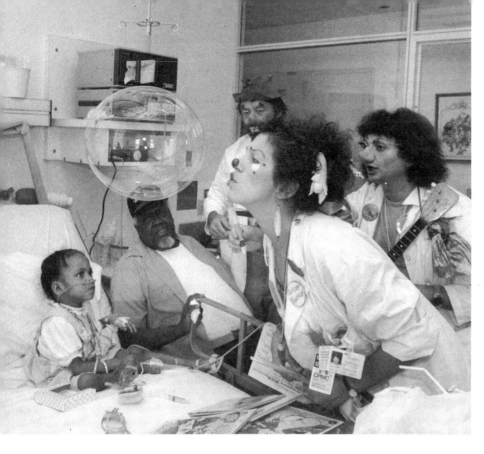

Merriment accompanies medicine when it's time for a visit from the Big Apple Circus's Clown Care Unit, a 30-member troupe that cheers up young patients in the pediatric wards of several New York City hospitals. The three clowns performing here are, left to right, Michael Christensen (also known as Dr. Stubs), Hilary Chaplain (Dr. Celery Trashcan), and Vladimir Olshansky (Dr. Bobo).

PEDIATRICS

New Drug Helps Premature Babies' Lungs • Transfusion Alternative for Anemic Infants • Hepatitis B Vaccine Recommended • How Poverty Affects Children's Health

Help for Premature Lungs

Three large studies published recently demonstrated that a substance called surfactant, when administered directly into the lungs of premature infants, reduced the number of deaths due to respiratory distress syndrome. This syndrome is the most common reason for death and disability among infants born prematurely. The immature lungs of such infants are not only very small, they also lack natural surfactant, which allows their tiny air pockets to reexpand easily once the air in them has been exhaled. Synthetically manufactured surfactant became available in 1990.

In one study, infants born weighing 700-1,100 grams (1.54-2.42 pounds) who did not receive surfactant were twice as likely to die before one year of age as patients who did. Another study demonstrated that when surfactant was given within 30 minutes of birth to premature infants born after 26 or fewer weeks of gestation, in anticipation of the development of lung problems, 75 percent survived; only 54 percent survived among infants who were not given surfactant

until they developed signs of respiratory problems. A third study in patients born weighing at least 1,250 grams (2.75 pounds) showed that two doses of surfactant reduced many of the other consequences of prematurity, as well as decreasing the likelihood of death due to respiratory disease.

Treating Anemia Without Transfusions

Another problem seen frequently in premature infants is anemia. They develop anemia partly because of the relatively large amounts of blood that must be drawn for the many laboratory tests done to assess their status, and partly because they do not produce adequate amounts of the hormone erythropoietin, which stimulates production of red blood cells. Recent research showed that treatment with genetically engineered erythropoietin provided a better solution to this type of anemia than blood transfusion. Premature infants given erythropoietin every other day for ten days had an increase in their red blood cell count equivalent to that in infants who received transfusions. Additionally, the infants who received erythropoietin maintained their level of red blood cells, while many of those who received transfusions developed signs of anemia again within two weeks.

Preventing Hepatitis B

With hepatitis B on the rise in the United States, the Advisory Committee on Immunization Practices recommended in early 1991 that universal immunization of all infants is the best way to halt the spread of the disease among all age groups. The committee, which functions under the auspices of the U.S. Department of Health and Human Services, said that two doses of vaccine should be given during the first 6 months of life and that a third should be administered between the ages of 6 and 18 months.

Hepatitis B is a viral infection transmitted through contact with blood and other secretions, but not through usual daily person-to-person contact. Most adults who become infected with hepatitis B develop an acute illness and then recover fully. Some adults (about 10 percent of those infected) develop chronic infection, with ongoing liver damage and a risk of developing cancer of the liver. For children under five, the risk of chronic infection is much higher, and for infants who are infected at the time of birth through contact with the blood and secretions of an infected mother, the risk of chronic infection and chronic liver disease may be as high as 90 percent. An effective vaccine against hepatitis B has been available since 1982.

In the past hepatitis B vaccine has been recommended only for selected individuals who could be expected to be exposed to hepatitis B virus through household contacts, life-style, or work-related activities. However, reported cases of hepatitis B in the United States increased by 37 percent from 1979 to 1989, with an estimated 200,000-300,000 newly infected individuals annually.

Vaccination programs similar to the one proposed by the Advisory Committee on Immunization Practices have been implemented among Alaskan natives, who have a high endemic rate of hepatitis B infection, and have resulted in a 99 percent decline in the incidence of infection.

Effects of Poverty

During the 1980s the number of children living in poverty in the United States increased, so that by 1990 approximately 20 percent of American children were poor. The effect of increasing poverty on the health of children was examined in several studies.

Water Intoxication Of Infants. In recent years physicians in the United States have noted an increase in the number of infants being admitted to hospitals because of water intoxication. Water intoxication results when a young infant's kidneys—which normally regulate the concentration of salt in the bloodstream and the level of fluid in the body—are overwhelmed by a sudden increase in the amount of water ingested. The resulting hyponatremia, or low sodium concentration, can result in convulsions, coma, and brain swelling. In healthy infants, hyponatremia resulting from water intoxication is normally extremely rare.

Physicians in St. Louis reported on 34 infants with water intoxication. All of the infants had previously been healthy. The most common reason given by their caretakers for giving the infants large amounts of water or very dilute infant formula was that they had exhausted, or nearly exhausted, their supply of formula and were trying to satisfy the infant's hunger as best they could.

Decline In Breast-feeding. A recent study of breast-feeding trends revealed that the number of mothers breast-feeding in the United States shrank in the late 1980s. Breast-feeding has been demonstrated to have significant nutritional and immunological advantages for infants, as well as emotional and psychological benefits for both mother and infant. Awareness of the advantages of breast-feeding led to a

The most common cause of death and disability of premature babies is immaturity of the lungs. Recent studies, however, have shown that treating the lungs with a substance called surfactant can greatly improve the infants' chances. Shown here, a premature baby who weighed 2 pounds at birth.

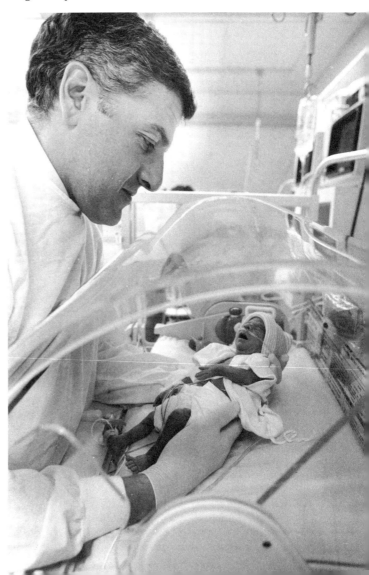

marked increase in the number of new mothers choosing to breast-feed during the years 1965-1982. The percentage of mothers who initiated breast-feeding during the years 1984-1989, however, declined by 13 percent (from 59.7 percent to 52.2 percent), and the percentage of mothers still breast-feeding when their infant was six months old declined by 24 percent (from 23.8 percent to 18.1 percent).

Though the decline was seen in all groups studied, it was more pronounced among women who were younger, less educated, black, working outside the home, or receiving infant formula from the Women, Infants, and Children supplemental food program, or who had given birth to an infant of low birthweight.

Measles Epidemic Update

U.S. physicians continued to see a disturbingly high number of measles cases in 1991, although the number of reported cases, more than 9,200, was considerably lower than in 1990, when more than 27,000 cases were reported. Physicians also reported seeing, some for the first time, serious complications of measles, including croup and life-threatening secondary bacterial infection of the trachea. Measles is easily preventable with proper immunization.

The ongoing measles epidemic has been called one of the most visible consequences of declining access to preventive health care for a large proportion of American children. Although approximately 90 percent of U.S. children have received a full series of immunizations—including vaccines to protect against infection due to tetanus, diphtheria, whooping cough (pertussis), polio, measles, mumps, and rubella (German measles)—by the time they reach school age, as many as 50 percent of the children in some American cities are now inadequately immunized at two years of age. Outbreaks of measles, which was thought to be nearly eradicated in the early 1980s, began to occur in increasing numbers in the late 1980s and are now commonplace again.

Long-term Effects of Iron Deficiency

Researchers reported in 1991 that iron deficiency in infancy can have long-lasting effects on mental and motor development. A group of Costa Rican children, who had been found to have iron deficiency anemia as infants and had been given adequate iron supplementation to correct the condition, were studied again at five years of age. All were found to be in excellent physical health and to have no evidence of iron deficiency at the time they were studied. Compared to children who had never been iron deficient, however, they had lower scores on tests of mental and motor functioning. Socioeconomic differences could not explain the disparity between the groups.

This study points up one of the advantages of breast-feeding during early infancy: iron absorption from breast milk is significantly more efficient than from infant formula. The amount of readily absorbable iron is frequently inadequate in the diets of infants and young children, particularly when intake of cow's milk is excessive. At least 20 to 25 percent of children in the world are iron deficient. Iron is necessary to prevent anemia, but iron deficiency results in behavior problems and poor learning, even if it is not severe enough to produce anemia.

JULIA A. McMILLAN, M.D.

PUBLIC HEALTH

Rise in Heterosexual AIDS Cases • Heavy Demand Depletes Flu Vaccine • New Lead Poisoning Standards Set • Resurgence in Tuberculosis • FDA Plans Faster Drug Availability

AIDS

The AIDS epidemic was well into its second decade when basketball star Earvin (Magic) Johnson disclosed in November that he was infected with the human immunodeficiency virus (HIV) that causes AIDS. For many Americans his announcement drove home the message that heterosexuals can get the disease, a fatal infection that slowly destroys the body's immune system. According to the U.S. Centers for Disease Control (CDC), the number of Americans requesting tests for HIV skyrocketed during the month after Johnson's announcement—in some cities to as much as ten times the normal number. AIDS is spread mainly through sexual intercourse, through shared hypodermic needles that are used to inject illegal drugs, and from infected mothers to their newborn babies.

Since 1990 heterosexuals have accounted for a rising proportion of new AIDS cases in the United States. Nevertheless, the disease is still transmitted primarily among homosexual men, and heterosexual transmission was responsible for only 6 percent of the total number of cases reported by the end of 1991.

As of January 31, 1992, the number of AIDS cases reported in the United States stood at 209,693, with a death toll of 135,434. Some 1 million Americans were believed to be infected with HIV. In Canada, 5,647 cases of AIDS and 3,432 deaths due to AIDS had been reported by January 1, 1992. Worldwide, more than 446,000 AIDS cases were reported in 162 countries, and an additional 11 million adults were believed to

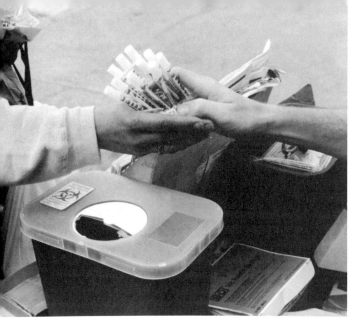

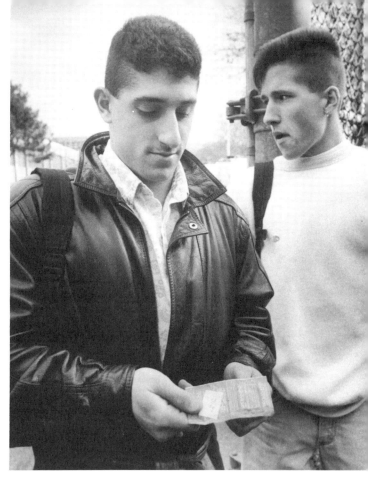

In order to check the spread of AIDS, public health officials have begun reaching out to vulnerable populations. Needle exchange programs, such as one in New Haven, Conn. (above), are targeted at intravenous drug users, and in New York City, some high schools have begun to distribute free packs of condoms. These students at John Dewey High School in Brooklyn (right) were among the first recipients.

be infected. Although the rate of increase in the spread of infection appeared to be slowing in the United States, the infection rate continued to increase in developing countries, especially in sub-Saharan Africa, South America, and the Caribbean.

The count of AIDS cases in the United States is expected to jump when the CDC's expanded definition of AIDS goes into effect. In August the CDC said that as of 1992, people will be considered to have AIDS if they are HIV-infected and have fewer than 200 CD4 cells per cubic millimeter of blood. (CD4 cells are white blood cells important in the immune system; the AIDS virus destroys them.) The previous definition of AIDS included only HIV-infected people who also had one or more of a variety of infections and cancers. The new definition means that many infected people will be counted earlier.

In September the National Commission on AIDS, a panel appointed by U.S. President George Bush and Congress to help establish national policy, issued a report saying that some progress against the disease had been made but that Bush and other federal officials had failed to provide either leadership or adequate funding for prevention efforts and treatment. The commission recommended that insurance coverage for medical costs be provided for everyone, that laws banning needle-exchange programs be eliminated, and that treatment for drug abuse should be made available to any who need it.

Prevention. The sharing of contaminated needles (and the syringes, water, and cotton balls used with them) by intravenous drug users is the main way the AIDS virus is transmitted in many U.S. cities. In several cities programs in which drug users may exchange used needles for clean ones have been reported to slow the spread of disease. Yale University researchers reported in July that such a program in New Haven, Conn., had reduced new HIV infections by one-third. Critics said that the programs encourage drug abuse.

In the fall, as part of an AIDS education and prevention effort, teachers at some New York City high schools began distributing condoms, which slow the spread of AIDS through sexual intercourse. The school system became the first in the United States to make condoms widely available to teenagers. Some parents, religious leaders, and members of the city's board of education protested the action.

Efforts to develop an AIDS vaccine continued. By the end of 1991, 11 experimental vaccines had been injected into some 600 uninfected human volunteers from low-risk populations to test the vaccines' safety and ability to provoke an immune response. None had yet been tested for the ability to protect against infection. In late 1991, World Health Organization officials drew up plans to begin such testing in Brazil, Rwanda, Thailand, and Uganda by 1993, bypassing the usual animal trials. U.S. and Thai Army officials studied the feasibility of vaccine trials among army recruits and civilians in Thailand. The CDC also explored the possibility of vaccine trials among high-risk Americans.

Treatment. In 1991 the U.S. Food and Drug Administration (FDA) approved three drugs for AIDS or AIDS-related conditions, bringing the total number of drugs for AIDS patients to nine. The newly approved drugs are:

• Dideoxyinosine (DDI) (brand name, Videx), an antiviral agent approved for use by AIDS patients who cannot tolerate or do not respond to zidovudine (formerly called AZT), the only other drug approved for treatment of AIDS. Like zidovudine, DDI slows replication of the AIDS virus and slows the decline of the immune system, but it does not cure AIDS. The drug was simultaneously approved in Canada by the Health Protection Branch of the Canadian Department of Health and Welfare.

• Foscarnet (brand name, Foscavir), a drug that delays progression of cytomegalovirus (CMV) retinitis, a sight-threatening condition that afflicts about 20 percent of AIDS patients. Many people cannot tolerate the side effects of the only other drug available for treating CMV retinitis in AIDS patients, ganciclovir. Moreover, study findings showed that foscarnet is more effective than ganciclovir and allows people with AIDS to live longer.

• Erythropoietin (brand name, Procrit), a genetically engineered version of a kidney hormone that stimulates the bone marrow to make red blood cells. A deficiency of red blood cells (anemia) is often caused by zidovudine and drugs that are taken for AIDS-related infections and cancers.

The FDA also authorized wider use of an experimental antiparasitic drug known as 566 for treatment of *Pneumocystis carinii* pneumonia (PCP) in people with AIDS who cannot tolerate the side effects of standard drug therapy. PCP, a potentially fatal infection, affects more than 80 percent of people with AIDS.

Healthcare Workers With AIDS. In December the CDC dropped a plan to publish a list of procedures that it considered too risky for HIV-infected healthcare workers to perform because of the risk of transmitting the virus to patients. Instead, the agency proposed putting more emphasis on identifying infected health workers who do not meet standards of infection control or whose stamina or mental state makes them unfit to practice. The CDC first called for a list of risky procedures in July, saying that healthcare workers who do certain "exposure-prone" surgical procedures should voluntarily be tested for HIV and hepatitis B. The agency also said that those infected with HIV should stop doing operations and invasive procedures unless they get permission from

local panels of health professionals and then tell patients they are infected. The CDC asked professionals groups to define procedures that posed the highest risks. But medical and dental groups—except the American Medical Association—refused to develop any lists, saying there was no significant risk of infecting patients and that guidelines would cause unnecessary alarm. According to the CDC, 6,000 healthcare workers have AIDS and perhaps 50,000 may be infected with HIV.

Concern about AIDS transmission from healthcare workers to patients was piqued by a highly publicized appeal for mandatory testing from 23-year-old Kimberly Bergalis, who was infected with the AIDS virus by her dentist. Bergalis died in December. The dentist, Dr. David Acer of Florida, was the only healthcare worker known to have infected patients. Five of his patients were found to be infected with the same strain of AIDS as killed him in 1990. CDC officials could not explain how the transmission had occurred but suspected that Acer may have used improperly cleaned instruments that were contaminated with blood from infected patients.

Cholesterol Screening

Because of strong evidence that coronary heart disease and high blood cholesterol run in families, the National Cholesterol Education Program in April recommended that certain children be tested for high cholesterol. Cholesterol, a fatty substance in the blood, contributes to clogging of the arteries, increasing the chances of getting heart disease.

According to the new guidelines, children should be tested if their parents or grandparents had heart attacks, atherosclerosis (clogging of the arteries with fat), or other cardiovascular disease at or before age 55 or if a parent has a cholesterol level over 240 milligrams per deciliter. The new recommendations could apply to as many as a quarter of American children. Most children found to have high cholesterol could be treated through low-fat, low-cholesterol diets, but some of them might also require drug treatment. According to earlier guidelines issued by the National Cholesterol Education Program, all adults over 19 should have their cholesterol levels measured.

Flu Vaccine Shortage

An unusually early start to the influenza season, along with predictions of severe outbreaks, created one of the heaviest demands ever for flu vaccine in the United States. By late November leading distributors and all four manufacturers of flu vaccine said they had run out of stock. Of 25 immunization programs surveyed by the CDC in early December, 17 needed more vaccine. The shortage was eased somewhat when one manufacturer was able to prepare some 500,000 additional doses. Flu vaccine is generally produced in a one-time process because it takes a month to make. New flu vaccine is made each year after experts predict which viral strains will predominate in the coming flu season. It is distributed in September. For the 1991-1992 flu season, vaccine manufacturers originally produced and distributed 32 million doses of vaccine—more than in previous years, the CDC said.

Federal health officials encourage vaccination for healthcare workers, for people aged 65 and older, and for anyone with a chronic lung or heart condition because they are especially susceptible to bacterial pneumonia and other serious complications of the flu that can lead to hospitalization and death. However, anyone over 6 months can get a flu vaccine to lessen the respiratory symptoms of flu.

By the end of December there were no reports of unusual rates of infection or flu-related deaths. Flu outbreaks had occurred in 28 states and involved mostly schoolchildren. More than twice as many patient visits as normal for flu-like illnesses were reported from the mid-Atlantic region (New York, New Jersey, and Pennsylvania) and the West South Central region (Louisiana, Texas, Arkansas, and Oklahoma).

Lead Poisoning

In 1991 federal health officials expressed a growing awareness of the hazards of lead at blood levels well below what was previously thought to be dangerous. Exposure to lead has been linked to kidney disease, nervous system damage, and hypertension in adults and to intelligence deficits and learning abilities in developing infants and children, who are particularly sensitive to lead. Young children are typically exposed to lead by eating chips of lead paint or breathing in dust from the paint.

In February the Department of Health and Human Services introduced a 20-year plan for eliminating childhood lead poisoning that would require removing lead paint from homes, installing new water pipes if old ones contain lead solder, and carrying away contaminated dirt from yards. The CDC in October lowered the threshold at which children are considered to have lead poisoning, from 25 to 10 micrograms per deciliter of blood. Under the agency's new guidelines, children under six should get an annual blood test to measure lead levels. A level over 10 micrograms per deciliter among several children within a specific area should act as a warning flag that a community may have a problem. For children with lead levels over 15 micrograms per deciliter, efforts should be made to identify and get rid of sources of lead exposure. Children with lead levels over 20 should be evaluated and

treated by a doctor, and those with levels over 45 should undergo a procedure for removing excess lead from the body. Seventeen percent of American children under the age of six are estimated to have lead levels higher than 15. The Bush administration, however, budgeted only half the amount requested for a testing program in 1992 and a fraction of the amount required for subsidized lead removal in homes.

Researchers reported in early 1991 that alcohol and some other liquids (especially those with a high acid content, such as fruit juice or vinegar) may leach lead from crystal decanters and other crystal containers. Crystal glassware may begin releasing lead within minutes of coming into contact with food or beverages, and eventually the amount of lead can rise to potentially dangerous levels. The FDA advised the public that pregnant women, infants, and children should not use crystal glassware and that foods or beverages should not be stored in crystal.

In September the FDA and the Bureau of Alcohol, Tobacco, and Firearms announced that use of lead foil caps on wine bottles would be banned and a limit set on lead in table wine. The action came two months after the federal government released findings showing that many wines sold in the United States contain lead in quantities up to three times the amount allowed for drinking water—currently 50 parts per billion. Much of the problem was attributed to residues on the rims of bottles capped by lead foil, which is used to protect the corks from being chewed by rodents in wine cellars. The FDA said table wines that contain lead levels above 300 parts per billion could be harmful to consumers. (Only 3 to 4 percent of table wines tested contained more than 300 ppb of lead.) In December most California wineries agreed to abandon the practice of capping wine bottles with lead foil by January 1, 1992.

The FDA also set lower limits for lead in ceramic dishware used to hold food. The agency advised consumers to avoid storing acidic foods such as fruit juices, wine, and vinegar in ceramic containers for long periods.

Smoking

The CDC estimated that about 28 percent of Americans smoked in 1988 (the latest year for which statistics are available), down from 29 percent in 1987 and 40 percent in 1964, when the U.S. Surgeon General first issued a warning against smoking. Smoking rates were highest among people who were separated or divorced and among less-educated Americans. The CDC also said that smokers are beginning the habit younger. Smokers born in the 1950s started smoking at age 17, compared with 18 for smokers born in the 1930s and 20 for smokers born from 1910 to 1919.

287

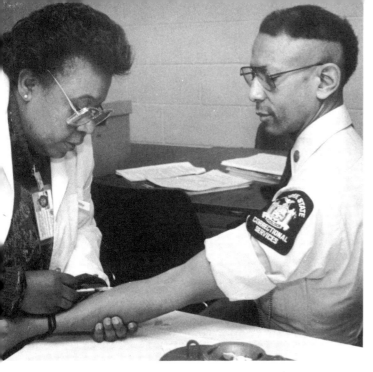

Tuberculosis, a disease once thought to be vanishing in the United States, instead was seen to be making a comeback, and one area in which its resurgence was most noticeable was in prisons. Here, an employee in a New York City correctional facility is tested for the disease.

Despite the declining smoking rate, the death toll worsened, reflecting the widespread habit of smoking during the 1950s and 1960s. In 1988 more than 430,000 Americans died from smoking, up 11 percent from the 390,000 deaths attributed to smoking in a 1985 study. Lung cancer deaths accounted for more than 110,000 of the total, other cancer deaths some 30,000, cardiovascular diseases for about 200,000, respiratory diseases like bronchitis and emphysema for over 80,000, and miscellaneous smoking-related problems for the rest. According to a draft report sponsored by the Environmental Protection Agency and other federal agencies, secondhand cigarette smoke kills 53,000 nonsmokers annually, including 37,000 from heart disease.

In July the National Institute for Occupational Safety and Health recommended that employers ban smoking in the workplace, offer classes to help workers stop smoking and offer incentives to encourage them to stop. The recommendations were submitted for consideration to the Occupational Safety and Health Administration, which is responsible for setting health rules in the workplace.

Tuberculosis

A resurgence of tuberculosis in the United States led a national panel of experts to conclude in December that Americans were not being adequately protected against the disease and infected patients were not being treated effectively. From 1989 to 1990 the num-

ber of tuberculosis cases increased 9.4 percent, to 25,701 cases. For 1991, a preliminary count showed that more than 23,500 cases had been reported. In November, New York City health officials said tuberculosis was out of control in their city. New York City's tuberculosis rate of 44.6 per 100,000 was five times as great as the national rate. Most of the cases occurred in people infected with the AIDS virus, who are susceptible to a variety of infections because of impaired immune systems. Tuberculosis in people who are infected with HIV is difficult to diagnose using standard tests.

Contributing to the seriousness of the outbreaks was the rising incidence of drug-resistant strains of tuberculosis, which are difficult to treat and often fatal. One in five cases in New York City was drug-resistant. Among several outbreaks reported in the United States during 1991, one of the worst was an outbreak of drug-resistant tuberculosis in New York prisons that left 13 inmates and 1 guard dead. Tuberculosis is caused by a type of bacterium. It primarily attacks the lungs but can also affect other parts of the body. It is most commonly transmitted from one person to another when a patient with tuberculosis of the lungs coughs the bacteria into the air to be inhaled by someone else. Tuberculosis spreads easily in crowded settings like prisons as well as shelters for the homeless. Many public health experts called for aggressive diagnosis and treatment efforts to control tuberculosis, particularly among people who are infected with the AIDS virus.

Speeding Drug Approvals

The FDA announced in November a plan to reform the drug approval process that would almost halve the time it takes—currently about ten years—to move important new drugs from laboratory to pharmacy. Priority would be given to drugs for incurable or life-threatening diseases like AIDS and cancer. The time savings would be accomplished in part by considering during the approval process the results of studies done in foreign countries as well as in the United States, contracting with outside experts to review drug applications for routine drugs like antibiotics and painkillers, and using private review boards to evaluate animal studies in order to relieve FDA staff of some of the burden. In addition, a formal program for harmonizing drug testing and approval criteria among the United States, the European Community, and Japan began to take shape in November.

Although Americans in general greeted the plan enthusiastically, Senator Edward Kennedy (D, Mass.) and Representatives John Dingell (D, Mich.) and Henry Waxman (D, Calif.) expressed concern that reliance on outside parties' evaluations might weaken the agency and lower its standards for drug approval. They asked the FDA to hold off implementing certain recommendations in the plan until Congress evaluated them.

The FDA had already taken a fast track approach to bring the AIDS drug DDI to the market. Because the need for the drug was so great, the FDA approved it before the completion of long-term safety and efficacy tests, on the grounds that patients in clinical trials had shown improvement. LINDA HIGGINS

TEETH AND GUMS

Water Fluoridation Defended • Safety of Fillings Affirmed • A Drug to Reduce Dental Anxiety • Teen Gum Disease

Safety of Fluoridation

The addition of small amounts of sodium fluoride to U.S. public water supplies to protect against tooth decay has over the years been branded by critics as everything from a Communist conspiracy to a mass poisoning operation. In 1991 fluoridation received scientific defense against its most substantive challenge to date.

The issue this time was safety. In half a century of large-scale water fluoridation, hundreds of studies have attested to fluoride's safety and effectiveness. However, a 1990 study conducted by the U.S. Public Health Service's National Toxicology Program, detected a rare form of bone cancer called osteosarcoma in four of 180 male rats given high levels of sodium fluoride in water. Although sodium fluoride was not found to cause cancer in female rats, or mice of either sex, that were studied, the Public Health Service established a special panel of scientists to review fluoride's benefits and risks.

The group's extensive final report, released in February 1991, showed no evidence of any cancer risk to humans in areas where the water had been fluoridated to a level of about one part per million. (This is the level generally considered optimal, since it is high enough to combat tooth decay but is low enough to pose little risk of causing the mottling of tooth enamel known as dental fluorosis.) The report also found no association between fluoride exposure and birth defects or digestive, genital, urinary, or respiratory problems.

There is evidence, however, that dental fluorosis has increased, both in communities with fluoridated water and those with nonfluoridated. The most likely reason for this is rising exposure to fluoride in dental products, mainly toothpastes. Dental fluorosis results

from an interaction between excess fluoride and the cells that form enamel as the teeth develop. Fluoride has no such effect after teeth come in, since the enamel-forming cells disappear when the tooth crowns are fully formed. Fluorosis can be reduced to a minimum by making sure that young children use only small (pea-sized) amounts of toothpaste, avoid swallowing toothpaste, and rinse thoroughly after they have finished brushing.

Fluoridated and nonfluoridated communities do not differ in their tooth decay rates as much as in the past, because of the availability of fluoride sources other than water. Nevertheless, the benefits of water fluoridation are still clearly evident. They apply to individuals of all ages and socioeconomic groups, but especially to poor children.

Safety of Dental Fillings

Also under challenge recently was dental amalgam, the mix of metal filings (mainly silver) and mercury that has been the major material used in tooth fillings for more than a century. A number of ills, from kidney disease to multiple sclerosis, have been blamed on amalgams because they release tiny but measurable levels of mercury vapor during chewing.

Alternatives to amalgam as filling materials either are more expensive (such as gold and porcelain inlays) or have a limited track record (in the case of tooth-colored composites). Accordingly, the Public Health Service set up a committee to review amalgam's benefits and risks, with a report expected in 1992. Meanwhile, expert panels established by the U.S. Food and Drug Administration and the National Institute of Dental Research examined many of the studies that had been done on dental amalgam. The FDA's Dental Devices Advisory Panel concluded "that none of the data presented show a direct hazard to humans from dental amalgam."

The National Institute of Dental Research panel reviewed all materials currently used in restoring decayed teeth, including, in addition to silver amalgam, plastic composites, ceramics, "glass ionomer" cements, and metal alloys. The general conclusion was that "although mercury vapor is released from dental amalgam, the quantities released are very small and do not cause verifiable adverse effects on human beings." The panel said that there was no evidence that any currently used restorative material caused significant side effects.

Medication for Dental Anxiety

Certain antianxiety drugs might help reduce some patients' fear of dental procedures, according to a recent study. Fear of dental treatment, known as dental phobia, keeps many people from seeking badly needed

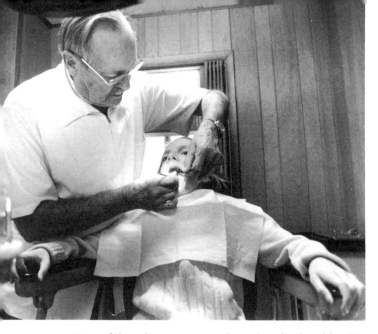

Fear of dental treatment, such as that displayed by this tense young patient, keeps many people from getting essential dental care. A new study, however, has found that the use of beta blockers—drugs commonly used to treat hypertension and irregular heart beat—can reduce anxiety in dental patients.

care. The problem can often be overcome through behavioral techniques for "retraining" the phobic patient, but these require a series of office visits. An effective anxiety-reducing medication could provide a shortcut.

The study, which was of a preliminary nature, involved a type of medication known as a beta blocker. Beta blockers are widely used for treating hypertension and abnormal heart rhythms, but they have also been prescribed for short-term use to counter acute anxiety in situations such as public speaking, artistic and athletic performances, and examinations. The study compared a beta blocker and a placebo (inactive substance) in a dental office situation where a local anesthetic was injected, a rubber dam (a protective rubber sheet) was positioned in the mouth, and a tooth was worked on with a high-speed drill. Patients who received the beta blocker reported less anxiety, perceived the pain as less intense, and felt less aversion to treatment.

Gum Disease in Teenagers

As part of a national survey of children's oral health, 11,000 adolescents between the ages of 14 and 17 were examined for two forms of severe gum disease: localized juvenile periodontitis (LJP), which affects lower front teeth and first molars, and generalized juvenile periodontitis (GJP), which can affect any of the teeth. In general, as expected based on previous studies, juvenile periodontitis was found to be relatively rare among U.S. teenagers. However, when the results are projected to the total U.S. population of ages 14 to 17,

the numbers are substantial: an estimated 70,000 cases of LJP and 17,000 cases of GJP.

These forms of gum disease affect different groups to different extents. The survey found that black teens were 15 times more likely to have LJP and 25 times more likely to have GJP than whites. Black males were three times as likely to have LJP as black females, but white females were at greater risk than white males.

Juvenile periodontitis first occurs around puberty and can have a very destructive effect on the soft tissues and bone supporting the teeth. With early detection and proper treatment, the teeth can be saved.

Preventing Decay and Gum Disease

New results from a study in Sweden confirmed that a program of regular hygiene can be of long-lasting value in preventing tooth decay and gum, or periodontal, disease in adults. The program involved oral hygiene to control plaque, a bacterial coating that builds up on teeth and along the gum line; daily use of a fluoridated toothpaste; and regularly repeated professional tooth cleaning.

Previous reports, after three and six years, had noted that the program had virtually prevented the progression of tooth decay and gum disease. The new results covered 15 years of continuous participation in the study. As in the past, most patients showed minimal loss of periodontal tissue support—that is, there was no progression of gum disease—and a continued low level of tooth decay.

Transmission of Decay-producing Bacteria

A recent study suggested that it might be possible to reduce tooth decay in some young children by treating their mothers. The bacteria known as *Streptococcus mutans* are generally considered to be the microorganisms most responsible for the initiation of tooth decay. Certain types of these bacteria are transmitted from mother to child and establish residence in the mouth sometime after the baby, or primary, teeth have begun to appear ("teething"). The study found that 75 percent of children infected with *S. mutans* from their mothers acquired the bacteria when they were between 19 and 28 months old. The rest were infected by 33 months. None of the uninfected children in the study developed tooth decay, whereas 29 percent of those infected did. The existence of such a well-defined "window of infectivity" suggests that treating mothers during this period with suitable antibacterial drugs might reduce the opportunity for bacteria transmission and thus prevent decay in their offspring.   IRWIN D. MANDEL, D.D.S.

FOR YOUR HEALTH

EATING RIGHT

LOW-FAT FOOD

Most nutrition experts recommend that no more than 30 percent of calories should come from total fat, no more than 10 percent from saturated fat. The following recipes all meet these 30/10 guidelines.

Main Course Dishes

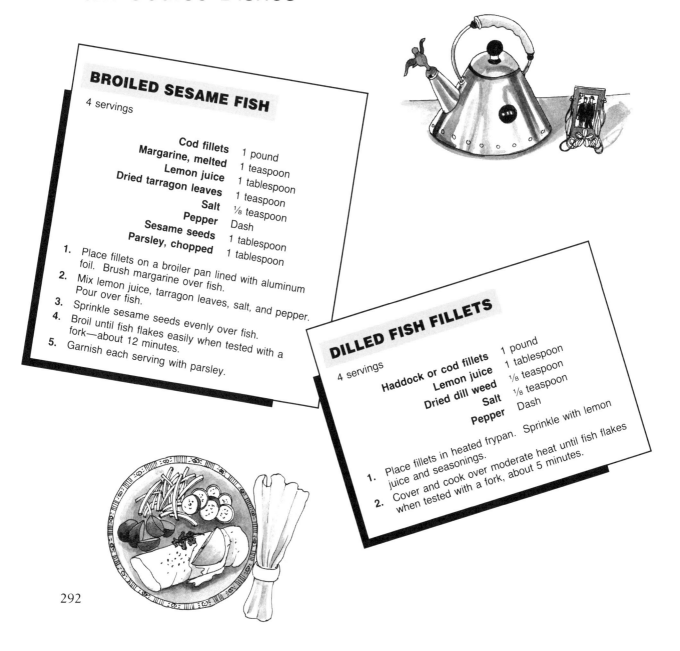

BROILED SESAME FISH

4 servings

Cod fillets	1 pound
Margarine, melted	1 teaspoon
Lemon juice	1 tablespoon
Dried tarragon leaves	1 teaspoon
Salt	⅛ teaspoon
Pepper	Dash
Sesame seeds	1 tablespoon
Parsley, chopped	1 tablespoon

1. Place fillets on a broiler pan lined with aluminum foil. Brush margarine over fish.
2. Mix lemon juice, tarragon leaves, salt, and pepper. Pour over fish.
3. Sprinkle sesame seeds evenly over fish.
4. Broil until fish flakes easily when tested with a fork—about 12 minutes.
5. Garnish each serving with parsley.

DILLED FISH FILLETS

4 servings

Haddock or cod fillets	1 pound
Lemon juice	1 tablespoon
Dried dill weed	⅛ teaspoon
Salt	⅛ teaspoon
Pepper	Dash

1. Place fillets in heated frypan. Sprinkle with lemon juice and seasonings.
2. Cover and cook over moderate heat until fish flakes when tested with a fork, about 5 minutes.

CHICKEN ITALIANO

4 servings, 1 chicken breast half and ¾ cup spaghetti mixture each

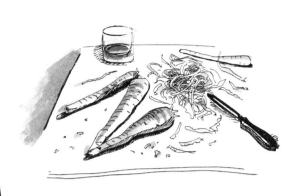

Chicken breast halves, skinned, boned	4
Oil	1 teaspoon
Thin spaghetti, broken into fourths	1½ cups dry
Onion, cut in wedges	1 small
Green pepper, cut in strips	1 small
Instant minced garlic	⅛ teaspoon
Oregano leaves	1 teaspoon
Salt	⅛ teaspoon
Pepper	⅛ teaspoon
Bay leaf	1
Tomatoes	16-ounce can
Water	¼ cup
Parsley, chopped	1 tablespoon, if desired

1. Pound chicken breasts with a metal meat mallet between sheets of plastic wrap until about ½-inch thick.
2. Heat oil in frypan. Brown chicken breasts on each side.
3. Add spaghetti, onion, and pepper strips around chicken. Sprinkle with seasonings.
4. Break up large pieces of tomatoes. Pour tomatoes and water over top of chicken.
5. Bring to boiling point. Reduce heat, cover, and cook until chicken and spaghetti are done, about 15 minutes.
6. Remove bay leaf. Garnish with parsley.

BEEF AND VEGETABLE STIRFRY

4 servings, about ¾ cup each

Beef round steak, boneless	¾ pound
Oil	1 teaspoon
Carrots, sliced	½ cup
Celery, sliced	½ cup
Onion, sliced	½ cup
Soy sauce	1 tablespoon
Garlic powder	⅛ teaspoon
Pepper	Dash
Zucchini squash, cut in thin strips	2 cups
Cornstarch	1 tablespoon
Water	¼ cup

1. Trim all fat from steak. Slice steak across the grain into thin strips about ⅛-inch wide and 3 inches long. (Partially frozen meat is easier to slice.)
2. Heat oil in frypan. Add beef strips and stirfry over high heat, turning pieces constantly, until beef is no longer red—about 3 to 5 minutes. Reduce heat.
3. Add carrots, celery, onion, and seasonings. Cover and cook until carrots are slightly tender—3 to 4 minutes.
4. Add squash; cook until vegetables are tender-crisp—3 to 4 minutes.
5. Mix cornstarch and water until smooth. Add slowly to beef mixture, stirring constantly.
6. Cook until thickened and vegetables are coated with a thin glaze.

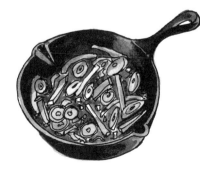

293

Recipes courtesy of the U.S. Department of Agriculture.

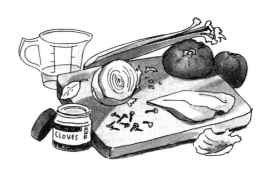

CHICKEN STEW

4 servings, about 1 cup each

Chicken breast halves, without skin	2
Water	1½ cups
Salt	¼ teaspoon
Whole cloves	2
Bay leaf	1
Frozen mixed vegetables	⅔ cup
Potatoes, pared, diced	⅔ cup
Onion, chopped	½ cup
Celery, sliced	¼ cup
Tomatoes	1 cup (½ 16-ounce can)
Ground thyme	¼ teaspoon
Pepper	⅛ teaspoon
Flour	¼ cup
Water	¼ cup

1. Cover and cook chicken in water with salt, cloves, and bay leaf until tender—about 45 minutes.

2. Remove chicken from broth. Separate meat from bones. Dice meat.

3. Skim fat from broth. Discard cloves and bay leaf. Add water to make 2 cups. Cook mixed vegetables, potatoes, onion, and celery in broth for 10 minutes.

4. Break up tomatoes; add tomatoes, thyme, and pepper to broth mixture. Cook slowly for 15 minutes. Add chicken.

5. Mix flour and water until smooth. Stir into chicken mixture. Cook, stirring constantly, until thickened—about 1 minute.

ENCHILADA CASSEROLE

4 pieces, 4 by 4 inches each

Filling	
Onion, chopped	½ cup
Green pepper, chopped	½ cup
Celery, chopped	¼ cup
Water, boiling	¼ cup
Chicken, cooked, diced	1 cup
Canned pinto beans, drained	1 cup
Tomato puree	½ cup
Corn tortillas	8

Sauce	
Tomato puree	1½ cups
Water	¾ cup
Chili powder	1 tablespoon
Ground cumin	⅛ teaspoon
Garlic powder	⅛ teaspoon
Salt	⅛ teaspoon

Topping	
Monterey Jack cheese, shredded	¼ cup

1. Preheat oven to 350°F (moderate)

2. Cook onion, green pepper, and celery in boiling water until tender. Drain liquid if necessary.

3. Add chicken, beans, and ½ cup of tomato puree. Mix gently.

4. Mix all sauce ingredients together thoroughly.

5. In an 8x8x2 inch baking pan, place four tortillas, one-half of the filling mixture, and one-fourth of the sauce. Add remaining filling mixture and another one-fourth of the sauce. Cover with four tortillas and remaining sauce.

6. Sprinkle cheese over top.

7. Bake until cheese is melted and sauce is bubbly—about 30 minutes.

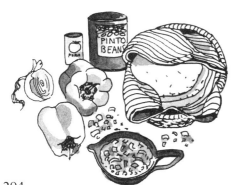

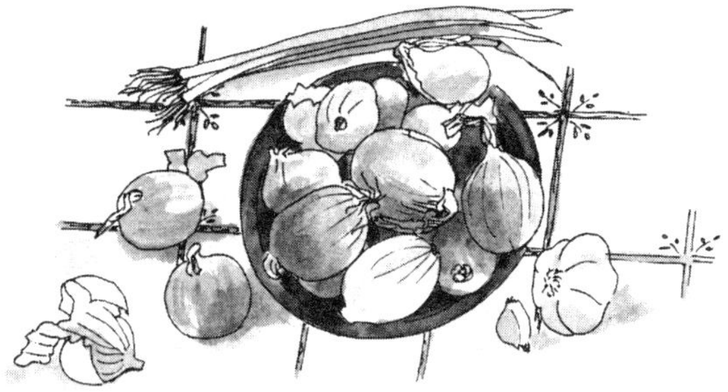

RICE-PASTA PILAF

4 servings, about ½ cup each

Uncooked brown rice	⅓ cup
Chicken broth, unsalted	1½ cups
Thin spaghetti, broken into 1/2- to 1-inch pieces	1/3 cup dry
Margarine	2 teaspoons
Green onions, chopped	2 tablespoons
Green peppers, chopped	2 tablespoons
Fresh mushrooms, chopped	2 tablespoons
Garlic, minced	½ clove
Savory	½ teaspoon
Salt	¼ teaspoon
Pepper	⅛ teaspoon
Slivered almonds, toasted (see Note)	1 tablespoon

1. Cook rice in 1 cup of the broth in a covered sauce-pan until almost tender—about 35 minutes.
2. Cook spaghetti in margarine over low heat until golden brown—about 2 minutes. Stir frequently; watch carefully.
3. Add browned spaghetti, vegetables, remaining ½ cup of chicken broth, and seasonings to rice.
4. Bring to boil, reduce heat, cover, and cook over medium heat until liquid is absorbed—about 10 minutes.
5. Remove from heat; let stand 2 minutes.
6. Garnish with almonds.

Note: Toast almonds in 350°F (moderate) oven until lightly browned—5 to 12 minutes. Or, toast in heavy pan over medium heat for 10 to 15 minutes, stirring fre-quently.

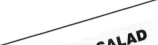

TUNA PASTA SALAD

4 servings, about 1 cup each

Elbow macaroni, uncooked	¾ cup
Tuna, water-pack, drained	6½-ounce can
Celery, thinly sliced	½ cup
Seedless red grapes, halved	1 cup
Salad dressing, mayonnaise type, reduced calorie	3 tablespoons

1. Cook macaroni according to package directions, omitting salt. Drain
2. Toss macaroni, tuna, celery, and grapes together.
3. Mix in salad dressing.
4. Serve warm, or chill until served.

PORK-SWEET POTATO SKILLET

4 servings, 1 chop and about ¾ cup vegetables each

Thin-cut pork chops	4 (about 1 pound)
Apple juice	1 cup
Onion, cut in ¼-inch slices	1 medium
Flour	1 tablespoon
Ground allspice	⅛ teaspoon
Salt	⅛ teaspoon
Sweet potatoes, vacuum packed	17-ounce can

1. Trim fat from chops. Brown on both sides in hot frypan. Add ¾ cup of the apple juice. Top with onion slices. Cover and cook 5 minutes at reduced heat.
2. Mix flour and seasonings. Stir into remaining ¼ cup apple juice. Stir into liquid in pan.
3. Arrange sweet potatoes around and over chops. Spoon sauce over potatoes.
4. Cover and cook about 10 minutes longer, until po-tatoes are hot and chops are done.

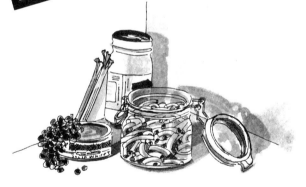

Snacks and Sandwiches

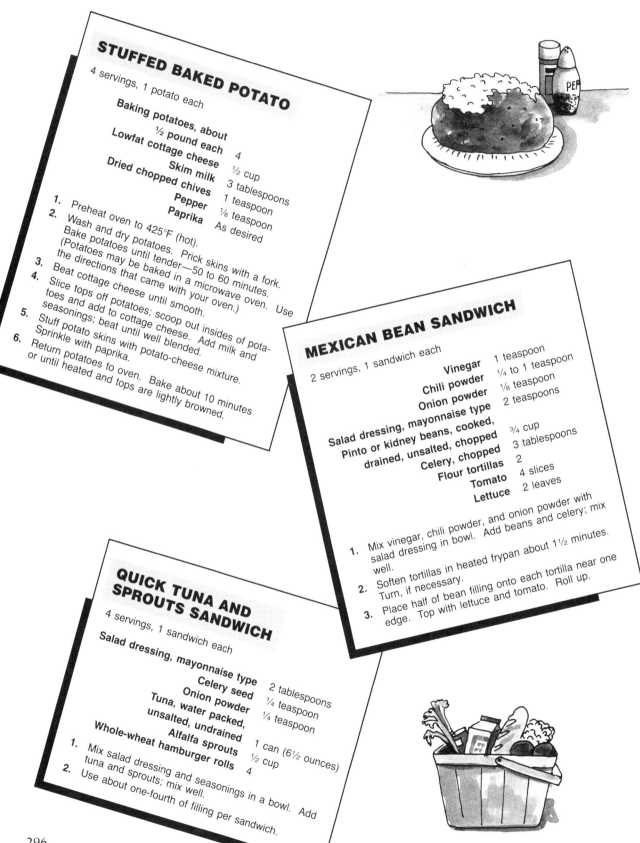

STUFFED BAKED POTATO

4 servings, 1 potato each

Baking potatoes, about ½ pound each	4
Lowfat cottage cheese	½ cup
Skim milk	3 tablespoons
Dried chopped chives	1 teaspoon
Pepper	⅛ teaspoon
Paprika	As desired

1. Preheat oven to 425°F (hot).
2. Wash and dry potatoes. Prick skins with a fork. Bake potatoes until tender—50 to 60 minutes. (Potatoes may be baked in a microwave oven. Use the directions that came with your oven.)
3. Beat cottage cheese until smooth.
4. Slice tops off potatoes; scoop out insides of potatoes and add to cottage cheese. Add milk and seasonings; beat until well blended.
5. Stuff potato skins with potato-cheese mixture. Sprinkle with paprika.
6. Return potatoes to oven. Bake about 10 minutes or until heated and tops are lightly browned.

MEXICAN BEAN SANDWICH

2 servings, 1 sandwich each

Vinegar	1 teaspoon
Chili powder	¼ to 1 teaspoon
Onion powder	⅛ teaspoon
Salad dressing, mayonnaise type	2 teaspoons
Pinto or kidney beans, cooked, drained, unsalted, chopped	¾ cup
Celery, chopped	3 tablespoons
Flour tortillas	2
Tomato	4 slices
Lettuce	2 leaves

1. Mix vinegar, chili powder, and onion powder with salad dressing in bowl. Add beans and celery; mix well.
2. Soften tortillas in heated frypan about 1½ minutes. Turn, if necessary.
3. Place half of bean filling onto each tortilla near one edge. Top with lettuce and tomato. Roll up.

QUICK TUNA AND SPROUTS SANDWICH

4 servings, 1 sandwich each

Salad dressing, mayonnaise type	2 tablespoons
Celery seed	¼ teaspoon
Onion powder	¼ teaspoon
Tuna, water packed, unsalted, undrained	1 can (6½ ounces)
Alfalfa sprouts	½ cup
Whole-wheat hamburger rolls	4

1. Mix salad dressing and seasonings in a bowl. Add tuna and sprouts; mix well.
2. Use about one-fourth of filling per sandwich.

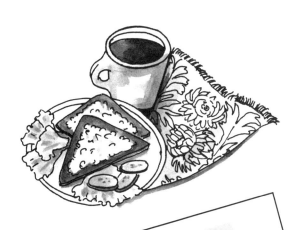

MEXICAN SNACK PIZZAS

4 servings

Whole-wheat English muffins	2
Tomato puree	¼ cup
Kidney beans, canned, drained, chopped	¼ cup
Onion, chopped	1 tablespoon
Green pepper, chopped	1 tablespoon
Oregano leaves	½ teaspoon
Mozzarella cheese, part skim milk, shredded	¼ cup
Lettuce, shredded	¼ cup

1. Split muffins; toast lightly.
2. Mix puree, beans, onion, green pepper, and oregano. Spread on muffin halves. Sprinkle with cheese.
3. Broil until cheese is bubbly, about 2 minutes.
4. Garnish with shredded lettuce.

CHICKEN SALAD SANDWICH

4 servings, 1 sandwich each

Salad dressing, mayonnaise type	2 tablespoons
Onion powder	⅛ teaspoon
Dried tarragon, crushed	⅛ teaspoon
Garlic powder	Dash
Chicken, without skin, cooked, chopped	1 cup
Celery, chopped	½ cup
Whole-wheat bread	8 slices
Lettuce leaves	4

1. Mix salad dressing and seasonings in a bowl. Stir in chicken and celery. Mix well.
2. Spread about ⅓ cup of the filling on each of four bread slices. Top with lettuce and remaining bread.

WHOLE-WHEAT CORNMEAL MUFFINS

8 muffins

Yellow cornmeal, degerminated	⅔ cup
Whole-wheat flour	⅔ cup
Sugar	1 tablespoon
Baking powder	2 teaspoons
Salt	⅛ teaspoon
Skim milk	⅔ cup
Egg, beaten	1
Oil	2 tablespoons

1. Preheat oven to 400°F (hot).
2. Grease 8 muffin tins or use paper liners.
3. Mix dry ingredients thoroughly.
4. Mix milk, egg, and oil. Add to dry ingredients. Stir until dry ingredients are barely moistened. Batter will be lumpy.
5. Fill muffin tins two-thirds full.
6. Bake until lightly browned—about 20 minutes.

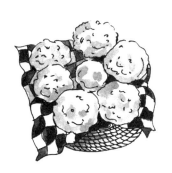

297

Desserts

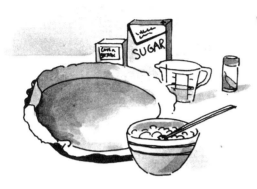

PINEAPPLE-APRICOT PIE

8-inch pie, 8 servings

Graham cracker crust	
Graham crackers, crushed	1 cup
Margarine	3 tablespoons

Filling	
Crushed pineapple, juice packed	15¼-ounce can
Apricot halves, juice packed	16-ounce can
Sugar	¼ cup
Cornstarch	3 tablespoons
Ground cinnamon	½ teaspoon
Juice from pineapple and apricots	1 cup
Lemon juice	2 teaspoons

To make crust:

1. Preheat oven to 375°F (moderate).
2. Mix graham cracker crumbs and margarine thoroughly. Save ¼ cup of crumb mixture for top of pie.
3. Press remaining crumb mixture into 8-inch pie pan so the bottom and sides are completely covered. Cool.
4. Bake until crust is firm, about 5 minutes. Cool.

To make filling:

5. Drain pineapple and apricots; save 1 cup juice. Coarsely chop apricots.
6. Mix sugar, cornstarch, and cinnamon in saucepan. Stir in fruit juice.
7. Cook over low heat, stirring constantly, until thickened. Remove from heat.
8. Add pineapple, apricots, and lemon juice. Mix well.
9. Spoon filling into crust. Sprinkle remaining crumb mixture over top of filling.
10. Chill until set.

ORANGE-APRICOT COOKIES

about 4 dozen cookies

All-purpose flour	1 cup
Whole-wheat flour	¾ cup
Sugar	¼ cup
Baking powder	2 teaspoons
Ground cinnamon	½ teaspoon
Salt	¼ teaspoon
Dried apricots, chopped	¾ cup
Orange juice, fresh	½ cup
Oil	¼ cup
Orange rind, grated	1 teaspoon
Egg, beaten	1

1. Preheat oven to 375°F (moderate).
2. Mix dry ingredients thoroughly.
3. Add remaining ingredients. Mix well.
4. Drop dough by teaspoonfuls onto ungreased baking sheet, about 1 inch apart.
5. Bake about 11 minutes or until lightly browned.
6. Remove from baking sheet while still warm.
7. Cool on rack.

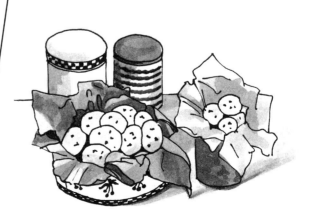

BOOKS OF THE YEAR

This section presents brief reviews of some of the more noteworthy books published in the United States in 1991 that deal with health and medical topics and are accessible to the general reader. The books are listed alphabetically by title under topic covered. The prices given may in some cases be preliminary and thus subject to change.

GENERAL/REFERENCE

**Dying at Home:
A Family Guide for Caregiving.**
Sankar, Andrea. Johns Hopkins. ISBN 0-8018-4230-1. $19.95.

Sankar, a medical anthropologist and coeditor of *The Home Care Experience: Ethnography and Policy* (Sage, 1990), has written a book on home death for those already caring for a terminally ill loved one at home or those considering it. The author examines the physical, social, and emotional toll involved and illuminates each topic—discharge to home, formal and informal support, care giving, signs of death, and after death—with apt and often moving observations made by people who experienced the home death of a child, parent, or spouse or companion.—*Anne C. Tomlin, Auburn Memorial Hospital Library, N.Y.*

Getting Back on Your Feet: How to Recover Mobility and Fitness After Injury or Surgery to Your Foot, Leg, Hip, or Knee.
Pryor, Sally R. Chelsea Green. ISBN 0-930031-38-5. $16.95.

This thorough and practical guide offers the kind of advice on using crutches, walkers, and other mobility aids that doctors, physical therapists, or other health professions might not but should have given patients. Covering the wide range of injuries from simple strains to severe disabilities, it provides a variety of tips on how to cope with stairs, how to manage in the kitchen, how to sit down and stand up, etc. There are also physical and mental exercises, a discussion of all forms of rehabilitation, and hints to helpful families and friends on what *not* to do or say.—*Edward R. Pinckney, M.D., Beverly Hills, Calif.*

Getting the Most for Your Medical Dollar.
Inlander, Charles B., and Karla Morales. Pantheon. ISBN 0-679-72781-7. $14.95.

This book, written by the directors of the Peoples' Medical Society, gives instruction on how to ask logical and informed questions about medical treatment, how the medical system works, and how it bills for services, to help people become active participants in their healthcare. It covers choosing a form of healthcare and a provider, medical insurance policies and payments, and dealing with Medicare paperwork and copayments. The nursing-home and alternative-care section answers what questions should be asked about services and payments, and saving money when making a selection. The book is filled with useful tables, which include medical abbreviations, insurance and Medicare work forms, names, addresses, and toll-free phone numbers for support organizations; medical, dental, and nursing-home licensing offices; state health departments; and Medicare carriers. A list of books on varied medical and health topics is followed by instructions for using local library resources.—*Betsy Kraus, New Mexico Technical Library, Socorro*

Living With It: Why You Don't Have To Be Healthy To Be Happy.
Szasz, Suzy. Prometheus Books. ISBN 0-87975-659-4. $22.95.

Szasz, an academic reference librarian, has written a mesmerizing account of her life as a sufferer of systemic lupus erythematosus, or lupus. She offers it as a counterpoint to accounts of people who have overcome medical or psychological tragedies and have returned to normal health. Szasz's life stopped being normal with her diagnosis at age 13. She will always be sick. She shares what she has learned in her 20 years as a chronically ill person: become as educated about the condition and its treatment as possible; choose doctors carefully and work with them, not against them; remain as independent as you possibly can; understand and be prepared for the financial battles; keep your mind active; and do as much as you can. One is impressed throughout the book with Szasz's intelligence, her willpower, and her joy in life's pleasures. "Life really is a crapshoot," she writes, and it is clear that Szasz has made the most of what she was thrown.—*Barbara Keen, Spokane Community College Library, Wash.*

The Outward Bound Wilderness First-Aid Handbook.
Isaac, Jeff, and Peter Goth, M.D. Lyons & Burford. ISBN 1-55821-106-3. $13.95

Simon & Schuster's Pocket Guide to Wilderness Medicine.
Gill, Paul G., Jr., M.D. Fireside: Simon & Schuster. ISBN 0-671-70615-2. $9.95.

Here are two new guides for the outdoors bound. Organization is the keystone on which Isaac, a physician's assistant, and Goth, a physician, base their handbook. After developing a standardized approach to all wilderness medical problems and drawing on the techniques used by Outward Bound, the authors use this methodology in each of the case studies they present in the text. The authors assume the reader knows basic human anatomy and physiology. Gill, a physician and sports medicine editor for *Outdoor Life*, has written a readable and humorous treatise, full of personal anecdotes, for the layperson. He provides advice on treating such ailments as snake and insect bites,

299

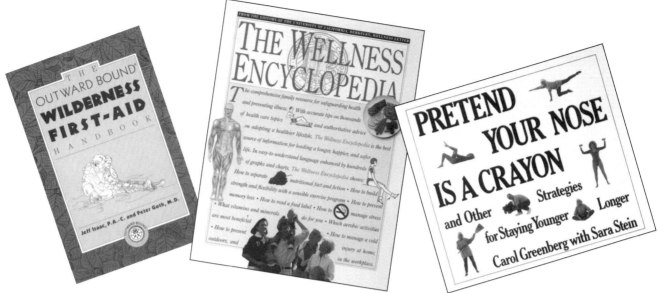

sprains and fractures, and heatstroke and hyperthermia. Gill's book, when compared to Isaac and Goth's, covers more situations that might arise in the outdoors (for example, lightning strikes), but the two titles usually prescribe similar treatments for situations discussed in both.—*Robert Jordan, University of Iowa, Iowa City*

The Wellness Encyclopedia: The Comprehensive Family Resource for Safeguarding Health and Preventing Illness.
Houghton. Edited by University of California at Berkeley Wellness Letter Editors. ISBN 0-395-53363-5. $29.95.

This excellent family healthcare guide, meant to be read cover to cover, draws on expanded and updated articles from the *Wellness Letter*—a newsletter begun in 1984 under the auspices of the School of Public Health at the University of California, Berkeley. Within five broad divisions—longevity, nutrition (especially well done), exercise, self-care, and environment and safety—information for making intelligent choices for a better, healthier life is presented in authoritative, easy-to-understand language. Illustrations and highlighted, boxed texts and charts are particularly praiseworthy. The detailed index gives access to both conventional and controversial topics: from choosing shoes to bottled water. With its preventive medicine and public health point of view, this complements similar sources such as the *Mayo Clinic Family Health Book* (Greenwillow, 1990). Highly recommended.—*James Swanton, Albert Einstein College of Medicine, New York*

When You're Sick and Don't Know Why: Coping With Your Undiagnosed Illness.
Hanner, Linda, and John J. Witek, M.D., with Robert B. Clift. DCI Publishing. ISBN 0-937721-83-2. $8.95.

This new book, written by the author of *Lyme Disease: My Search for a Diagnosis* (Kashan Publishing, 1991) with the aid of a physician and a practicing psychologist, is one of the best self-help books to come along in some time. Hanner estimates that almost one-third of the adults in the United States suffer from chronic illnesses, many of which are difficult to impossible to diagnose in a timely manner. Hanner discusses how to relate to the medical profession as well as how to deal with your family and friends when you are sick but don't know why. Her own experiences as well as those of others shine with her desire to help the unfortunate undiagnosed.—*Barbara Kormelink, Bay Medical Center Library, Bay City, Mich.*

AGING AND THE AGED

Biomarkers: The 10 Determinants of Aging You Can Control.
Evans, William, and Irwin H. Rosenberg with Jacqueline Thompson. Simon & Schuster. ISBN 0-671-68457-3. $21.95.

Pretend Your Nose Is a Crayon and Other Strategies for Staying Younger Longer.
Greenberg, Carol, with Sara Stein. Houghton. ISBN 0-395-55741-0. $17.95. Paper: ISBN 0-395-55742-9; $9.95.

Many aches and pains that accompany growing older are not a natural result of the aging process but are caused by the sedentary life-style of many older people. Stiff joints, sore backs, and fatigue can be reversed by regular aerobic, stretching, and muscle-building exercises. These two books offer sensible programs to increase fitness and vitality in almost everyone aged 50 to 80. *Pretend Your Nose Is a Crayon*, written by a physical therapist, offers a gentle, humorous, "user friendly" approach to fitness. It presents basic principles of physiology to introduce the ten-minute-a-day, three-times-a-week routine that utilizes strength-building weights. Exercises are illustrated with photos of "models" ranging in age from the early 50s to 94. Other chapters detail special exercises for those with arthritis, chronic back problems, or other injuries, along with tips for starting a walking program and incorporating exercises into household and garden chores.

"Biomarkers," developed by two Tufts University researchers, are ten indicators of physical function that influence well-being. These indicators, including muscle mass, strength, blood pressure, and aerobic capacity, can be controlled by almost anyone of any age through regular aerobic and isotonic exercise. This book discusses each biomarker in detail, with references to recent scientific literature, and provides two self-tests to determine fitness levels. Programs, presented as charts illustrated with drawings, are geared for a variety of fitness levels. Tips on diet and motivation accompany the charts. Exercises aren't that much different from those in Greenberg's book but may appear a bit daunting for the over-50 group who may never before have participated in a regular exercise or fitness program.—*Karen McNally Bensing, Benjamin Rose Institute Library, Cleveland*

The Caregiver's Guide: Helping Older Relatives and Friends With Health and Safety Concerns.
Rob, Caroline, with Janet Reynolds. Houghton. ISBN 0-395-50086-9. $22.95. Paper: ISBN 0-395-58780-8; $12.95.

Rob, a medical writer who has done geriatric nursing, and geriatric nurse practitioner Reynolds have written a valuable handbook designed to answer questions about aging and health. Clearly written, their guide covers changes in vision and hearing, skin, digestion, heart and lungs, bones, kidney and bladder, as well as depression, memory loss and nervous system disorders, cancer, and diabetes. Chapters on medication safety, convalescent home care, and getting help from social service agencies complete the work. Recommended because of its comprehensive coverage, practical tips, and sound advice.—*Anne C. Tomlin, Auburn Memorial Hospital Library, N.Y.*

AIDS

The Guide to Living With HIV Infection.
Bartlett, John G., M.D., and Ann K. Finkbeiner. Johns Hopkins. ISBN 0-8018-4193-3. $38.95. Paper: ISBN 0-8018-4194-1; $15.95.

Bartlett, professor of medicine and director of the Infectious Diseases Division of the Johns Hopkins Medical Institutions, and Finkbeiner, a science writer, have written this authoritative, plain-spoken book to let people with HIV infection, AIDS-related complex (ARC), or AIDS "know what they're up against" and to help them deal thoroughly and positively with the medical and emotional problems the infection presents. Aimed at teaching HIV-infected people "how to live as long and full and satisfying a life as possible," this guide offers practical advice on such topics as what to do when diagnosed, how to prevent transmission, and how to maintain positive attitudes. The glossary is especially helpful in understanding

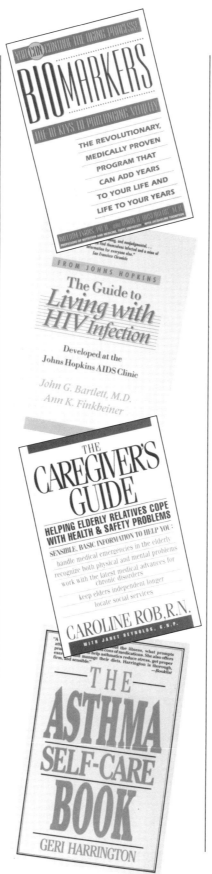

HIV/ARC/AIDS terminology. With more than 1 million Americans living with HIV infection, this book is recommended to the broadest readership as one of the best AIDS popular handbooks. The paperback is a good buy.—*James Swanton, Albert Einstein College of Medicine, New York*

ASTHMA

The Asthma Self-Care Book: How to Take Control of Your Asthma.
Harrington, Geri. HarperCollins. ISBN 0-06-016584-7. $19.95.

Breathing Easy: A Parent's Guide to Dealing With Your Child's Asthma.
Stevens, Maryann. Prentice-Hall. ISBN 0-13-083692-3. $9.95.

An asthma attack is a terrifying event to experience, a frightening one to witness. Because one feels so helpless in the face of an attack, having information and strategies to cope with it can only benefit the asthmatic as well as the onlooker. Harrington nearly died from an asthma attack and writes from firsthand experience. She stresses that knowledge is power for an asthmatic, since understanding the disease and its triggers, and knowing what action to take when, can prevent or control some attacks. Having a doctor you respect and trust, managing your asthma with medications, and recognizing and coping with the triggers or stimuli that initiate breathing difficulties are essential to living with asthma. A useful appendix includes information on medications and organizations devoted to asthma education, plus complete data on lung associations and asthma rehabilitation centers and programs.

Stevens addresses asthma from a parent's view, with an eye toward prevention. This practical approach answers basic questions about triggers, environment, medications, and living with asthma day by day. Ideas on ways to make hospitalization less traumatic are reassuring to both parent and child. A discussion of government and private organizations provides essential information, as does a geographic listing of accredited programs in allergy/immunology. There is a reading list and suggested exercises. Both books make valuable contributions to self-help methods in coping with this chronic disease that afflicts over 10 million people and is on the rise.—*Janet M. Coggan, University of Florida Libraries, Gainesville*

CANCER

Courage: The Testimony of a Cancer Patient.
Creaturo, Barbara. Pantheon. ISBN 0-394-58077-X. $23.

While ovarian cancer is relatively rare (18,000 women diagnosed each year), deaths caused by it exceed those of cervical and endometrial cancers combined. Creaturo, who died after she finished this book, chronicles her battle with this deadly disease. Her journey is reflected in her chapter titles: Discovery, Panic, Experiment, Struggle, and a fleeting Victory. Creaturo's medical odyssey convinces her not to accept passively the recommendations given her but to investigate all available treatments from the standard to experimental, while educating herself about her illness. In describing her search for a cure, she reveals strength and perseverance, and her fighting spirit is awesome. The afterword, written by Ezra Greenspan, the chairman and medical director of the ChemoTherapy Foundation, has useful data on new drugs, recent strides in immunotherapy, and a new advocacy group. Read with Mary-Ellen Siegal's *The Cancer Patient's Handbook* (Walker, 1986), Creaturo's book provides a strategy for coping with cancer.—*Janet M. Coggan, University of Florida Libraries, Gainesville*

Everyone's Guide to Cancer Therapy: How Cancer Is Diagnosed, Treated, and Managed on a Day-to-Day Basis.
Dollinger, Malin, M.D., and others. Somerville House Book: Andrews & McMeel. ISBN 0-8362-2418-3. $29.95. Paper: ISBN 0-8362-2417-5; $19.95.

Written by two oncologists for the layperson, this authoritative but readable reference stands out in the literature as a uniquely comprehensive, thorough source of up-to-date information about cancer generally and individual common cancers. Similar in scope,

but with a much fuller, more complete treatment than the American Cancer Society's *Cancer Book* (Doubleday, 1986), this affordable guide offers an understanding of current diagnosis and treatment, therapy and management, supportive care, and developments in assessment. In an easy-to-use format in four parts, the authors answer myriad questions about every aspect from early detection and stages to risk factors and genetics, with a chapter highlighting the role of the National Cancer Institute in sponsoring clinical trials. Useful appendixes include a glossary of medical terms, a list of anticancer drugs and their side effects, and a directory of cancer centers, associations, and support groups.—*Marilyn Rosenthal, Nassau Community College Library, Garden City, N.Y.*

Managing the Side Effects of Chemotherapy and Radiation, revised edition.
Dodd, Marilyn J. Prentice-Hall. ISBN 0-13-547480-9. $12.95.

Dodd, an oncology nurse and professor, has compiled a much-needed and easy-to-use resource for cancer patients and their families. Since chemotherapy and radiation treatments can cause severe and debilitating side effects, it becomes vital to learn how to cope and overcome those effects. Education is a key to that process. Part 1 defines chemotherapy, lists the 48 most common chemotherapeutic drugs and their side effects, and sug-

gests ways to manage those effects. Especially useful and practical is a nutrition section with ideas on food intake and recipes. Radiation treatment, side effects, and ways to deal with them form the second part. The third section consists of a self-care log and worksheet. Expanded from its initial edition (Appleton & Lange, 1987), this book makes a significant contribution to patient education and should be required reading for all oncology patients.—*Janet M. Coggan, University of Florida Libraries, Gainesville*

CEREBRAL PALSY

Children With Cerebral Palsy: A Parents' Guide.
Woodbine House. Edited by Elaine Geralis. ISBN 0-933149-15-8. $14.95.

Cerebral palsy affects 1 in every 500 children. This lifelong disability resulting from damage to the brain before, during, or soon after birth encompasses a wide variety of disorders that affect one's ability to control muscles and posture. This volume, featuring contributions from professional care givers, therapists, and parents, provides a thorough description of cerebral palsy, its diagnosis and treatment, and its effects on development. Practical hints on the daily care of the afflicted child are offered, as well as help in seeking out and understanding the role of occupa-

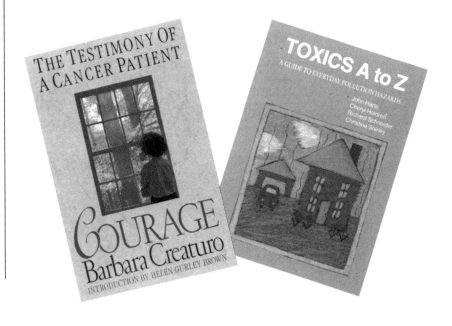

tional, physical, and speech therapy. A guide to early intervention, special education, and an outline of legal rights are included. The extensive listing of federal, state, and local government agencies as well as parent and professional groups is especially useful.—*Jodith Janes, Cleveland Clinic Foundation*

DIABETES

The Diabetic Man: A Guide to Health and Success in All Areas of Your Life.
Lodewick, Peter, M.D., and others. Lowell House, distributed by Contemporary Books. ISBN 0-929923-24-3. $19.95.

June Biermann and Barbara Toohey, whose numerous books (for example, *The Diabetic's Book*, J. P. Tarcher, 1990) have inspired many newly diagnosed diabetics, join a renowned diabetologist to focus on issues faced by the diabetic man. They suggest diabetes is either "Type U," or uncontrolled, or "Type C," or controlled, with control being not only desirable but the only way to sidestep the well-publicized but avoidable complications of this chronic disease. In a lively, conversational format, the authors reassure and help the diabetic man gain control of his life through careful management. Medicine, nutrition, sports, sex (impotence being a particular concern), and traveling are all discussed. Women will find this book helpful in learning how to support the diabetic man or male child in their lives.—*Anne Washburn, Smith, Helms, Mulliss, and Moore Library, Greensboro, N.C.*

DIGESTIVE SYSTEM

Gastrointestinal Health.
Peikin, Steven R., M.D. HarperCollins. ISBN 0-06-016497-2. $19.95

Peikin, director of gastrointestinal nutrition at Thomas Jefferson University Hospital, states in his introduction that more than 8 million Americans, many between the ages of 25 and 40, suffer from chronic digestive problems. This book addresses the many gastrointestinal (GI) problems in a clear, easy-to-understand style; most importantly, each specific ailment is thoroughly explained, including diagnostic procedures, drug and dietary therapy, and prognosis. Peikin stresses his self-help nutritional program, not necessarily as a cure-all, but as a method of alleviating and reducing many of the symptoms of gastrointestinal distress. Included are an excellent list of "flag foods," a two-week master diet program, and, best of all, well-written recipes that will appeal to everyone, including those without gastrointestinal problems. This is highly recommended for its thorough coverage, sound advice, and healthy suggestions.—*Debra Berlanstein, Towson State University Library, Baltimore*

ENVIRONMENT AND HEALTH

Healthy Homes, Healthy Kids: Protecting Your Children From Everyday Environmental Hazards.
Schoemaker, Joyce M., and Charity Y. Vitale. Island Press. ISBN 1-55963-057-4. $19.95. Paper: ISBN 1-55963-056-6; $12.95.

Children are particularly vulnerable to environmental hazards, and the home is a place where parents have greater control to reduce or eliminate such hazards. This book provides well-presented and thoughtful information on the dangers of lead, radon, asbestos, pesticides, food additives, household chemicals, and electromagnetic fields, to name a few. Each chapter begins with a brief overview of problem, risk, and what to do and ends with a resources section of products and services and sources of information. Although books such as Ellen Greenfield's *House Dangerous* (Vintage, 1987), Linda Hunter's *The Healthy Home* (Rodale, 1989), and Gary Null's *Clearer, Cleaner, Safer, Greener* (Villard, 1990), cover some of the same material, they don't focus on the environmental impact on children's health. This highly accessible book provides a needed resource with reasonable approaches for action.—*Kathleen L. Atwood, Pomfret School Library, Conn.*

Toxics A to Z: A Guide to Everyday Pollution Hazards.
Harte, John, and others. University of California Press. ISBN 0-520-07223-5. $75. Paper: ISBN 0-520-07224-3; $29.95.

For the average individual trying to manage in a polluted world, this is an eminently readable guide to the toxins we live with. The first part of the book includes an overview of toxic issues, discusses the major sources of toxic exposure (air, water, food, and consumer products), and deals with special groups of toxics like petrochemicals and radiation. Part 2 is an alphabetical listing of over 100 commonly occurring toxic substances. Each entry addresses properties, health effects, and protection and prevention methods. A cross-reference to entries by exposure ("workplace contaminants") is a useful aid.—*Linda Knaack, Mount Ida College, Newton, Mass.*

Your Health and the Indoor Environment: A Complete Guide to Better Health Through Control of the Indoor Atmosphere.
Dunford, Randall Earl, with Kevin G. May, M.D. NuDawn Publishing. ISBN 0-9628093-3-0. $19.95.

In a reassuring style that offers food for thought and action without being alarmist, Dunford discusses the dozens of allergens that are everywhere (particularly indoors), health problems they can cause, where they are most prevalent, how to prevent them, and how to "cure" them. He provides in 16 readable chapters and 7 appendixes a vast amount of information on the usual and unusual sources of allergens and offers good general instructions on alleviating a difficult problem.—*Aletha Kowitz, Bureau of Library Services, American Dental Association, Chicago.*

HEART DISEASE

The Female Heart: The Truth About Women and Coronary Artery Disease.
Legato, Marianne J., M.D., and Carol Colman. Prentice Hall Press. ISBN 0-13-321811-2. $19.95

Because women, according to popular belief, are much less prone than men to develop cardiovascular disease, their heart problems, when they do develop, often are ignored or made light of. However, as Legato, a physician who specializes in cardiac care for women, points out, 500,000 women suffer from cardiac disease of some sort each year. Women seem more inclined than men to play down warning signs and to ignore sound medical advice. Stress, heredity, and poor living habits can have the same deleterious effect on the female heart as on the male. The author points out the ways in which diagnosis, treatment, and prognosis of cardiovascular disease differ in females. However, the sound principles of regular medical checkups, proper eating, and exercise habits apply equally to men and women.—*Eleanor Maass, Maass Assocs., New Milford, Pa.*

Heart to Heart:
A Guide to the Psychological
Aspects of Heart Disease.
Budnick, Herbert N., with Scott Robert Hays. Health Press. ISBN 0-929173-07-4. $22.95.

Severe cardiovascular disease can be emotionally crippling. Budnick, a psychotherapist specializing in patients with heart disease and their families, addresses this highly original study to those who must grapple with the uncertainties and fears created by a life-threatening disorder. In simple, readily comprehensible language, he provides reassurance and offers coping mechanisms for adjusting to the many changes necessitated by the illness. Drawing on both personal (having witnessed his father and sister succumb to heart disease) as well as professional experience, Budnick offers succinct advice regarding the changing roles of each family member.—*Carol R. Glatt, VA Medical Center Library, Philadelphia.*

MEDICATIONS AND DRUGS

Drug Interactions Guide Book.
Harkness, Richard. Prentice-Hall. ISBN 0-13-219601-8. $24.95. Paper: ISBN 0-13-219619-0; $12.95.

Harkness, a pharmacist, has written a book for laypersons that is well organized and easy to comprehend. Each

entry lists the uses of the drugs involved, which drug's action is increased or decreased by an interaction with another drug, and the possible consequences. Graphs showing the possibility and severity of each interaction are useful. There is also a "What to Do" section on preventing or minimizing the interaction. The introductory pages of the book state this section is a guide for health professionals and caution the reader not to try to manage the interaction themselves. Considering people do not always read instructions, this warning should have been repeated in the text. Few drug information books published for consumers provide this much detail on drug interactions.—*Kathleen Smith, Philadelphia College of Pharmacy and Science.*

MEN'S HEALTH

Male Sexual Health.
Baldwin, Dorothy. Hippocrene. ISBN 0-87052-955-2. $19.95.

British-born biologist Baldwin has compiled a breezy guide to men's sexual organs and their health, covering functional, preventive, and disease issues. Less earthy in her language than James Gilbaugh's *A Doctor's Guide to Men's Private Parts* (Crown, 1989) and less technical than Yosh Taguchi's *Private Parts* (Doubleday, 1989), she covers concerns from birth to old age, including circumcision, maintenance and care, hormones and drugs, sexual dysfunction, sexually transmitted diseases (including AIDS), and stress management. This work is a good middle-ground choice for its readability (although it's occasionally superficial and cutesy) and avoidance of street terminology.—*Robert Aken, University of Kentucky Libraries, Lexington.*

MENTAL HEALTH

The Dinosaur Man: Tales of Madness and Enchantment From the Back Ward.
Baur, Susan. HarperCollins. ISBN 0-06-016538-3. $19.95.

Everyone has a story. The stories that make up this book are neither ordi-

nary nor extraordinary. They derive from Baur's work with schizophrenic patients, many of whom have been hospitalized for years at a place disguised for this telling as "Mountain Valley Hospital." Some patients are painfully aware that they are ill. Many are unable to distinguish between experienced and imagined events (the subject of Baur's dissertation was memory). Throughout the work, Baur (*Hypochondria: Woeful Imaginings*, University of California, 1988) is both participant and observer, as she brings into focus those among us who are frequently forgotten. This sensitively written book is recommended. It was optioned by Orion Pictures for a film produced by and featuring Jodie Foster.—*Marlene Charnizon, New York*

The Enigma of Suicide.
Colt, George Howe. Summit Books, distributed by Simon & Schuster. ISBN 0-671-50996-9. $24.95.

Written by a writer for *Life* magazine, this well-researched book covers all aspects of suicide, including its social, cultural, and legal history; the biological and psychological research available; attempts at prevention; the right-to-die movement; and the effects on survivors. Interspersing interviews with factual information, the author provides the reader with a deeper understanding of the study of suicide and points out that for some people suicide may be the only choice. Some of the stories are depressing, but this book will probably be comforting to survivors who are trying to make sense of why their loved ones succumbed to this dreaded persuasion.—*Lucy Patrick, Florida State University Library, Tallahassee*

NUTRITION AND DIET

The American Heart Association Cookbook, 5th edition.
Times Books. Edited by Rodman D. Stark, M.D., and Mary Winston. ISBN 0-8129-1895-9. $25.

Many of the recent slew of health-conscious cookbooks base their recipes on the American Heart Association guidelines; now there's a new edition from the source. Half the recipes were revised, many new ones were added, and much information was updated. There are special sections on shopping and cooking, health concerns, and other related topics. Overall, the recipes are a mixed bag of very traditional family fare and some upscale dishes, international specialties, and Americanized versions of ethnic favorites—with more canned and frozen ingredients than one might expect from the book's orientation.—*Judith C. Sutton, Sutton's Place Cuisine, New York*

Defensive Dining: How to Stay Trim & Healthy While Eating in Virtually Any Restaurant.
Sindell, Cheryl. Knightsbridge Publishing Company. ISBN 1-56129-072-6. $12.95.

Written by a nutritionist with extensive knowledge of ethnic foods, this indispensable guide to restaurant dining is divided into three parts. Part 1 describes common problems faced by dieters when eating out and offers practical solutions. Part 2 discusses in detail French, American, Italian, Mexican, Chinese, Japanese, Indian, and Greek cuisines, listing healthy, low-calorie dishes to order and unhealthy, fatty, or salty dishes to avoid. Part 3 recommends ordering special meals when flying (at no extra cost) and provides a plan to help minimize jet lag. The author urges diners to order with confidence and not to feel intimidated when asking for the foods and preparation methods they need to eat healthfully in restaurants.—*Linda Chopra, Cleveland Heights-University Heights Public Library, Ohio*

The Duke University Medical Center Book of Diet and Fitness.
Hamilton, Michael, and others. Columbine: Fawcett: Ballantine. ISBN 0-449-90526-0. $19.95.

Here is a safe, sensible diet book. Based upon the first residential weight-loss program in America, this book does not rely on gimmicks or fads but provides sound emotional guidance, good nutritional advice, interesting meal plans and recipes, and a reasonable exercise program. Logically divided into four sections stressing the above fundamentals, it is interspersed throughout with engaging case histories. There are many fill-in charts, graphs, lists, etc. The book is an antidote to the plethora of dangerous diets.—*Linda Chopra, Cleveland Heights-University Heights Public Library, Ohio*

Power Foods:
High Performance Nutrition for High-Performance People.
Applegate, Liz. Rodale Press. ISBN 0-87857-967-2. $18.95.

Recipes for Runners:
Nutritional Diets to Improve Every Athlete's Performance.
Green, Sammy. Avery Publishing Group. ISBN 0-572-01499-6. $7.95.

Compiled by a British marathon runner and health food specialist, *Recipes for Runners* contains a manageable number of recipes divided into chapters for breakfast, snacks, carbohydrates, legumes, nuts, vegetables, fish, meat and poultry, salads, and desserts. All are prepared from fresh, natural ingredients with a low-fat, high-fiber content. Clear, concise instructions and metric, imperial, and American measurements are given for each. Preceding each section of recipes is a very brief, one-page nutritional overview of the foods included. Although British spellings and expressions are used throughout, this short, easy-to-read cookbook should appeal to most American readers.

Power Foods, on the other hand, is a rather comprehensive nutrition reference incorporating the latest scientific research about diet and exercise. Applegate, the nutrition editor of *Runner's World* magazine, packs a lot of detailed but not too technical information into this useful guide. Organized into chapters covering drinks, carbohydrates, proteins, fats, vitamins and minerals, eating management, calories, power-eating strategies, high-performance menus, and meal planning, the book contains numerous tables that break down complex information into less intimidating, bite-sized pieces. Meal plans, but not recipes, are interspersed throughout.

Although these two books basically deal with the same subject, their approach and focus are very different. Whereas *Recipes for Runners* is basically a cookbook, *Power Foods* is a compendium on nutrition.—*Linda Chopra, Cleveland Heights-University Heights Public Library, Ohio*

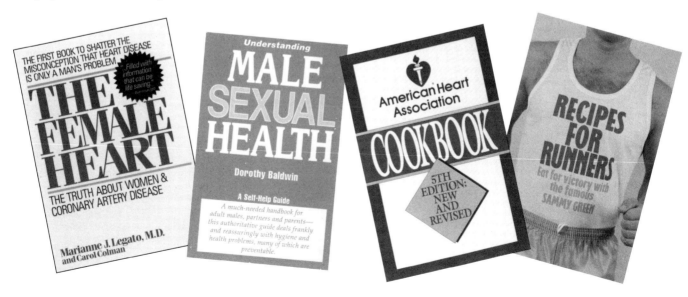

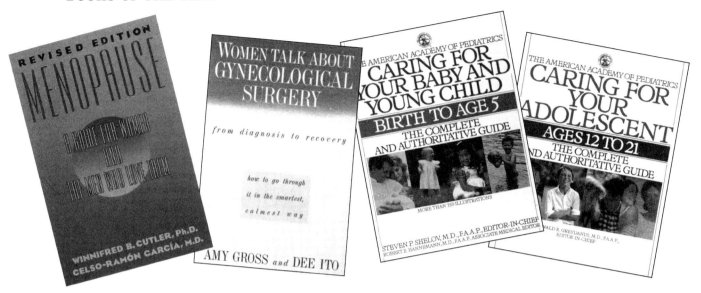

The Real Life Nutrition Book.
Finn, Susan, M.D., and Linda Stern Kass. Penguin. ISBN 0-14-013174-4. $15.

Now here's a nutrition book you can really sink your teeth into. Finn, president-elect of the American Dietetic Association, and Kass, a medical writer, address the practical aspect of how to fit good nutrition into a life jam-packed with activities that all too frequently impinge on good intentions: two-career families, health club workouts, eating on the run. They also consider personal factors: controlling weight and cholesterol levels, the effects of stress on over- or undereating. This book is chock full of suggestions for incorporating good nutrition and healthy eating habits into everyday life. The authors evaluate fast foods and prepared supermarket dishes as well as cookbooks. Menu plans and recipes are included.—*Carol Spielman Lezak, General Learning Corporation, Northbrook, Ill.*

Safe Food:
Eating Wisely in a Risky World.
Jacobson, Michael F., and others. Center for Science in the Public Interest and Living Planet Press, distributed by Publishers Group West. Foreword by Ralph Nader. ISBN 1-879326-01-9. $8.95.

Are we eating pesticides, bacteria, veterinary drugs, or industrial pollutants in our family dinner? The authors, health and nutrition experts connected with the Center for Science in the Public Interest (CSPI), offer tips

for selecting, handling, storing, and preparing safe and healthy food. They suggest ways for the educated consumer to help bring about reforms and improve government regulations for safer food. They also cite extensive scientific studies including CSPI's *Nutrition Action Healthletter*. There is some overlap of material with Geri Harrington's *Real Food, Fake Food* (Macmillan, 1987), though this has a different format and is more current. The general reader and informed layperson will like this book.—*Loraine F. Sweetland, Rebok Memorial Library, Silver Spring, Md.*

OBSTETRICS AND GYNECOLOGY

Breast Care Options for the 1990's.
Kuehn, Paul, M.D. Newmark Publishing Company. ISBN 0-938539-04-3. $19.95.

An updated, revised edition of *Breast Care Options* (Newmark, 1986), this book discusses prevention strategies, new diagnostic and treatment methods, and types of ongoing innovative research. A woman with breast cancer faces many medical choices, from mammography and magnetic resonance imaging to mastectomy or limited surgery. This guide provides women with up-to-date data to make the best possible decision for their particular stage of breast disease.

Special features of the book include a useful medical glossary, a listing of cancer centers and organizations, plus a question-and-answer section at the end of each chapter. For those wanting further information, *Dr. Susan Love's Breast Book* (Addison-Wesley, 1990) investigates breast diseases in greater depth, as well as from a more academic perspective.—*Janet M. Coggan, University of Florida Libraries, Gainesville*

How to Get Pregnant With the New Technology.
Silber, Sherman J., M.D. Warner. ISBN 0-446-51498-5. $21.95.

In the more than ten years since Silber published *How To Get Pregnant* (1980) there have been remarkable advances in the treatment of infertility. With compassion and thoroughness, Silber provides infertile couples with an easy-to-read guide to the bewildering maze of new reproductive technologies: surrogate pregnancy, egg donation, in vitro fertilization (IVF), gamete intrafallopian transfer (GIFT), and microsurgery. Honest, compassionate, and sometimes critical, he also exposes misleading diagnoses that, in his view, have caused couples great anxiety and sometimes needless expense. His discussion on the causes of and therapies for infertility will provide couples considering treatment the information that they need in order for them to make thoughtful decisions.—*Jodith Janes, Cleveland Clinic Foundation*

Menopause: A Guide for Women and the Men Who Love Them, revised edition.
Cutler, Winnifred, and Celso-Ramon Garcia, M.D. Norton. ISBN 0-393-02922-0. $25.

As the baby boom generation ages, more books dealing with aspects of that process are starting to appear. This revised edition of *Menopause* (Norton, 1983) reflects the most recent findings about the role of hormone replacement therapy in the lives of menopausal women. The authors, a biologist and a physician who advocate its use, explain the physiological changes that occur during this time and offer detailed information about the benefits and risks of hormone replacement therapy. They emphasize the prevention of osteoporosis and heart disease. They also offer sound advice about nutrition and exercise for maintaining good health and information about alternatives for those women who do not wish to take hormones. The book is equipped with a glossary of terms, along with an extensive bibliography that provides access to the medical literature for further research.—*Barbara M. Bibel, Oakland Public Library, Calif.*

Recovering From a C Section.
Blackstone, Margaret, with Tahira Homayun, M.D. Longmeadow Press. ISBN 0-681-41154-6. $6.95.

A well-written and much-needed guide for pregnant women who might face a C section. The authors, a cesarean mother and a gynecologist, address every aspect of this method of delivery, both physical and emotional, pointing out that a successful delivery is defined by a healthy mom and healthy baby, not by how that was achieved. Too many women feel like failures because they didn't have a "normal" delivery. This book dispels the myths surrounding C sections giving encouragement, tips for coaches, advice on caring for your body after the surgery, and generally informing readers about a subject that is usually treated peripherally in pregnancy handbooks. It may be news to some that many women who have delivered both vaginally and by C section report that they prefer surgery!—*Anne Washburn, Smith Helms Mulliss & Moore Library, Greensboro, N.C.*

Women Talk About Gynecological Surgery From Diagnosis to Recovery: How to Go Through It in the Calmest, Smartest Way.
Gross, Amy, and Dee Ito. Potter, distributed by Crown. ISBN 0-517-58055-1. $22.95.

A companion volume to the authors' *Women Talk About Breast Surgery* (Potter/Crown, 1990), this covers the most common gynecological surgical procedures with a refreshingly candid outlook. Repeating the previous book's question-and-answer format, it features interviews with several women who talk about their personal experiences with gynecological surgery. The interviewees share the specifics of their diagnosis and treatment, their interactions with medical personnel, and their feelings regarding surgery and recovery. They are completely honest, acknowledging unpleasant experiences while emphasizing more positive aspects of treatment. Specialists and medical personnel in gynecological fields were also consulted to clarify procedures and explain new techniques that have proven helpful for some patients. The personal perspectives will help women make informed decisions about healthcare, while at the same time providing ammunition against fear and uncertainty.—*Deborah Emerson, Monroe Community College Library, Rochester, N.Y.*

Your Pregnancy Companion.
Graham, Janis. Pocket Books. ISBN 0-671-68557-0. $9.95.

In this month-by-month account of pregnancy's progress, the author addresses pregnancy's impact on such key dimensions of a woman's life as her body, diet, workouts, feelings, and life-style, including work life. Within this framework, she covers a diverse series of common concerns ranging from normal fetal development, prenatal tests, and RH factor to calf cramps, maternity leave, and premature labor. The result is a delight to read, as the material presented is remarkably well organized, thoroughly researched, and presented in a no-nonsense factual manner that never is condescending or oversimplified. Additional readings are suggested.—*Kathryn Hammell Carpenter, University of Illinois, Chicago*

PEDIATRICS AND CHILDCARE

Caring for Your Adolescent: Ages 12 to 21.
American Academy of Pediatrics. Bantam. Edited by Donald E. Greydanus and others. ISBN 0-533-07556-X. $24.50.

Less conclusive than the first volume in this three-part series on parenting (*Caring for Your Baby and Young Child*), this handbook explores in an objective but compassionate manner all aspects of adolescent development and experience. The introduction apprises parents of the challenges faced in raising teenagers—a substantive list of 13 items—but consoles them with a brief account of the rewards involved. A short section on legal and health rights of adolescents advises parents of limits to their authority. Other chapters underscore the individual pace of psychological, social, physical, and sexual development in adolescents. Readable, often listing recommended readings, this text occasionally disappoints because the sections are so brief, for example, on dating, friendships, and sexual preference.—*Kathryn Hammell Carpenter, University of Illinois, Chicago*

Caring for Your Baby and Young Child: Birth to Age 5.
American Academy of Pediatrics. Bantam. Edited by Steven P. Shelov and others. ISBN 0-553-07186-6. $32.50.

Subject to extensive review by academy members, this handbook on the early years of a child's life is comprehensive, authoritative, and interesting. In section 1, chapters divided according to developmental stages track physical, mental, emotional, and verbal growth, basic care, health and safety concerns, and family issues. Section 2 covers child health hazards and treatment. In contrast to the frank, informative, reassuring, but somehow frantic and intimidating personal accounts of parents found in such books as Frances Burck's *Babysense: A Practical and Supportive Guide to Baby Care*, 2nd edition (St. Martin, 1991), this survey is cool, confident, and reassuring if somewhat impersonal. This volume was to be

307

followed by *Caring for Your Adolescent: Ages 12 to 21* (1991) and by *Caring for Your School-Age Child: Ages 5 to 12* (1992).—*Kathryn Hammell Carpenter, University of Illinois, Chicago*

The Complete Guide to Choosing Child Care.
Berezin, Judith. Random. ISBN 0-679-73100-8. $12.95.

This well-organized handbook, "prepared under the auspices of the National Association of Child Care Resource and Referral Agencies [NACCRRA] and Child Care, Inc.," offers excellent advice to parents, guardians, or anyone in need of connecting, formally or informally, with others for care-giving help. Checklists of pertinent questions; diverse personal observations; suggested considerations and sampler forms related to in-home family day care; infant/toddler/early childhood centers; *in loco parentis* for school-age children; and summer camps are all included, plus a section on child abuse issues. A final chapter suggests ways in which individuals can encourage quality child care and education on their own or through public or private institutions. The appendix has a starter list of useful references: *au pair* agencies and state and national agency affiliates of the NACCRRA. A very useful book indeed.—*Suzanne W. Wood, State University of New York College of Technology, Alfred*

Feeding Your Baby: From Conception to Two Years.
Lambert-Lagace, Louise. Surrey Books. ISBN 0-940625-37-7. $10.95.

Written by a registered dietician and mother of three, this updated Americanized version of her earlier Canadian editions is easy to read and down to earth. It offers sound nutritional advice starting from preconception through pregnancy, from birth to the toddler years. Coupling the author's own philosophies with scientific research findings, this guide covers such topics as the benefits of breastfeeding, introducing solids, vegetarian diets, and food allergies. The charts and diagrams summarizing such factors as caffeine intake, the ideal weights for mom, and the benefits of various nutrients, vitamins, and minerals are very useful. Menus and reci-

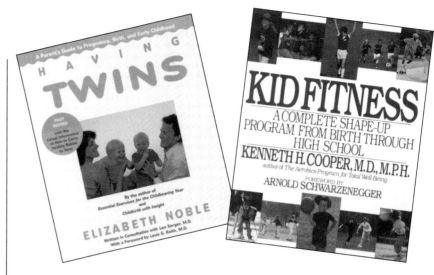

pes for baby food are also included.—*Angela Washington-Blair, Brookhaven College Learning Resource Center, Farmers Branch, Texas*

Having Twins: A Parent's Guide to Pregnancy, Birth, and Early Childhood, 2nd edition.
Noble, Elizabeth, with Leo Sorger, M.D. Houghton. ISBN 0-395-51088-0. $24.95. Paper: ISBN 0-395-49338-2; $12.95.

The well-received first edition (1980) served as a core book on the topic for many years. Now, Noble has revised and expanded this indispensable tool on the history and physiology of twinning. New material on prenatal care, birthing, bonding, and emotional coping provides updated information. The excellent section on nutrition has been enhanced to include modern, alternative choices, and the section on exercise remains unchanged and one of the best for multiple-birth mothers. Both physical and emotional needs are equally considered by Noble, as her realistic treatment of possible complications is balanced by her sensitive, and at times personal, insights. There is a bibliography and source list.—*Mary Hemmings, University of Calgary Law Library, Alberta*

Kid Fitness: A Complete Shape-Up Program From Birth to High School.
Cooper, Kenneth H., M.D. Bantam. ISBN 0-553-07332-X. $19.50.

Cooper, a physician and preventive medicine specialist, has raised our fitness consciousness by popularizing aerobic exercises in five books including *The Aerobics Program for Total Well-Being* (Evans, 1982). Cooper's

concern with the declining fitness levels of today's youth has prompted this book aimed at parents who want to teach their children the basics of sound exercise and good nutrition. He offers wise advice on how to motivate kids and test their fitness and recommends a system of aerobic, strength, and flexibility training keyed to the child's developmental level. Cooper doesn't include as many exercises with photographs as Bonnie Prudden's *Fitness From Six to Twelve* (Ballantine, 1987) nor does he cover the individual sports and school programs found in Bob Glover and Jack Shepard's *Family Fitness Handbook* (Penguin, 1989), but neither title has recipes and as good nutritional focus.—*Sandra Math, St. John's University Library, Staten Island, N.Y.*

A Parents' Guide to Attention Deficit Disorders.
Bain, Lisa J., with Children's Hospital of Philadelphia. Delta: Dell. ISBN 0-385-30031-X. $10.

This is the first in a new series sponsored by the Children's Hospital of Philadelphia. Bain, a medical journalist, attempts to help parents understand attention deficit-hyperactivity disorder. (ADHD). She writes in clear, understandable prose, resulting in a comprehensive study of ADHD, its diagnosis, history, possible causes, methods for management, and issues of family stress and school-home relationships. Bain addresses the controversies surrounding not only ADHD treatment, but also the arguments regarding its definition. She acknowledges the lack of absolute solutions, the variations in cases, and the need for parental decisions. As a parent resource, Bain's book is especially thorough and well balanced.—*Kay Brodie, Chesapeake College, Wye Mills, Md.*

Safe Kids: A Complete Child Safety Handbook and Resource Guide for Parents.
Fancher, Vivian Kramer. Wiley. ISBN 0-471-52973-7. $12.95.

An amazing amount of clear, commonsense information is packed into this safety book for parents and others working with children from infant to high-school age. Chapters focus on identification, on school and street safety, on care givers, on medical, fire, recreational, cycle, and transportation safety, on sexual abuse, and more. All have checklists and additional current resources. Drugs are not covered, but good sources for information on this subject are included.—*Annette V. Janes, Hamilton Library, Mass.*

Your Child Has a Disability: A Complete Sourcebook of Daily and Medical Care.
Batshaw, Mark L., M.D. Little, Brown. ISBN 0-316-08369-0. $27.95. Paper: ISBN 0-316-08368-2; $16.95.

Dividing his handbook into five parts, Batshaw, a pediatrician who works with children with developmental disabilities, discusses the diagnosis of a handicap, genetic and other causes of developmental disabilities, practical information on individual diseases and syndromes, approaches to therapy, and social, legal, and educational decisions with a disabled child. Additional readings amplify and enhance the content of each chapter. Batshaw presents a significant amount of material in a clear and concise manner, and his supportive approach will help parents meet the challenge of caring for a child with greater needs.—*Kathryn Hammell Carpenter, University of Illinois, Chicago*

TEETH AND GUMS

The Mount Sinai Medical Center Family Guide to Dental Health.
Klatell, Jack, and others. Macmillan. ISBN 0-02-563675-8. $24.95.

The recent revolution in dental technology and treatment has made a visit to the dentist something no one need fear and promises that teeth can last a lifetime. This guide discusses that revolution, presenting a large amount of scientifically sound information in a clear and easy-to-read text. While it does not offer a "Pollyanna" view of dental care and disease, it takes a reassuring but factual tone in describing what diseases affect the mouth, how to care for the teeth and gums, and what to expect in the dentist's office. Nothing comparable is available.—*Aletha Kowitz, Bureau of Library Services, American Dental Association, Chicago*

TRANSPLANTS

Organ Transplants: A Patient's Guide.
Massachusetts General Hospital Organ Transplant Team and H. F. Pizer. Harvard University Press. ISBN 0-674-64235-X. $24.95.

This is essentially a very practical and useful guide for a specialized but growing audience. (Over 14,000 people had organ transplants in 1990.) Its only major limitation is that, with any luck, this title will be quickly out of date as technology and drug regimens improve. Basically comprehensible to a knowledgeable layperson, the book describes transplants of the heart, lung, kidney, pancreas, liver, and bone marrow. In the discussion of the careful balancing of immunosuppression, which tries to avoid both rejection and infection, the depth of information on the biology of the immune system and immunosuppressant drugs may be more than some readers want or need. Psychosocial aspects could have benefited from more attention, and information on further resources such as self-help groups and other organizations would have also been useful. Heavy going at times, but recommended.—*Mary Chitty, Massachusetts College of Pharmacy and Allied Health Sciences Library, Boston*

Sweet Reprieve: One Couple's Journey to the Frontiers of Medicine.
Maier, Frank, with Ginny Maier. Crown. ISBN 0-517-58161-2. $20.

Frank Maier, *Newsweek*'s Chicago bureau chief, writes with wit, style, and grace about his liver transplant, the most complex single-organ operation of its kind. The first journalist to undergo this surgery and the only transplant patient to write of the experience, he describes the sudden onset of odd symptoms—vertigo, confusion, fatigue—and his subsequent denial of the possibility of illness. His determined wife, Ginny, took over, scheduling Frank at the Mayo Clinic, where tests showed chronic viral hepatitis C had ravaged his liver. Facing a terminal situation, Frank was given a second chance with the transplanted liver of a teenage boy in Louisiana. Although Frank lost his final battle on December 31, 1990, he left a legacy of inspiration and triumph; his son Michael added a postscript to the finished book. This sad but uplifting memoir fills a gap in the available literature.—*Janet Coggan, University of Florida Libraries, Gainesville*

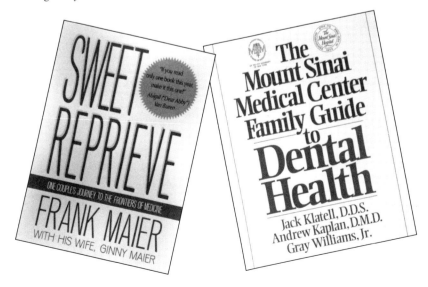

WHERE TO GET HELP

Listed here are some of the major organizations in the United States providing information about good health practices generally or about specific conditions and how to deal with them. The first four sources below are general ones. The rest are listed under the condition or disease they are concerned with; these conditions are in alphabetical order. Most organizations can be reached at a toll-free telephone number (identifiable by the 800 prefix). Where there isn't a toll-free number, an address is also given when possible.

GENERAL SOURCES

Centers for Disease Control Voice Information System
Tape-recorded information about public health topics, such as AIDS, Lyme disease, and chronic fatigue syndrome. Also, you can request to talk with a CDC expert during business hours, Eastern Standard Time.
404-332-4555

National Health Information Center
Provides phone numbers for more than 1,000 health-related organizations and offers various printed materials.
800-336-4797; in Maryland, 301-565-4167

National Institutes of Health
Bethesda, MD 20892
Free information, including the latest research findings, on a wide range of diseases.
301-496-4000

Tel-Med
Tape-recorded information on over 600 health topics. Sponsored by local medical societies, health organizations, or hospitals.
Check the phone book for local listings or call Tel-Med headquarters at 714-825-6034

AGING

National Council on the Aging
800-424-9046

AIDS

National AIDS Hotline
800-342-AIDS; in Spanish, 800-344-SIDA; for the hearing impaired, 800-AIDS-TTY

ALCOHOLISM AND DRUG ABUSE

Alcohol Abuse Emergency
800-ALCOHOL

National Clearinghouse for Alcohol and Drug Abuse
P.O. Box 2345
Rockville, MD 20852
301-468-2600

National Cocaine Hotline
800-COCAINE

National Council on Alcoholism and Drug Dependence Hopeline
800-475-HOPE

National Institute for Drug Abuse
800-662-HELP; in Spanish, 800-66-AYUDA

ALZHEIMER'S DISEASE

Alzheimer's Association
800-621-0379; in Illinois, 800-572-6037

ARTHRITIS

Arthritis Foundation
800-283-7800

ASTHMA AND ALLERGIES

Asthma and Allergy Foundation Patient Information Line
800-7-ASTHMA

Asthma Information Line
800-822-ASMA

National Jewish Center for Immunology and Respiratory Medicine Information Service
800-222-LUNG

AUTISM

National Autism Hotline
304-525-8014

BLINDNESS AND EYE CARE

American Foundation for the Blind
800-AF-BLIND; in New York State, 212-620-2147

Blind Children's Center
800-222-3566; in California, 800-222-3567

National Eye Care Project Helpline
800-222-EYES

NSPB (National Society to Prevent Blindness) Center for Sight
800-221-3004

CANCER

American Cancer Society
800-ACS-2345

National Cancer Institute's Cancer Information Service
800-4-CANCER

CEREBRAL PALSY

United Cerebral Palsy Associations
800-USA-5UCP; in Washington, D.C., 202-842-1266

CHILD ABUSE

Childhelp's National Child Abuse Hotline
800-4-A-CHILD

National Child Safety Council Childwatch
800-222-1464

National Center for Missing and Exploited Children
800-843-5678; for the hearing impaired, 800-826-7653; in Arlington, Va., 702-235-3900

Parents Anonymous Hotline
800-421-0353; in California, 800-352-0386

CYSTIC FIBROSIS

Cystic Fibrosis Foundation
800-FIGHT-CF; in Maryland, 301-951-4422

DIABETES

American Diabetes Association
800-ADA-DISC; in Virginia and Washington, D.C., 703-549-1500

Juvenile Diabetes Foundation Hotline
800-223-1138; in New York City, 212-889-7575

DOWN SYNDROME

National Down Syndrome Congress
800-232-6372; in Illinois, 312-823-7550

National Down Syndrome Society
800-221-4602; in New York City, 212-460-9330

DYSLEXIA

Orton Dyslexia Society
800-ABCD-123; in Maryland, 301-296-0232

EATING DISORDERS

Bulimia/Anorexia Self-Help Hotline
800-227-4785

National Anorexic Aid Society
1925 East Dublin-Granville Road
Columbus, Ohio 43229-3517
614-436-1112

EPILEPSY

Epilepsy Foundation of America
800-332-1000

HEADACHES

National Headache Foundation
800-843-2256; in Illinois, 800-523-8858

HEAD INJURIES

National Head Injury Foundation
800-444-NHIF

HEARING

American Speech-Language-Hearing Association Helpline
800-638-8255; in Maryland call collect, 301-897-0039

Hearing Helpline
800-327-9355; in Virginia, 703-642-0580

HEART DISEASE

American Heart Association National Center
7272 Greenville Avenue
Dallas, TX 75231
214-373-6300

National Heart, Lung, and Blood Institute Information Office
9000 Rockville Pike
Building 31-4A21
Bethesda, MD 20892
301-496-4236

HOSPICES

Hospice Education Institute Hospicelink
800-331-1620; in Connecticut, 203-767-1620

IMPOTENCE

Impotence Information Center
800-843-4315

KIDNEY DISEASES

National Kidney Foundation
800-622-9010

LIVER DISEASES

American Liver Foundation
800-223-0179; in New Jersey, 201-256-2550

LUNG DISEASES

American Lung Association
Check the phone book for local listings or call the national office at 212-315-8700

National Jewish Center for Immunology and Respiratory Medicine Information Service
800-222-LUNG

LUPUS

Lupus Foundation of America
800-558-0121; in Rockville, Md., 301-670-9292

MENTAL HEALTH

American Mental Health Fund
800-433-5959; in Illinois, 800-826-2336

National Foundation for Depressive Illness
800-248-4344

MULTIPLE SCLEROSIS

National Multiple Sclerosis Society
800-624-8236

NUTRITION

USDA Food Safety and Inspection Service Meat and Poultry Hot Line
800-535-4555

University of Alabama at Birmingham Nutrition Information Service
800-231-DIET

ORGAN DONATION

Organ Donor Hotline
800-24-DONOR

The Living Bank
800-528-2971; in Texas, 713-528-2971

PAIN

National Chronic Pain Outreach Association
7979 Old Georgetown Road
Suite 100
Bethesda, MD 20814-2429
301-652-4948

PARKINSON'S DISEASE

Parkinson's Educational Program
800-344-7872; in California, 714-250-2975

National Parkinson's Foundation
800-327-4545; in Florida, 800-433-7022; in Miami, 305-547-6666

PROSTATE PROBLEMS

Prostate Information Line
800-543-9632

RARE DISEASES

National Information Center for Orphan Drugs and Rare Diseases
800-456-3505; in Maryland, 301-565-4167

National Organization for Rare Disorders
800-999-NORD; in Connecticut, 203-746-6518

REHABILITATION

National Rehabilitation Information Center
800-34-NARIC; in Maryland, 301-588-9284

SEXUALLY TRANSMITTED DISEASES

American Social Health Association's National STD Hotline
800-227-8922

SICKLE CELL DISEASE

National Association for Sickle Cell Disease
800-421-8453; in California, 213-736-5455

SPINAL INJURIES

American Paralysis Association's Spinal Cord Injury Hotline
800-526-3456

National Spinal Cord Injury Association
800-962-9629; in Massachusetts, 617-935-2722

STROKE

National Stroke Association
800-787-6537

SUDDEN INFANT DEATH SYNDROME

American Sudden Infant Death Syndrome Institute
800-232-SIDS; in Georgia, 800-847-7437

NEW MEDICATIONS AND DRUGS

Prescription medications and drugs cannot be sold in the United States unless they have been approved by the Food and Drug Administration. The following pages describe notable ones that have recently gone on the market after FDA approval. Products are listed in alphabetical order under the type of condition for which they are used; conditions are also listed in alphabetical order. The drug or medication's generic name is given first, followed by the brand name in parentheses.

Cancer

Name: Altretamine (Hexalen)
Usage: This anticancer drug recently received FDA approval for use as second-line treatment of women with advanced **ovarian cancer**. Some patients whose cancer persisted or recurred after treatment with the current first-line combination of cisplatin (Platinol) and two other standard chemotherapeutic agents have improved for a time when treated with altretamine alone. Women with this hard-to-treat type of cancer who respond to this drug have shown a decrease in size of tumor masses, reduced disease symptoms, and increased ability to carry on their daily activities.
Side Effects: Nausea and vomiting often occur but can usually be controlled by antiemetic drug treatment. Drug-induced effects on sensory and motor nerve fibers sometimes cause numbness, tingling, pain, and muscle weakness. Bone marrow damage may reduce the number of white and red blood cells and platelets circulating in the bloodstream.
Comments: This drug was first found active against ovarian cancer more than a quarter of a century ago. However, its use was almost abandoned because of severe toxicity caused by the excessively high doses then employed. Recent studies sponsored by the National Cancer Institute have shown that when altretamine is given in lower doses at intervals of two weeks or longer, it is both better tolerated than and just as effective as the earlier, toxic, high doses.

Name: Filgrastim (Neupogen)
Usage: This biological product prepared by genetic engineering was approved for use in preventing **infections** that tend to develop in cancer patients receiving anticancer drugs. It is used specifically in feverish patients with very low levels of a type of white blood cell called neutrophils, or granulocytes, that attack foreign invaders. This condition, called neutropenia, or granulocytopenia, occurs as a result of bone marrow damage by the cancer chemotherapy drugs. Filgrastim stimulates the growth of bone marrow cell colonies that develop into new neutrophils, or granulocytes, that then circulate in the cancer patient's bloodstream.
Side Effects: The most common side effect of filgrastim is pain that has its origin in the patient's bones. It can usually be controlled by nonnarcotic pain killers.

Name: Fludarabine (Fludara)
Usage: This new anticancer drug is used to treat patients with B-cell **chronic lymphocytic leukemia (CLL)**

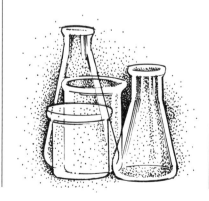

that has not responded to standard leukemia therapy. Patients treated in clinical trials had complete remissions in 13 percent of cases. Others with partial responses showed reduced size of lymph nodes, liver, and spleen, plus improved blood cell counts and fewer bone marrow abnormalities. Survival time in some patients unresponsive to other drugs doubled after several 5-day treatment courses repeated every 28 days.
Side Effects: Bone marrow suppression often followed by chills and fever caused by infections occurs commonly. Loss of appetite, nausea and vomiting, and fatigue and weakness are other complaints.

Name: Gallium nitrate (Ganite)
Usage: This salt of the element gallium helps lower excessively high levels of calcium in the blood of patients with various kinds of cancer. This lessens the discomforting and dangerous symptoms of cancer-caused **hypercalcemia**, an often life-threatening complication of breast cancer and other solid tumors in the ovaries, lungs, and other organs.
Side Effects: This drug can adversely affect kidney function, especially in patients whose kidneys are already impaired by hypercalcemia and who have lost a lot of body fluids. All patients must be adequately rehydrated with salty fluids before being given gallium nitrate solution by intravenous infusion. This drug should not be used by patients with severely damaged kidneys, and it should not be given if the patient is taking certain antibi-

otics that can also affect kidney function adversely.

Name: Ondansetron (Zofran)
Usage: This drug prevents the **nausea and vomiting** that occur in up to 90 percent of patients who receive chemotherapy for treating cancers of the ovaries, bladder, lungs, or head and neck. It is claimed safer and more effective than any of the antiemetic drugs that have previously been available to prevent or relieve this distressing condition.
Side Effects: Most of the side effects that occur in close to half the patients who are treated with ondansetron before they receive cancer chemotherapy are minor ones—consisting mainly of headache and diarrhea.

Name: Pamidronate (Aredia IV)
Usage: This drug, one of a class of chemicals that bind to bones and affect their calcium content, is highly effective for lowering excessively high blood calcium levels to normal in patients with cancer-associated **hypercalcemia**. It helps both patients with cancers that have spread to their bones and those with tumors that secrete substances able to break down bony tissue and release its calcium into the bloodstream. By blocking this calcium-releasing action, each pamidronate treatment brings about a remission of hypercalcemia-caused symptoms for two or three weeks. This improves patients' kidney function and reduces the risk of bone fractures and other symptoms.
Side Effects: The drug's most common side effect is mild fever that usually develops on the day after it is first given. Some patients also lose their appetite and become nauseated. Tissue around the vein into which this drug is dripped for 24 hours often becomes red, swollen, and painful to the touch.
Comments: Before infusing pamidronate, doctors must administer salt solution to overcome dehydration caused by hypercalcemia. Their goal is to keep the patient's urine output at about two quarts daily while the pamidronate is reducing blood calcium levels.

Name: Pentostatin (Nipent)
Usage: This drug recently received FDA approval for use in patients with **hairy cell leukemia** that had failed to respond to treatment with the standard drug alpha interferon (Intron A; Roferon-A). In clinical trials of pentostatin in this rare type of leukemia, 58 percent of patients responded with complete clearing of leukemic cells from their circulating blood and bone marrow and a decrease in size of enlarged lymph nodes and other organs. Another 28 percent of patients had a partial response to drug therapy—a decrease of 50 percent or more in blood and bone marrow cancer cells and in the size of lymph nodes and other organs. These responses lasted close to three years in some cases before relapses occurred.
Side Effects: Most drug reactions were mild to moderate, and only 11 percent of patients withdrew from trials because of adverse events. Most common were decreases in white and red blood cells and in platelets as a result of bone marrow suppression by the drug or the disease. Kidney function is checked before the start of treatment and periodically during drug therapy. If patients with impaired renal function are treated at all, they receive lower doses so that the drug will not accumulate to toxic levels.

Name: Sargramostim (Leukine; Prokine)
Usage: This genetically engineered biological product is used to speed the growth of **bone marrow transplants**. Administered by intravenous infusion to patients with such cancers as Hodgkin's disease, non-Hodgkin's lymphoma, or acute lymphoblastic leukemia, sargramostim stimulates development of two types of infection-fighting white blood cells—granulocytes, or neutrophils, and macrophages. Its use in the period after bone marrow has been transplanted reduces the length of infection episodes and the number of days patients have to be hospitalized and receive antibiotics.
Side Effects: In clinical trials, this drug rarely caused more side effects than an injected placebo (inactive

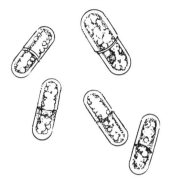

medication). The only events that occurred slightly more often with sargramostim were diarrhea, rash, and feelings of weakness or general discomfort.

Cardiovascular Disorders

Name: Benazepril (Lotensin)
Usage: This drug is effective for lowering **high blood pressure** in patients of all ages and is claimed especially safe for patients aged 55 or over. A member of the fast-growing class of antihypertensive drugs called angiotensin-converting enzyme (ACE) inhibitors, benazepril acts by blocking conversion of angiotensin I, an inactive substance circulating in the blood, to angiotensin II, a powerful pressure-raising hormone. This leads to the desired drop in patients' blood pressure.
Side Effects: Most patients tolerate this drug quite well, but about 1 in 20 discontinued taking it during clinical trials because of cough, headache, dizziness, or fatigue. In about 1 of every 200 patients treated, swelling of the lips and face develops. If such sudden edema extends to the tongue and throat tissues, emergency measures must be promptly employed to prevent potentially deadly obstruction of the airway.

Name: Bepridil (Vascor)
Usage: This is a new member of the calcium channel blockers, a class of drugs that dilate, or widen, blood vessels in the heart and elsewhere. It is reserved for patients with **chronic angina pectoris** whose episodes of chest pain persist despite treatment with other safer antianginal drugs. Taken alone, or added to

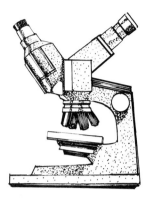

the treatment plan of patients already taking a beta blocker such as propranolol (Inderal) or a nitrate like nitroglycerin (both types of drugs used to lower high blood pressure), bepridil reduces the frequency of anginal attacks and improves patients' ability to perform the activities of their daily lives. Unlike other calcium antagonists, bepridil is not recommended for treating high blood pressure.

Side Effects: The most common side effects are nausea and complaints of stomach discomfort or abdominal pain and diarrhea. Dizziness, headache, and feelings of fatigue, weakness, and nervousness are also often reported. Much more serious is this drug's tendency to set off dangerous heart rhythm irregularities. For this reason, use of bepridil is not recommended for relief of chest pains in patients recovering from a recent heart attack.

Comments: This drug is best not given to patients who are taking other drugs that also affect the heart's rate and rhythm. Its tendency to affect cardiac rhythm adversely is also increased in patients with low blood serum levels of potassium. So before treatment is begun, patients' potassium levels are checked, and if these are low, the potassium deficiency is first corrected.

Name: Felodipine (Plendil)
Usage: A single daily dose of this drug for treating **high blood pressure** keeps patients' blood pressure under control for 24 hours when taken alone or combined with other pressure-reducing drugs. Like other drugs of its class, this calcium chan-

nel blocker widens blood vessels by blocking passage of calcium ions into the smooth muscle cells of arterial walls. The resulting reduction in resistance to blood flow lowers high blood pressure.

Side Effects: The most common side effect seen during clinical trials was swelling of the feet and ankles. It occurred most commonly in elderly patients taking high doses, but only about 1 in every 25 patients discontinued treatment. Other reasons for withdrawing felodipine were headache, flushing, and dizziness caused by excessive dilation of blood vessels in the head and face. On rare occasions, too great a fall in blood pressure may make a patient faint. Patients are advised to practice good dental hygiene to prevent drug-induced swelling of their gums, a reaction reported in less than 0.5 percent of patients.

Name: Fosinopril (Monopril)
Usage: A single daily dose of this new ACE inhibitor, a type of drug that blocks the production of a pressure-raising hormone in the blood, is enough to keep most patients' **high blood pressure** down for 24 hours. Those in whom its effects do not last that long may divide the drug's total daily dose in two and take it twice daily. Patients whose blood pressure is not fully controlled by fosinopril alone may respond with a further drop in pressure when a diuretic-type antihypertensive agent, which helps remove excess fluid from the body, is also taken.

Side Effects: In clinical trials, side effects were mild and transient and occurred no more often with fosinopril than in patients taking an inactive tablet (placebo). Among symptoms that have led to the drug's being discontinued in about 4 percent of patients are headache, cough, fatigue, diarrhea, nausea, and vomiting. Some patients become lightheaded and may even faint if their blood pressure drops too far and too fast.

Name: Isradipine (DynaCirc)
Usage: This calcium channel blocker reduces **high blood pressure** by widening blood vessels when

taken twice daily alone or together with a diuretic such as hydrochlorothiazide, which helps rid the body of excess fluids. Its artery-dilating action brings pressure down to normal in two out of three patients with high blood pressure. Doubling the daily dosage raises the number of responding patients to four out of five.

Side Effects: This drug is generally well-tolerated, and its side effects are mostly mild and transient. Most common are headache, dizziness, fluid retention, fever, and abdominal discomfort. Patients with normal heart function do not develop heartbeat irregularities or reduced pumping power. However, a too sudden drop in blood pressure has on rare occasions set off heart palpitations and fainting. Caution is required in patients suffering from congestive heart failure, especially when they take isradipine together with a heart-slowing beta blocker drug.

Comments: To keep this drug from making a patient's blood pressure drop too quickly, it is best taken with food to slow its absorption into the bloodstream. This also lessens the likelihood of the patient's developing dizziness and feelings of fatigue and weakness.

Name: Pravastatin (Pravachol)
Usage: This drug lowers **elevated blood cholesterol** levels when added to the treatment of patients who have failed to respond fully to a low-fat, low-cholesterol diet alone. Taken once daily at bedtime, it significantly reduces total blood cholesterol and low-density lipoprotein (LDL or "bad") cholesterol while raising high-density lipoprotein (HDL) cholesterol, the type that is often called "good" cholesterol because of its ability to remove excess cholesterol from the walls of arteries. These actions slow development of artery blockage in the heart, brain, and other organs. This reduces the patient's risk of heart attacks and strokes.

Side Effects: Patients occasionally complain of muscle aches and weakness. If this is accompanied by fever and a marked increase in blood levels of an enzyme that is released from injured skeletal muscles, this drug may have to be discontinued. A more common reason for stopping treatment is a rise in blood serum levels of liver enzymes, especially if the patient also complains of abdominal discomfort and loss of appetite. Pravastatin must not be taken by patients with liver disease or by pregnant women and nursing mothers. Drug-induced interference with biosynthesis of cholesterol and essential hormones and other substances made from it can harm the developing fetus or slow down infant growth rates.

Name: Quinapril (Accupril)
Usage: This ACE inhibitor, which lowers blood pressure by inhibiting the production of a pressure-raising blood hormone, was the fourth drug of this class to become available in 1991 for treating **high blood pressure**. It is recommended for use alone once a day as first-line treatment of hypertension. Many patients respond to such so-called monotherapy with a drop of their blood pressure to normal levels as the drug's dosage is gradually adjusted upward to an amount that is optimally tailored to each individual's needs.

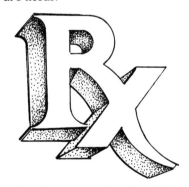

Side Effects: As with other ACE inhibitors, the frequency of side effects is relatively low, and most drug-induced discomfort is mild and transient, with fewer than 5 percent of patients withdrawing from clinical trials. The most common side effects are headache, dizziness, fatigue, cough, nausea, and abdominal pain. A potentially serious side effect is angioedema, or development of swelling of the face, lips, tongue, and, most dangerously,

of the voice box, or larynx, a condition that on rare occasions has led to patients choking to death.

Name: Ramipril (Altace)
Usage: This ACE inhibitor is used to treat mild to moderately **high blood pressure**; this type of drug inhibits the production of a pressure-raising blood hormone. To avoid too sudden a drop in pressure, treatment is begun with a single small daily dose that is then gradually adjusted upward to the optimal level for keeping the patient's blood pressure under control for 24 hours. Ramipril is recommended as a first-line drug for initiating treatment of high blood pressure. However, it is also sometimes used as a second drug that is added to the treatment schedule of patients who were first started on a diuretic-type antihypertensive drug, which helps the body get rid of excess fluid.
Side Effects: Among side effects most frequently reported are headache, dizziness, and fatigue. In one clinical trial, 12 percent of patients developed a dry, tickly cough that became annoying enough to make one-third of them withdraw from the study. As happens with other ACE inhibitors, some patients taking ramipril develop swelling of the voice box after taking their very first dose. Although such reactions are rare, all patients starting treatment are advised to stop taking their medication and report this symptom to their doctor right away, as fatal asphyxiation can occur.

Name: Ticlopidine (Ticlid)
Usage: This drug reduces the risk of patients suffering a brain-damaging **stroke** caused by a blood clot that blocks a brain artery. It acts by preventing blood particles called platelets from sticking together to form clots in blood vessels narrowed by cholesterol-containing growths on their inner walls. Ticlopidine is used to treat two types of patients: those with symptoms that suggest they are at risk of a first major stroke, and those who have already had a clot-induced stroke and show signs that they are threatened by another similar event.

Side Effects: More than half the patients treated complain of at least one side effect. Most common are gastrointestinal symptoms such as diarrhea, nausea or vomiting, and abdominal pain. These or a rash or a marked reduction in white blood cells led one of every four patients in clinical trials to discontinue treatment.
Comments: Ticlopidine is reserved for patients who cannot take aspirin, which, in small, regular doses, also decreases the risk of stroke. Patients taking this new drug must have their blood tested every two weeks during the first three months of treatment to detect any significant drop in white blood cell counts. They are also taught to report such early signs of infection as chills, fever, or a sore throat.

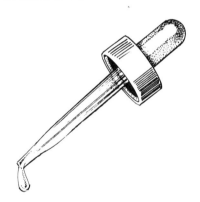

Eyes

Name: Dapiprazole Ophthalmic Eyedrops (Rev-Eyes)
Usage: Eye doctors can now use these drops to reverse the action of other drops that were applied previously to dilate a patient's pupils. Such dilation is needed to help ophthalmologists detect a detached retina, tumor, or other abnormalities at the back of the eyeball. However, drug-induced dilation of the pupil persists for several hours after the eye exam has ended and often causes discomfort and inconvenience. So dapiprazole drops are used right after the diagnostic procedure is completed to make the dilated pupils contract and return to normal size in 30 minutes to an hour. This relieves blurry vision and glare discomfort (photophobia).

315

Side Effects: Soon after dapiprazole drops are applied, blood vessels in the whites of the eyes of over 80 percent of patients become congested for about 20 minutes, and about half the patients feel some transient burning or itching. Between 10 and 40 percent of patients show some redness and swelling of their eyelids or other mild signs and symptoms.

Comments: Patients are cautioned not to drive at night soon after treatment with dapiprazole drops, as drug-induced constriction of the previously dilated pupils may make it difficult for their eyes to adapt to darkness and may also reduce their field of vision.

Infections

Name: Azithromycin (Zithromax)
Usage: A new antibiotic in the same chemical class as erythromycin, which has been in use for 40 years, is claimed safer and more effective than that well-known antibacterial drug. It acts against a wider spectrum of bacterial pathogens, including *Hemophilus influenzae*, a common cause of respiratory infections in children and others. It is approved for use in pediatric middle ear infections. Because the drug concentrates within cells that have been invaded by bacteria such as *Mycoplasma pneumoniae* and *Legionella pneumophila*, azithromycin is effective for treating the unusual types of pneumonia caused by these intracellular microbes. A single-dose treatment is also effective for treating infections of the genitourinary tract caused by *Chlamydia trachomatis*, the cause of the most common sexually transmitted disease (called chlamydia) in the United States.
Side Effects: The most common side effects involve the gastrointestinal tract, but these occur only about half as often as with erythromycin and tend to be transient and mild.

Name: Ciprofloxacin Ophthalmic Solution (Ciloxan)
Usage: This is an antimicrobial drug for treatment of bacterial infections involving the outer lining of the eye (conjunctivitis) and of ulcers on the cornea.
Side Effects: The solution may cause transient irritation, stinging, and redness.
Comments: This is the first quinoline-class antimicrobial drug that has been approved in the form of drops for the eye.

Name: Clarithromycin (Biaxin)
Usage: This new antibiotic, a chemical relative of the standard antibacterial agent erythromycin, has been approved by the FDA for use mainly in treating bacterial infections of the **respiratory tract**. Among infections of upper respiratory structures for which it is effective are sore throat (pharyngitis), tonsillitis, and sinusitis. The drug and the bactericidal by-product to which it is converted in the body also reach high concentrations in lower respiratory tract tissues such as the lungs and bronchial tubes. This accounts for their effectiveness in treating pneumonia and the acute bacterial infections that often develop suddenly in patients with chronic bronchitis.
Side Effects: Most of the side effects of clarithromycin are mild and transient, and only about 3 percent of patients have to discontinue treatment. Most commonly reported complaints are an abnormal taste, nausea, abdominal discomfort, diarrhea, and headache. The percentage of patients with gastrointestinal side effects is much lower than with erythromycin.

Name: Didanosine (DDI; Videx)
Usage: This antiviral drug slows replication of the **human immunodeficiency virus** (HIV), the cause of AIDS. It is approved for treating patients with AIDS who cannot tolerate zidovudine (AZT; Retrovir) or whose condition has continued to

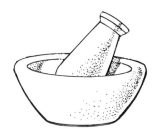

deteriorate during treatment with that drug, the only antiviral agent previously approved for treatment of AIDS.
Side Effects: This drug does not cause the severe anemia or persistent nausea that make many AIDS patients discontinue zidovudine. However, some patients taking didanosine have developed dangerous inflammation of the pancreas. So doctors watch patients for early signs and symptoms of pancreatitis that may make it necessary to discontinue this drug. More commonly reported side effects are numbness, tingling, and pain in the hands and feet. Other discomforting drug effects are diarrhea, headache, dizziness, and mental changes such as nervousness and confusion.
Comments: The FDA has been criticized for approving didanosine before its efficacy and safety were fully proven. The agency cleared the drug for general use against AIDS on the basis of its ability to boost patients' blood counts of T-4 type immune cells. However, unlike zidovudine, this second anti-HIV drug has not yet been shown to lengthen the lives of AIDS patients. Neither drug is a cure for AIDS.

Name: Foscarnet (Foscavir)
Usage: This drug received FDA approval for treating an AIDS-related eye infection that can cause blindness. It suppresses a herpesvirus called cytomegalovirus (CMV) that often attacks the retinas of people whose immune system has been impaired by AIDS. Foscarnet, like ganciclovir, a drug approved earlier for treating **CMV retinitis**, does not cure this AIDS complication. However, it lessens inflammation of this eye structure that is essential for sight and slows the progressive retinal damage.
Side Effects: The most common side effects of foscarnet are fever, nausea and vomiting, and diarrhea. More serious is drug-induced kidney damage and possible seizures, anemia, and reduced blood levels of calcium and other essential elements.
Comments: Within one month after FDA approval of foscarnet for treating CMV retinitis, the National Eye

Institute announced the results of a study showing that patients taking the drug were also living longer than those who were being treated with ganciclovir. The lengthened survival time suggests that foscarnet may control HIV, the AIDS virus, as well as CMV, the virus responsible for retinitis.

Name: Interferon gamma-1b (Actimmune)
Usage: This genetically engineered human immune system protein is used to reduce the frequency and severity of serious infections in patients with **chronic granulomatous disease** (CGD). This is a rare inherited disorder that usually begins in early childhood and leads to death from infection by pus-producing bacteria such as *Staphylococcus aureus* or by other pathogens, including the parasites responsible for toxoplasmosis and leishmaniasis. The drug is injected under the skin three times a week by a doctor, a nurse, or a family member who has been trained to give it correctly at home.
Side Effects: The most common side effects are fever, chills, headache, muscle pain, and fatigue. These flu-like symptoms may be minimized by giving the injections at bedtime. Acetaminophen (Tylenol and other brand names) helps to prevent the fever and relieve the headache.

Name: Norfloxacin Ophthalmic Solution (Chibroxin)
Usage: This solution of the fluoroquinoline-class antibacterial is dropped into the eyes of children or adults to treat "pink eye" (**conjunctivitis**, or inflammation of the mucous membranes lining the eyelid and covering the visible part of the eye) caused by a wide range of bacteria including *Hemophilus influenzae*, a common cause of eye infections in youngsters who are one year of age or older.
Side Effects: The most frequently reported side effect is local burning or discomfort. Conjunctival swelling and redness are also sometimes seen, and patients may complain of a bitter taste when the drug solution is absorbed into the bloodstream from the surface of the eye.

Name: Ofloxacin (Floxin)
Usage: This new fluoroquinolone-class antibacterial is effective against a broad spectrum of pathogens responsible for respiratory and urinary tract infections and the sexually transmitted diseases gonorrhea and chlamydia. Taken orally twice daily at 12-hour intervals, this drug reaches high concentrations in the blood, urine, and infected organs such as the lungs and hard-to-penetrate prostate gland tissues. It is the first drug of its class given FDA approval to treat chronic bacterial prostatitis caused by *Escherichia coli*, a common infection in older men. Treatment of prostatitis takes six weeks, but acute urinary tract infections can be cleared up in three days, and a single dose of ofloxacin cures acute gonorrhea.
Side Effects: The most commonly reported side effects are nausea, headache, insomnia, dizziness, and diarrhea.
Comments: While most side effects are mild, serious and sometimes fatal allergic reactions have occurred. This drug should not be used by people known to be allergic to other quinoline-type anti-infective drugs, nor by pregnant women or nursing mothers.

Name: Podofilox (Condylox)
Usage: The active ingredient of this drug is isolated from the plant extract podophyllin resin; it became available in a low concentration alcoholic solution for application to external **genital warts** caused by strains of the human papillomavirus (HPV). Patients apply the solution once in the morning and once in the evening for three days in a row, and then stop using it for the next four days. After three treatment weeks most of the patients' warts have cleared. However, about 30 percent of the warts tend to recur, so, as with all other types of treatment for genital warts, these courses of topical application must often be repeated.
Side Effects: Most patients feel some itching, burning, or pain in the treated areas. These symptoms and associated redness, soreness, and tenderness are usually transient. However, if inflammation,

swelling, bleeding, or excessive pain occur, patients are instructed to stop any further applications and contact the doctor.

Insomnia

Name: Estazolam (ProSom)
Usage: This central nervous system depressant drug received FDA approval for short-term treatment of **chronic insomnia**. Clinical trials comparing it with other sleep-producing drugs of the same chemical class and with a placebo proved that estazolam was effective for putting patients to sleep more quickly when they had difficulty in falling asleep. It also increased the total sleep time of patients with severe anxiety and depression who were prone to frequent awakenings during the night and to wakening too early in the morning. Sleep lab scientists noted marked to moderate improvement, and some patients reported that they felt refreshed upon arising.
Side Effects: The most commonly reported side effects are some degree of drowsiness or lethargy during daytime waking hours. Some patients complain of headaches and nervousness. While patients taking bedtime doses nightly for up to 12 weeks in clinical trials did not become tolerant to estazolam or show signs that the drug was accumulating in the brain or body, some who discontinued it abruptly suffered withdrawal signs and symptoms including generalized feelings of discomfort (dysphoria) and increased anxiety.
Comments: Estazolam is a close chemical cousin of triazolam (Halcion), a widely used hypnotic that was banned in Britain in October 1991 after reports of psychiatric reactions including depression and memory impairment. The FDA labeling for this new drug warns that amnesia and impaired thinking and motor coordination are possible with all drugs of this class.
MORTON J. RODMAN, PH.D.

Morton J. Rodman is Professor Emeritus of Pharmacology, Rutgers University, New Brunswick, N.J.

Index

Page number in *italics* indicates the reference is to an illustration.

A

Abortion
free speech issue, 245
multiple pregnancy fetus
reduction, 280
Accidents
air travel (avoidance), 50
head injuries, 212
oil industry contract workers,
255
see also Safety
Accupril, *see* Quinapril
Accutane, *see* Isotrentinoin
ACE inhibitors
antihypertensive drugs, 313,
314, 315
ACEP, *see* American College of
Emergency Physicians
Acer, David
HIV-infected healthcare workers
issue, 286
Acetaminophen
osteoarthritis, 164
pain relief, 54-55, 56, 57
Acetazolamide
smell/taste disorders, 148
Acidity
water, 32
Acne
cause and treatment, 205
Actimmune, *see* Interferon gamma-
1b
Acute lymphoblastic leukemia
gene therapy, 313
Acute promyelocytic leukemia
retinoic acid, 248
Acyclovir
herpes, 238
Addiction, *see* Alcoholism; Drug
abuse
Additives
foods and cosmetics, 276
Adenomatous polyposis coli (APC)
colon cancer, 249, 257
Adenosine
food-fuel conversion, 259
Adkins, Janet
Alzheimer's disease, 272
Adolescents
AIDS prevention, 285
bacterial meningitis, 182
gum disease, 290
skin problems, 205
suicide, 266
wrestlers' herpes, 238
Adult seborrheic dermatitis
cause and treatment, 205
Advertising
cereal claims, 104
convenience food claims, 278
nutrition claims, 277
pharmaceutical, 276
Advil, *see* Ibuprofen
**Advisory Committee on
Immunization Practices**
hepatitis B vaccine, 282

**Advisory Council on Social
Security**
healthcare costs, 258
Aerobic exercise
fibromyalgia, 208
muscle-mass loss, 81
protein needs, 100
Africa
AIDS, 285
protein deficiencies, 106
Afterloss
grief support group, 198
Aging and the aged, 241-242
bone loss, 83
cataracts, 232-233
constipation, 193
flu vaccine recommendation,
287
hospital day-care, 211
hypertension treatment, 266
injury from falls, 212, 214
middle age, 215-218
music therapy, 209-211
prostate cancer, 223
septicemia, 174
skin problems, 205, 206
strength loss and training, 83,
87
taste and smell, 147
women's health study, 261
Agriculture, U.S. Department of
dietary guidelines, 74, 79, 277,
278
food nutrition labeling, 277
yogurt benefits, 200
AIDS
boarder babies, 64-71
Canadian policies, 261
drug approval speed-up, 288,
289
drugs, 261, 286, 316
heterosexuals, 284
infected healthcare workers,
245, 251, 286
Magic Johnson, 269
public health, 284-286
tuberculosis cases, 288
Air pollution
exercise concerns, 178
eye redness, 202
lead, 253
mercury, 252
Air travel
health tips, 44-53
**Albert and Mary Lasker
Foundation**
award, 270
Alcohol consumption
air travel, 47-48, 51, 52
beneficial cardiac effects, 264,
279
lowered pancreatic cancer risk,
250
panic disorder, 226
postconcussion syndrome linked
to lowered tolerance, 214
see also Wine

Alcoholism
liver disease, 12
protein deficiency, 106
Allergies
conjunctivitis, 202, 203
fluoroquinolone-class
antibacterials, 317
nonprescription painkillers, 55
sinus problems, 234, 235
skin disorders, 205, 206
smell and taste disorders, 146
Allogenic transplantation
organs and tissues, 8
Alpha interferon
hairy cell leukemia, 313
Alpha-thalassemia
research, 271
ALS, *see* Amyotrophic lateral
sclerosis
Altace, *see* Ramipril
Altretamine
cancer drug, 312
Altruism
in middle years, 218
Alzheimer's disease
genetic defect, 255
medication, 242
music therapy, 210, 211
right to die case, 272
sensor bracelet tags, 281
AMA, *see* American Medical
Association
**American Association for the
Advancement of Science**
online journal, 244
American Cancer Society
colonoscopic examinations, 250
prostate cancer, 224
American College of Cardiology
bypass surgery criteria, 134
**American College of Emergency
Physicians**
emergency care overcrowding,
126, 128, 130
**American College of Sports
Medicine**
workouts, 82
American Heart Association
bypass surgery criteria, 134
American Medical Association
basic food groups issue, 279
Medicare physicians' fees, 259
Physician Advisory Panel on
Radio, Television, and Motion
Pictures, 27
physician self-referral, 260
risk procedures list, 286
Amino acids
proteins, 99, 101, 102, 103
Amitriptyline
pain relief, 60
Amniocentesis
prenatal test, 271
Amyloid precursor protein
Alzheimer's disease, 256
Amyotrophic lateral sclerosis
constipation, 193

personal experience with, 187-
189
Analgesics
pain relief, 54-62
Anaphylactic shock
swelling, 206
Anderson, R. Rox
laser surgery, 90
Androgens
prostate cancer, 224
Anemia
AIDS drug side effect, 316
air travel precautions, 49-50, 53
dietary iron link, 75
iron-deficiency, 284
premature infants, 282
screening test, 271
Angina pectoris
heart attack risk, 134
new drug, 313
Syndrome X factor, 266
Angioedema
antihypertensive drug side
effect, 315
Angioplasty, balloon, *see* Balloon
angioplasty
Angiotensin-converting enzyme,
see ACE inhibitors
Animal products, *see* Fat, dietary;
Fish; Meats; Poultry
Animals
child safety tips, 124-125
guide dogs, 53
Lyme disease, 114
organ transplants into humans,
20
Antianxiety drugs
dental phobia treatment, 289,
290
see also specific names
Antibiotics
bacterial meningitis, 180, 181
Group A streptococcal
infections, 171, 172, 173,
174
Lyme disease, 109, 110, 113,
114
new medications, 316
scar tissue formation, 237
sinusitis, 234
skin problems, 205
taste disorders, 147, 149
yogurt culture, 201
see also specific names
Antibodies
Lyme disease diagnosis, 108
proteins, 99
Antidepressant drugs
constipation side effect, 193
osteoarthritis, 165
pain relief, 60
panic disorder, 227
Prozac side effects, 268
smell and taste disorders, 149
Antigens
organ/tissue transplants, 10, 18
prostate-associated, 224, 247

Photo/Art Credits